ATLAS OF
INTRAOPERATIVE TRANSESOPHAGEAL ECHOCARDIOGRAPHY

ATLAS OF INTRAOPERATIVE TRANSESOPHAGEAL ECHOCARDIOGRAPHY

Surgical and Radiologic Correlations

Donald C. Oxorn MD
Professor of Anesthesiology
Adjunct Professor of Medicine
Department of Anesthesia,
Division of Cardiothoracic Anesthesia
School of Medicine
University of Washington
Seattle, WA
USA

Catherine M. Otto MD
Professor of Medicine
J. Ward Kennedy-Hamilton Endowed
   Professorship in Cardiology
Adjunct Professor of Anesthesiology
Department of Medicine
School of Medicine
University of Washington
Seattle, WA
USA

SAUNDERS

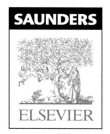

ELSEVIER

SAUNDERS
ELSEVIER

An imprint of Elsevier Inc.

©2007, Elsevier Inc. All rights reserved.

First published 2007

ISBN 10: 0-7216-5356-1
ISBN 13: 978-0-7216-5356-3

British Library Cataloguing in Publication Data
A catalogue record for this book is available from the British Library

Library of Congress Cataloging in Publication Data
A catalog record for this book is available from the Library of Congress

Notice
Medical knowledge is constantly changing. Standard safety precautions must be followed, but as new research and clinical experience broaden our knowledge, changes in treatment and drug therapy may become necessary or appropriate. Readers are advised to check the most current product information provided by the manufacturer of each drug to be administered to verify the recommended dose, the method and duration of administration, and contraindications. It is the responsibility of the practitioner, relying on experience and knowledge of the patient, to determine dosages and the best treatment for each individual patient. Neither the Publisher nor the author assume any liability for any injury and/or damage to persons or property arising from this publication.

The Publisher

ELSEVIER your source for books, journals and multimedia in the health sciences

www.elsevierhealth.com

Working together to grow libraries in developing countries

www.elsevier.com | www.bookaid.org | www.sabre.org

ELSEVIER   BOOK AID International   Sabre Foundation

The publisher's policy is to use paper manufactured from sustainable forests

Printed in China

Last digit is the print number: 9 8 7 6 5 4 3 2 1

Commissioning Editor:
Natasha Andjelkovic

Project Development Manager:
Laurie Anello

Project Manager:
Alan Nicholson

Designer:
Stewart Larking

Marketing Manager:
Laura Meiskey

Contents

Foreword

Recent advances in cardiology and cardiac surgery have had the effect that the typical cardiac surgery patient today is remarkably more complex than was the case even a few years ago. As coronary artery disease has been increasingly treated with medication and percutaneous interventions, coronary artery bypass grafting, while still important, has become a less prominent part of cardiac surgical practice. Meanwhile, more complex operations for cardiac transplantation, implantation of ventricular support devices, valvular heart disease, primary and reoperative treatment of adult congenital heart disease, and the treatment of thoracic aortic disease constitute a much greater portion of adult cardiac surgical practice.

Intraoperative transesophageal echocardiography (TEE) has emerged from a technological curiosity 20 years ago to an invaluable tool in the operating room of most cardiac surgical centers. No new anesthetic technique, pharmacologic intervention, intraoperative monitoring device, nor surgical advance has had such a profound impact on the conduct of cardiac surgery since the introduction of cardiopulmonary bypass. Anatomic, physiologic, and pathologic information is provided in real time to the surgeon, anesthesiologist and perfusionist while the patient is under anesthesia. On a daily basis, such critical information fosters clarity of early surgical results, and better clinical outcomes for our patients.

With the increasing complexity of heart surgery in the modern era, TEE will continue to be an essential diagnostic and monitoring tool.

Drs Donald Oxorn and Catherine Otto have led our efforts at the University of Washington to better define the utility and effectiveness of transesophageal echocardiography. This atlas reflects the quality of their work and their leadership in this important, emerging field of perioperative medicine. It has been a pleasure for all of us to watch this endeavor bear educational fruit. It has been an even more important pleasure for all of us to work with these excellent clinicians in the operating room on a daily basis.

T. Andrew Bowdle, MD PhD
Professor of Anesthesiology and Pharmaceutics
Chief of Cardiothoracic Anesthesiology
University of Washington
Seattle, Washington

Edward D. Verrier, MD
William K. Edmark Professor of
Cardiothoracic Surgery
Chief of Cardiothoracic Surgery
University of Washington
Seattle, Washington

Preface

As the complexity of cardiac surgical procedures has increased, transesophageal echocardiography (TEE) has become pivotal in intraoperative clinical decision making. In light of this evolution, the TEE practitioner is often called upon to confirm or refute a pre-existing diagnosis or to evaluate a previously unsuspected abnormality. In addition, TEE is used to evaluate the success and detect complications of cardiac surgical treatments.

This atlas will be of interest to all health care providers involved in the preoperative, intraoperative and postoperative care of patients undergoing cardiac surgical procedures. In addition to cardiac anesthesiologists, this book will be useful to cardiac surgeons seeking to understand echocardiography, cardiologists and cardiology fellows interested in expanding their knowledge of cardiac surgery, radiologists with a particular interest in cardiovascular disease, and to the rest of the cardiac team including cardiac sonographers, cardiac perfusionists, nurse practitioners and physician assistants, especially those who are not familiar with what actually transpires in the operating room. Primary care physicians with an interest in cardiology also will find this atlas helpful.

In the operating room, the TEE practitioner does not just acquire echocardiographic images, but is actively involved in clinical decision making. Thus, the TEE practitioner needs to be knowledgeable about the clinical presentation of cardiac conditions, the indications for surgical intervention and the expected surgical outcomes. In addition, supplemental information from other imaging and diagnostic modalities, reviewed before surgery, assists the practitioner in the interpretation of intraoperative TEE.

The impetus to write this book came out of our personal experiences of practice of TEE in the setting of cardiac anesthesia and surgery, and acute care medicine. What we found lacking was a method of conveying to students and colleagues the correlation between findings on TEE, results of other diagnostic modalities, and what was actually seen in the operating room. This book provides a unique integration of the clinical presentation, intraoperative transesophageal echocardiographic images, other diagnostic modalities, the surgical procedure and the cardiac pathology.

This atlas uses a case based format, organized into 12 chapters, each with a different clinical focus. Chapters include coronary artery disease, mitral valve disease, aortic valve disease, endocarditis, prosthetic valves, right sided valve disease, adult congenital heart disease, hypertrophic cardiomyopathy, pericardial disease, diseases of the great vessels, masses, and devices and catheters.

In each chapter, approximately 15 cases – some common, some esoteric – are presented. Each case includes the clinical presentation, multiple TEE images and images from other diagnostic modalities such as radiographs magnetic resonance imaging, computed tomography, cardiac catheterization, nuclear cardiology, and ECG. In addition, still and video images of the surgical procedure and intraoperative findings are shown, and where applicable, images from gross and microscopic pathology. TEE and cardiac surgery are not static entities; therefore the DVDs that accompany the book provide TEE clips and intraoperative footage. Each case is accompanied by an explanatory text discussing the acquisition, interpretation and clinical significance of the TEE findings, along with suggestions for further reading.

(Continued)

This atlas is not a substitute for training in TEE performance and interpretation, instead it is designed to serve as an adjunct in furthering or testing the individual's knowledge. The case-based format allows integration of multiple types of data but does not provide a comprehensive coverage of all topics in echocardiography. We expect that readers already have studied standard textbooks of clinical echocardiography and have some clinical experience with echocardiography. Readers are encouraged to review the American Society of Echocardiography and Society of Cardiovascular Anesthesiologists (http://scahq.org) guidelines for training in intraoperative TEE.

Donald C. Oxorn, MD
Professor of Anesthesiology
Adjunct Professor of Medicine
University of Washington, Seattle, WA

Catherine M. Otto, MD
J Ward Kennedy-Hamilton Chair in Cardiology
Professor of Medicine
Adjunct Professor of Anesthesiology
Director, Cardiology Fellowship Program
University of Washington, Seattle, WA

Acknowledgments

We acknowledge the contributions of our colleagues in Pathology: Dennis Reichenbach; in Cardiothoracic Anesthesiology: T Andrew Bowdle, Krishna Natrajan, Jorg Dziersk, Mark Edwards, Stephan Lombaard, Ray Liao; in Cardiothoracic Surgery: Edward Verrier, Gabriel Aldea, Christopher Salerno, Christopher King, Douglas Wood, Michael Mulligan; in Cardiology: Edward Gill for provision of the three-dimensional TEE images and clips; Valerie Oxorn and Starr Kaplan for their artwork, and to Angie Frederickson for secretarial support.

The patience and encouragement of our families, my wife Susan Murdoch and my children, Jonathan Oxorn, Sean Murdoch-Oxorn, and Alexandra Murdoch-Oxorn was ever present and much appreciated.

I (D.C.O), would like to thank two individuals from the University of Toronto; my friend and mentor Gerald Edelist, and Cam Joyner, my first and foremost teacher in echocardiography.

Abbreviations

A1, A2, A3	anterior leaflet sections		OR	operating room
A-COM	anterior commissures		P1, P2, P3	posterior leaflet sections
AML	anterior mitral leaflet		PA	pulmonary artery
Ao	aorta		P-COM	posterior commissures
AP	anteroposterior		PDA	patent ductus arteriosus
AR	aortic regurgitation		PE	pericardial effusion
ARDS	adult respiratory distress syndrome		PFO	patent foramen ovale
AS	aortic stenosis		PG	pressure gradient
ASA	atrial septal aneurysm		PISA	proximal isovelocity surface area
ASD	atrial septal defect		PM	papillary muscle
ATL	anterior tricuspid leaflet		PML	posterior mitral leaflet
AV	aortic valve; atrioventricular		PMN	polymorphonuclear leukocytes
CS	coronary sinus		PR	pulmonic regurgitation
CT	computed tomography		PTL	posterior tricuspid leaflet
CW	continuous wave (Doppler)		PV	pulmonic valve
CVA	cerebrovascular accident		PW	pulsed wave (Doppler)
Cx	circumflex coronary artery		RA	right atrium
DA	descending aorta		RAA	right atrial appendage
ECG	electrocardiogram		RBC	red blood cells
ICD	implantable cardioverter defibrillator		RCA	right coronary artery
IVC	inferior vena cava		RCC	right coronary cusp
IVS	interventricular septum		RLPV	right lower pulmonary vein
LA	left atrium		ROA	regurgitant orifice area
LAA	left atrial appendage		RPA	right pulmonary artery
LAD	left anterior descending coronary artery		RUPV	right upper pulmonary vein
LCC	left coronary cusp		RV	right ventricle
LCX	left circumflex artery		RVH	right ventricular hypertrophy
LIMA	left internal mammary artery		RVOT	right ventricular outflow tract
LLPV	left lower pulmonary vein		SAM	systolic anterior motion
LMCA	left main coronary artery		STJ	sinotubular junction
LPA	left pulmonary artery		SV	stroke volume
LUPV	left upper pulmonary vein		SVC	superior vena cava
LV	left ventricle		TEE	transesophageal echocardiography
LVOT	left ventricular outflow tract		TMR	transmyocardial revascularization
MAIVF	mitral aortic intervalvular fibrosa		TR	tricuspid regurgitation
MI	myocardial infarction		TTE	transthoracic echocardiography
MR	mitral regurgitation		TV	tricuspid valve
MRI	magnetic resonance imaging		VSD	ventricular septal defect
MV	mitral valve		VTI	velocity time integral
NCC	non-coronary cusp			

1

Coronary Artery Disease

Visualization of the Coronary Arteries and Regional Wall Motion

Case 1-1
Normal Coronary Arteries

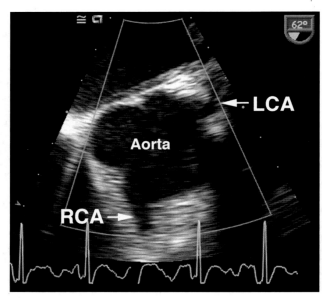

Fig 1-1. In a magnified short-axis view of the aorta slightly cephalad to the valve plane, the right coronary artery (**RCA**) and left coronary artery (**LCA**) ostia are seen arising from the right and left coronary sinuses of Valsalva, respectively. The left main coronary artery is easily visualized in nearly all patients. The right coronary is visualized less often.

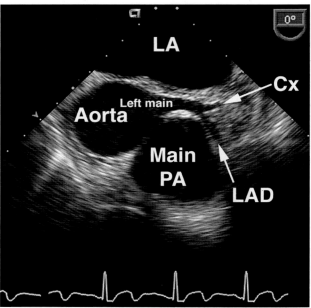

Fig 1-2. Transesophageal echocardiography (**TEE**) images in a different patient demonstrate the course of the left main coronary artery as it passes behind the main pulmonary artery and bifurcates into the posteriorly directly circumflex (**Cx**) and more anteriorly directly left anterior descending (**LAD**) coronary artery. This view was obtained starting in a short-axis view of the aorta to visualize the left main coronary ostium and then rotating the image plane until the bifurcation was seen.

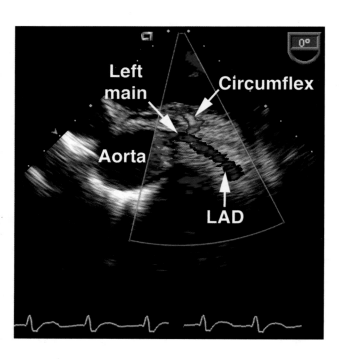

Fig 1-3. In the same view as shown in **Fig 1-2**, color Doppler demonstrates the predominantly diastolic flow in the left main, circumflex and left anterior descending (**LAD**) coronary arteries.

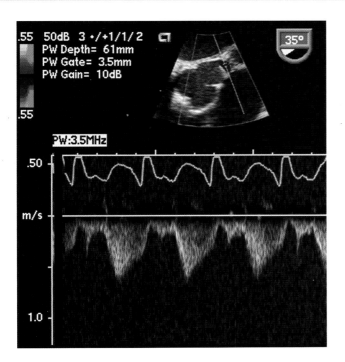

Fig 1-4. A pulsed Doppler sample volume is positioned in the left anterior descending coronary artery. The spectral tracing shows low-velocity diastolic flow, with small systolic component, typical for normal coronary blood flow.

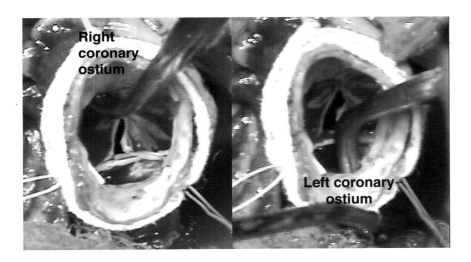

Fig 1-5. In this intraoperative photograph of the aortic valve from the aortic root side, the forceps tip is at the ostium of the right coronary artery (*left*). The right coronary ostium is anterior and slightly more cephalad than the left main coronary artery (*right*). The photograph is taken from the head of the operating table, and is therefore rotated 180° from what is seen on TEE imaging.

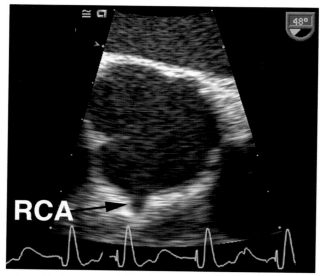

Fig 1-6. In a magnified short-axis TEE image, the ostium of the right coronary artery (**RCA**) is seen.

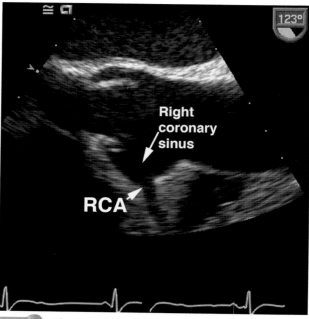

Fig 1-7. The right coronary artery (**RCA**) is often more easily visualized in a long-axis view of the aortic root, as shown in this example.

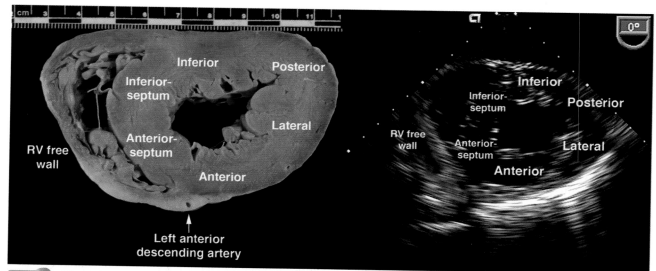

Fig 1-8. The left ventricular wall segments are shown for an anatomic specimen in the same orientation as a transgastric short-axis view of the ventricle. The ventricle is divided into six segments at the base and midventricular level, as shown. The posterior wall is also called the inferior–lateral wall, using the standard nomenclature for regional wall motion analysis.

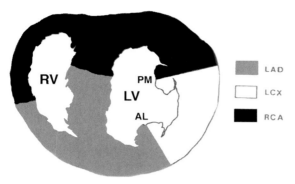

Fig 1-9. This schematic diagram of a short-axis view of the left (**LV**) and right ventricle (**RV**) in the same orientation as the transgastric short-axis views illustrates the correlation between coronary anatomy and regional myocardial function. There is some variability in the region supplied by the left circumflex artery (**LCX**), even at the base and midventricular levels. The apical region of the ventricle may be supplied by either the left anterior descending (**LAD**) or the right coronary artery (**RCA**) so that identification of the culprit vessel is problematic when only an apical abnormality is present. (Reproduced with permission from Oxorn D, Edelist G, Smith MS. An introduction to transoesophageal echocardiography: II Clinical applications. Can J Anaesth 1996; 43:278–294. ©1996 Canadian Journal of Anaesthesia.)

Comments

As shown in these examples, the proximal coronary arteries can often be visualized on TEE. The left main coronary artery arises from the left coronary sinus of Valsalva, is easily visualized in over 85% of patients and has a normal diameter of 4.2 ± 0.7 mm, with a slightly smaller average diameter in women (3.5 mm) compared with men (4.3 mm). The left main coronary artery bifurcates into the left anterior descending coronary, with a normal proximal diameter of 3.5 ± 1.0 mm, which supplies the anterior wall and anterior septum, and the circumflex coronary artery, with a normal diameter of 3.0 ± 0.6 mm, which supplies the lateral left ventricular wall. The right coronary artery arises from the right coronary sinus, with an average diameter of 3.6 ± 0.8 mm. The right coronary artery gives rise to the posterior descending coronary artery, supplying the inferior and posterior walls, in about 80% of patients (e.g. a right-dominant coronary circulation). The right coronary artery is not always visualized on TEE, being seen in about 50% of cases in one series.

The apical segments of the ventricle are often supplied by the left anterior descending artery, although the posterior descending coronary artery may extend to the inferior apex in some cases. The posterior (or inferior–lateral) left ventricular wall is variably supplied by either the circumflex or the posterior descending coronary artery. Coronary blood flow can be recorded using pulsed Doppler in many patients, with the typical pattern showing prominent diastolic flow, with a velocity about 0.6 cm/s, with little flow in systole. Although an increased velocity (>1 m/s) suggests stenosis and Doppler evaluation of coronary flow reserve is possible, these data are rarely used clinically.

TEE evaluation of the coronary arteries is most useful for detection of coronary artery aneurysms, coronary fistula and anomalous origins from a different sinus of Valsalva or from the pulmonary artery. Although some studies have shown that TEE evaluation is sensitive and specific for detection of significant left main or proximal coronary stenosis, TEE has not gained clinical acceptance as an approach to evaluation of atherosclerotic coronary disease. In addition to variable image quality, the inability to visualize distal vessel anatomy is a major limitation. Echocardiographic evaluation of coronary disease currently relies on evaluation of regional myocardial function at rest and with stress.

Suggested Reading

1. Lenter C (ed.) Geigy Scientific Tables, Volume 5: Heart and Circulation. CIBA-GEIGY Limited, Basel, Switzerland, 1990: 173–81.

2. Neishi Y, Akasaka T, Tsukiji M et al. Reduced coronary flow reserve in patients with congestive heart failure assessed by transthoracic Doppler echocardiography. J Am Soc Echocardiogr 2005; 18(1):15–19.

3. Dawn B, Talley JD, Prince CR et al. Two-dimensional and Doppler transesophageal echocardiographic delineation and flow characterization of anomalous coronary arteries in adults. J Am Soc Echocardiogr 2003; 16(12):1274–86.

Case 1-2
Coronary Artery Aneurysm

This 63-year-old man presented with atrial fibrillation. On his initial evaluation he was found to have a circumflex coronary artery aneurysm and fistula. On serial examinations over 6 years, the aneurysm showed a progressive increase in size. He was referred for magnetic resonance imaging (MRI) scanning and consideration of elective repair of the aneurysm, in conjunction with a Maze procedure for atrial fibrillation.

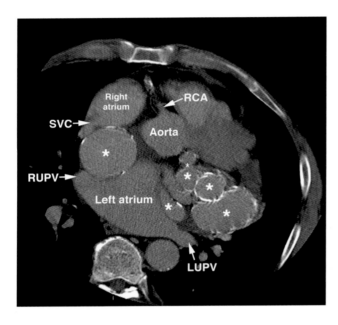

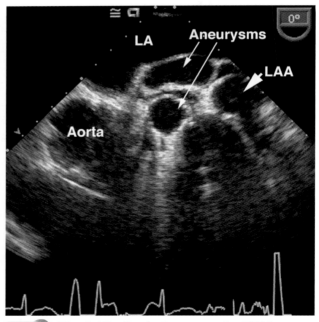

Fig 1-10. A tomographic MRI at the level of the left atrium demonstrates multiple aneurysms (**asterisks**) along the tortuous course of the left circumflex coronary to the left atrial fistula. The superior vena cava (**SVC**) is partially compressed by an aneurysm with a diameter of 5 cm that lies just anterior to the right upper pulmonary vein (**RUPV**). Other aneurysms lie just anterior to the left upper pulmonary vein (**LUPV**). The right coronary (**RCA**) ostium shows the normal size of the proximal coronary artery.

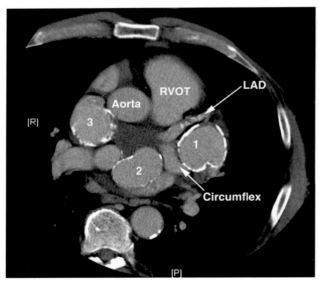

Fig 1-11. An MRI just superior to **Fig 1-10** demonstrates three calcified aneurysms (numbered 1, 2, 3) along the length of the fistula. The left anterior descending coronary (**LAD**) and circumflex arteries are seen.

Fig 1-12. On the intraoperative TEE image at 0 degrees turned slightly towards the patient's left side, there are two additional echo-free spaces between the aorta and left atrium. On further examination, these appear to be aneurysms along the course of the circumflex artery fistula.

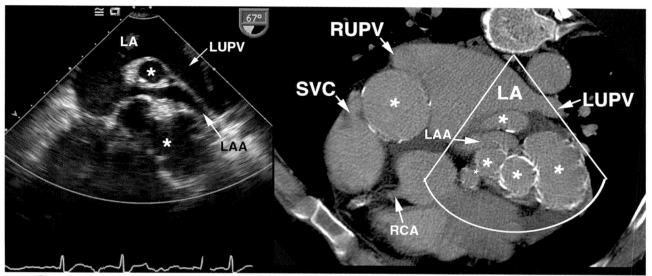

DVD **Fig 1-13.** In this view at 67 degrees rotation (*left*), there is an additional echolucent space (**asterisk**) between the entrance of the left upper pulmonary vein (**LUPV**) into the left atrium (**LA**) and the left atrial appendage (**LAA**). Another aneurysm (**second asterisk**) is seen anterior to the LAA. The relationship of this echocardiographic view to the MRI is shown (*right*) with the MRI reoriented, and an "ultrasound sector" superimposed.

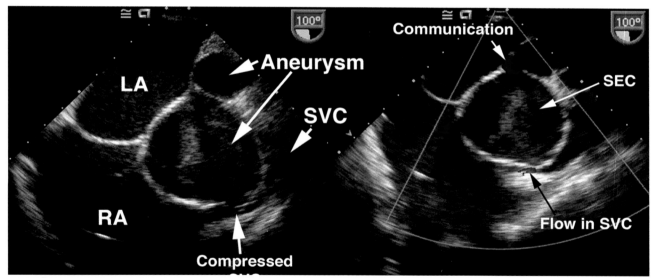

DVD **Fig 1-14.** In the long-axis view rotated to the patient's right side, which usually yields a "bicaval" view of the right atrium (**RA**), inferior and superior vena cava (**SVC**), there are two additional large echo-free spaces consistent with coronary aneurysms. The SVC is compressed by the larger aneurysm. Color Doppler (*right*) demonstrates flow in the compressed SVC, communication between aneurysms and spontaneous echo contrast (**SEC**) within the aneurysms.

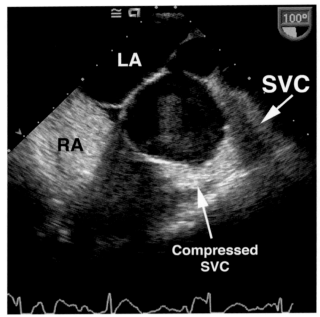

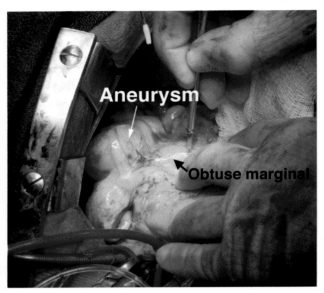

DVD **Fig 1-15.** In the same view as **Fig 1-14**, injection of agitated saline in a peripheral vein to opacify the right heart confirms the identity of the superior vena cava as it fills with contrast before the right heart opacifies.

Fig 1-16. On direct inspection at surgery, the patient was found to have a very enlarged circumflex artery, which was calcified from just beyond the pulmonary artery, throughout the length of the artery in the left atrioventricular groove, with extension into a fistula into the superior vena cava. There were several large, globular aneurysms, which were calcified and non-compressible.

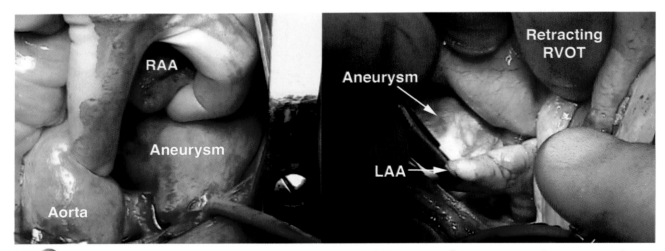

DVD **Fig 1-17.** Retraction of both atrial appendages revealed large circumflex aneurysms. The entry into the left atrium was closed and the circumflex artery was ligated proximally. The patient had an uneventful hospital course and he was in sinus rhythm at discharge.

Comments

Coronary artery aneurysms, defined as a localized area of dilation with a coronary diameter >1.5 times normal, may be due to a variety of systemic and arterial disease processes, including arteriosclerotic disease, Kawasaki disease, other types of vasculitis (Takayasu's arteritis, syphilis), connective tissue disorders (Ehlers–Danlos syndrome), coronary dissection and as a complication of a percutaneous intervention. Dilation of the coronary arteries also occurs in response to any chronic increase in coronary blood flow, such as left ventricular hypertrophy, an anomalous coronary arising from the pulmonary artery, or a coronary fistula, as in this case.

Coronary artery aneurysms are identified on echocardiography as relatively echo-free spaces, often with a swirling pattern of spontaneous contrast due to low-velocity blood flow, that can be connected to the coronary artery as the image plane is slowly rotated.

Coronary aneurysms may show progressive enlargement, sometimes rupture, and are prone to thrombus formation with resultant myocardial ischemia.

Suggested Reading

1. Dubel HP, Gliech V, Borges A et al. Images in cardiovascular medicine. Singular coronary artery aneurysm: imaging with coronary angiography versus 16-slice computed tomography, transesophageal echocardiography, and magnetic resonance tomography. Circulation 2005; 111(2):e12–13.

2. Gottesfeld S, Makaryus AN, Singh B et al. Thrombosed right coronary artery aneurysm presenting as a myocardial mass. J Am Soc Echocardiogr 2004; 17(12):1319–22.

3. Shiraishi J, Harada Y, Komatsu S et al. Usefulness of transthoracic echocardiography to detect coronary aneurysm in young adults: two cases of acute myocardial infarction due to Kawasaki disease. Echocardiography 2004; 21(2):165–9.

Case 1-3
Right Coronary Artery Dissection

This 71-year-old man had severe symptomatic calcific aortic stenosis. While undergoing diagnostic coronary angiography, he suffered a spiral dissection of the right coronary artery which was initially treated with multiple stents. Despite efforts to reperfuse the right coronary distribution, he suffered a ventricular fibrillation arrest. TEE at the outside hospital showed a proximal ascending aortic dissection. He was airlifted to our medical center and brought directly to the operating room.

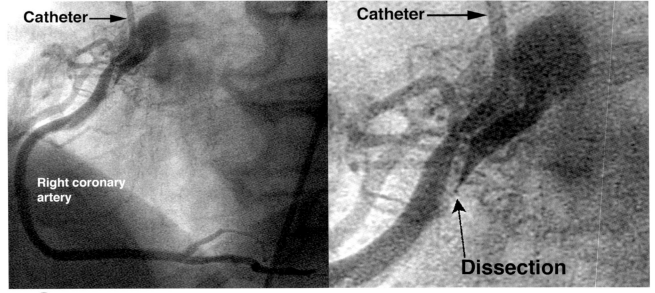

DVD **Fig 1-18.** The right coronary angiogram demonstrates extravasation of contrast near the vessel origin in the proximal aorta. The close-up view (*right*) shows the spiraling echolucency in the right coronary consistent with a dissection.

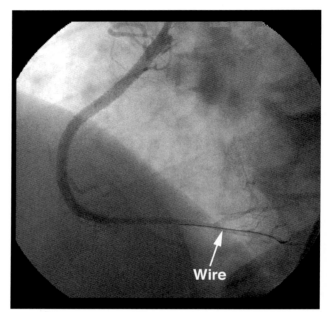

DVD **Fig 1-19.** After completion of the angioplasty, the right coronary artery appears widely patent, with the distal end of the guidewire seen in the posterior descending coronary branch.

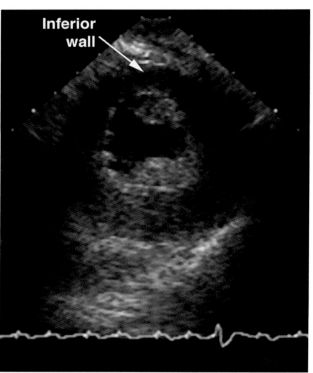

DVD **Fig 1-21.** The transgastric short-axis view of the left ventricle shows severe hypokinesis of the inferior wall, consistent with ischemia in the distribution of the right coronary artery.

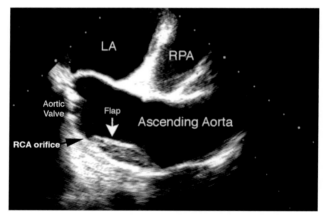

Fig 1-20. On intraoperative TEE, the long-axis view of the ascending aorta demonstrates a luminal flap, originating near the right coronary ostium. The echo density in the false lumen suggests thrombus formation. Note that the aortic valve is heavily calcified.

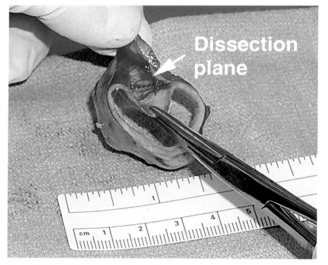

Fig 1-22. The patient underwent replacement of the aortic valve and ascending aorta with a composite valve and conduit. The left main coronary artery was reimplanted into the graft and a bypass graft was placed to the distal right coronary artery, with the proximal right coronary artery oversewn. A small segment of the resected aorta shows the dissection plane between the endothelium and media of the vessel. The patient had an uneventful hospital course and was discharged home on the 6th postoperative day.

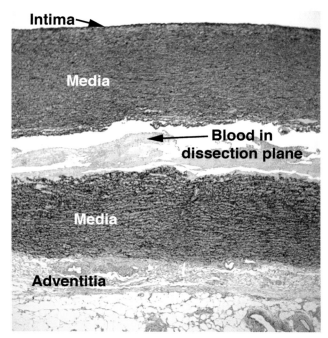

Intima

Media

Blood in dissection plane

Media

Adventitia

Fig 1-23. Microscopic examination of the aortic specimen shows the dissection plane through the media, filled with blood.

Comments

Coronary artery dissection can occur spontaneously or as a complication of cardiac catheterization. Coronary dissection is a rare cause of acute myocardial infarction in younger patients. Although there are no specific clinical predictors of spontaneous coronary dissection, it is more common in women than in men and the risk is increased during pregnancy.

Coronary dissection owing to diagnostic cardiac catheterization is rare but can result in acute severe myocardial ischemia, as in this case. The overall incidence of myocardial infarction with diagnostic coronary angiography is 0.06%, with infarction more often due to vessel thrombosis or embolization rather than to coronary dissection. When coronary dissection complicates a diagnostic or therapeutic percutaneous coronary procedure, the dissection flap may propagate retrograde, into the aorta, as in this case.

Suggested Reading

1. Leone F, Macchiusi A, Ricci R et al. Acute myocardial infarction from spontaneous coronary artery dissection: a case report and review of the literature. Cardiol Rev 2004;12(1):3–9.

2. Basso C, Morgagni GL, Thiene G. Spontaneous coronary artery dissection: a neglected cause of acute myocardial ischaemia and sudden death. Heart 1996; 75(5):451–4.

3. Johnson LW, Krone R. Cardiac catheterization 1991: a report of the Registry of the Society for Cardiac Angiography and Interventions (SCA&I). Cathet Cardiovasc Diagn 1993; 28(3):219–20.

4. Maiello L, La Marchesina U, Presbitero P, Faletra F. Iatrogenic aortic dissection during coronary intervention. Ital Heart J 2003; 4(6):419–22.

Case 1-4
Calcified Left Main Coronary Artery

This 63-year-old man, with a history of hypertension and hypercholesterolemia, presented with congestive heart failure symptoms. He was found to have severely reduced left ventricular systolic function with an ejec-tion fraction of 35%, a bicuspid aortic valve with moderate aortic insufficiency and stenosis, and severe three-vessel coronary disease. He also had chronic renal insufficiency and severe peripheral vascular disease.

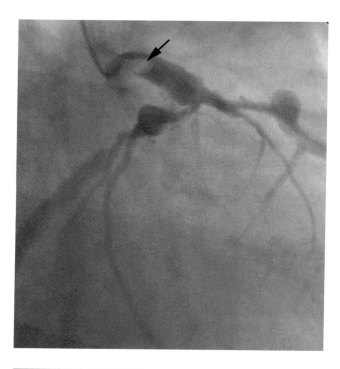

Fig 1-24. Coronary angiography shows a dilated left main coronary with a filling defect (**arrow**) near the ostium of the vessel. There is diffuse atherosclerosis with focal small aneurysms of the circumflex and left anterior descending coronary arteries.

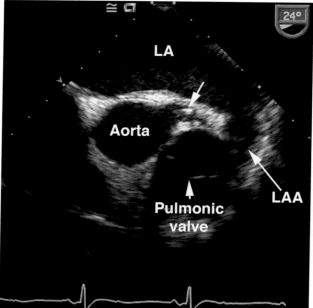

DVD **Fig 1-25.** The TEE short-axis view of the aortic valve at 24 degrees rotation shows an echo-dense mass in the dilated left main coronary. The orifice of the vessel measures 1.3 mm.

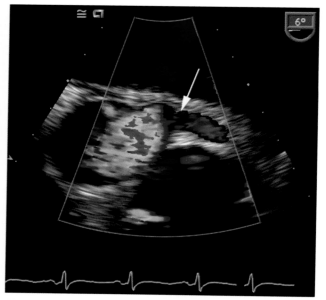

Fig 1-26. Color flow Doppler of the left main coronary demonstrates blood flow around the mass in the vessel (**arrow**).

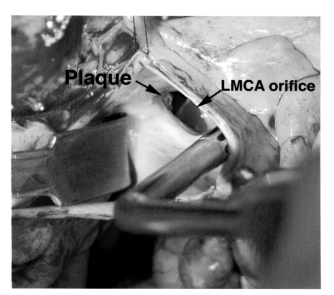

Fig 1-27. At surgical inspection, the atherosclerotic plaque within the dilated left main coronary artery (**LMCA**) orifice is seen. The patient underwent aortic valve replacement and coronary bypass grafting, including a left internal mammary artery (**LIMA**) graft to the left anterior descending coronary artery. He had an uneventful hospital course and was discharged on the 5th postoperative day with an ejection fraction of 43%.

Comments

This case demonstrates visualization of a large atherosclerotic plaque in the left main coronary artery and atherosclerotic-related aneurysms of the coronary vessels. Although TEE is *not* the procedure of choice for evaluation of coronary anatomy, it is sensitive and specific for detection of severe left main coronary stenosis. Thus, the echocardiographer should be alert to abnormalities of the proximal coronary arteries, especially in cases when preoperative coronary angiography was not performed.

Suggested Reading

1. Firstenberg MS, Greenberg NL, Lin SS et al. Transesophageal echocardiography assessment of severe ostial left main coronary stenosis. J Am Soc Echocardiogr 2000; 13(7):696–8.

2. Samdarshi TE, Nanda NC, Gatewood RP Jr et al. Usefulness and limitations of transesophageal echocardiography in the assessment of proximal coronary artery stenosis. J Am Coll Cardiol 1992; 19(3):572–80.

3. Yoshida K, Yoshikawa J, Hozumi T et al. Detection of left main coronary artery stenosis by transesophageal color Doppler and two-dimensional echocardiography. Circulation 1990; 81(4):1271–6.

Case 1-5
Right coronary artery air

Following cardiac surgery (especially when cardiac chambers have been opened), and in preparation for separation from cardiopulmonary bypass, the cardiac chambers are imaged to determine the presence of intracardiac air. If substantial air is present, there is concern that air entering the coronary ostia might interrupt coronary blood flow, resulting in myocardial ischemia. The surgeon will therefore make attempts to "de-air" the heart by applying suction to the ascending aorta in order to evacuate air as it passes through the aortic valve, and before it enters the coronary ostia. In extreme cases, actual needle aspiration of the left ventricular cavity may be undertaken.

DVD **Fig 1-28.** In the TEE four-chamber view at 0 degrees rotation, there are multiple bright mobile echodensities (termed echocardiographic contrast) in all four chambers of the heart, suggesting that microbubbles are present in the left- and right-sided circulations. A pocket of air (**arrow**) is frequently enmeshed in the left ventricular apex.

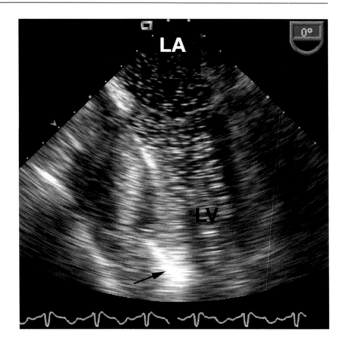

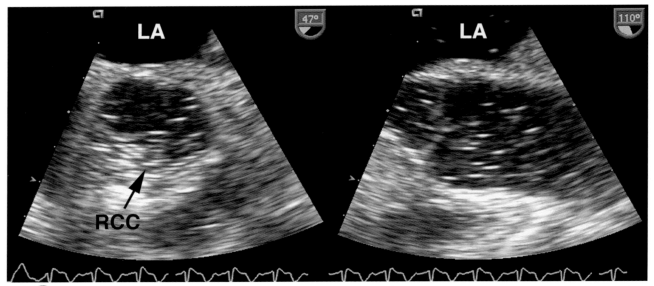

DVD **Fig 1-29.** In both short- (*left*) and long-axis (*right*) views of the aortic valve, microbubbles are seen in the aortic root. Microbubbles tend to accumulate in the sinus of Valsalva adjacent to the right coronary cusp (**RCC**), with preferential flow into the right coronary artery; this is because when the patient is lying supine, the right coronary artery is the most superior.

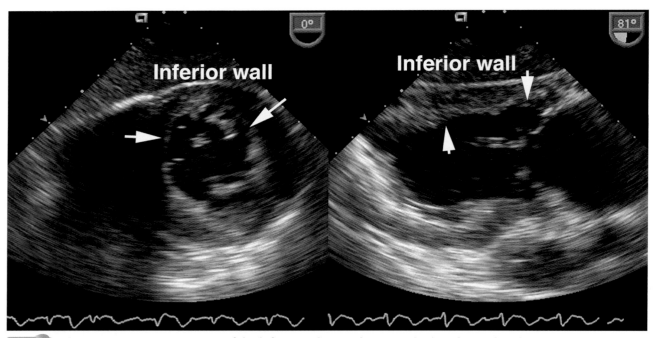

DVD **Fig 1-30.** Transgastric views of the left ventricle in a short-axis (*left*) and two-chamber (*right*) view show that the inferior wall segments between the arrows are akinetic, but not thinned.

Comments

On echocardiography, air in the cardiac chambers appears as mobile echodensities, e.g. echo contrast. The echocardiographer may be asked to evaluate residual air as the patient is weaned from cardiopulmonary bypass. Air detected by TEE is associated with transient ST-segment elevation on the electrocardiogram (ECG) and wall motion abnormalities on two-dimensional (2D) imaging. The association between intracardiac air and neurologic events after cardiac surgery is less clear, with some studies suggesting that left-sided microbubbles are not predictive of neurologic recovery, but other studies showing better postoperative cognitive function in patients with fewer microbubbles after surgery.

In a study of 417 patients undergoing intraoperative TEE at the time of valve surgery, the postoperative TEE findings changed therapy by detection of valve dysfunction in 3.6%. However, in an additional 11.3%, the TEE showed residual air, prompting additional removal of air before weaning from cardiopulmonary bypass.

Suggested reading

1. Shapira Y, Vaturi M, Weisenberg DE et al. Impact of intraoperative transesophageal echocardiography in patients undergoing valve replacement. Ann Thorac Surg 2004; 78(2):579–83.

2. Orihashi K, Matsuura Y, Sueda T et al. Pooled air in open heart operations examined by transesophageal echocardiography. Ann Thorac Surg 1996; 61:1377–80.

3. Borger MA, Peniston CM, Weisel RD et al. Neuropsychologic impairment after coronary bypass surgery: effect of gaseous microemboli during perfusionist interventions. J Thorac Cardiovasc Surg 2001; 121:743–9.

4. Dalmas JP, Eker A, Girard C et al. Intracardiac air clearing in valvular surgery guided by transesophageal echocardiography. J Heart Valve Dis 1996; 5:553–7.

Myocardial Infarction

Case 1-6
Anterior Myocardial Infarction

This 56-year-old man with no prior cardiac history presented with a 3-hour history of intermittent chest pain and anterior ST-segment elevation on ECG. He was taken directly to the cardiac catheterization laboratory where he was found to have an occluded proximal right coronary artery, with filling of the distal vessel by left-to-right collaterals, and an acute occlusion of the left anterior descending coronary artery. The left anterior descending occlusion could not be crossed. An intraaortic balloon pump was placed and he was referred for emergency coronary bypass grafting surgery. Preoperative echocardiography demonstrated a left ventricular ejection fraction of 29% with severe hypokinesis of the inferior wall and akinesis of the mid and apical segments of the anterior wall.

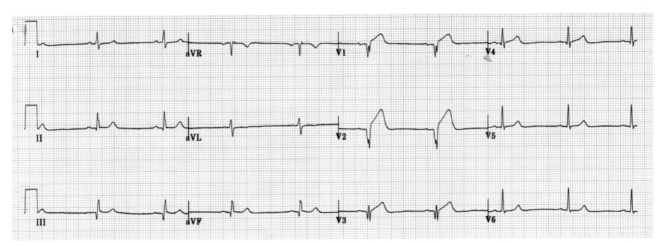

Fig 1-31. The ECG demonstrates Q waves and ST elevation in leads VI-V3 consistent with an acute anteroseptal myocardial infarction. There also are small Q waves in III and AVR without associated ST changes.

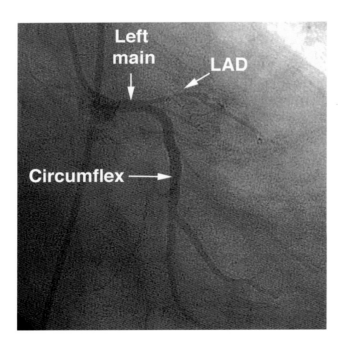

DVD **Fig 1-32.** At coronary angiography there was an old occlusion of the right coronary artery. The left main and left circumflex showed only mild diffuse disease but there was a complete proximal occlusion of the left anterior descending coronary (**LAD**) with contrast filling only a small diagonal branch to the basal anterior wall.

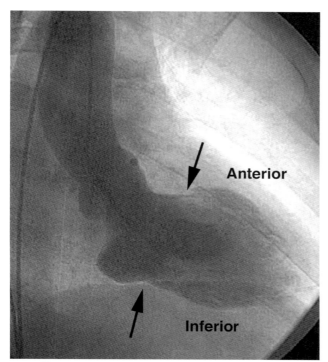

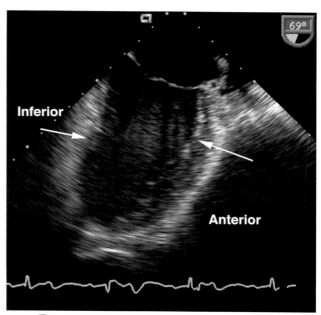

DVD **Fig 1-35.** The image plane is rotated to 69 degrees to obtain a two-chamber view. The arrows indicate 'hinge points' in the inferior and anterior walls; the myocardium below these points is akinetic.

DVD **Fig 1-33.** The left ventriculogram in a right anterior oblique view demonstrates normal endocardial motion at the ventricular base (**arrows**) with akinesis of the anterior wall, consistent with the acute event and akinesis of the inferior wall, consistent with the old myocardial infarction.

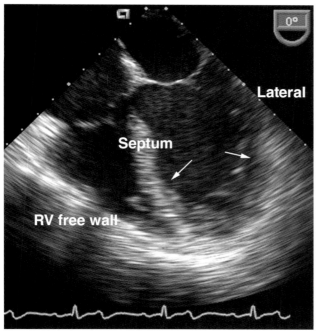

DVD **Fig 1-34.** In the TEE four-chamber view at 0 degrees, the apical segments of the lateral wall and septum below the arrows are severely hypokinetic.

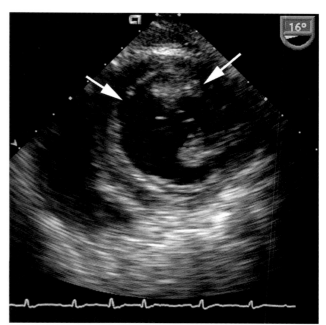

DVD **Fig 1-36.** In the transgastric short-axis view, the area of basal akinesis of the inferior wall (**arrows**) is seen.

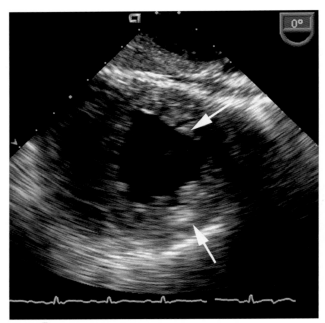

Fig 1-37. In a short-axis view slightly more apical than in **Fig 1-36**, the lateral wall is the only functioning segment of the heart (between the **arrows**).

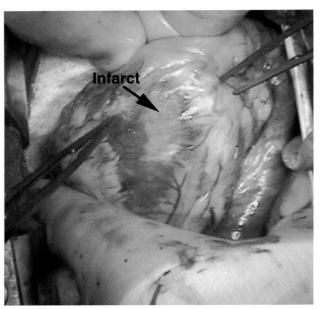

Fig 1-39. At surgical inspection, the infarct of the anterior wall is seen as an area of pallor, or "bulls-eye." The patient underwent three-vessel coronary bypass grafting. His postoperative course was complicated by atrial fibrillation and a prolonged need for inotropic support. However, by the 10th postoperative day, he had an ejection fraction of 45% on oral medications and was discharged home.

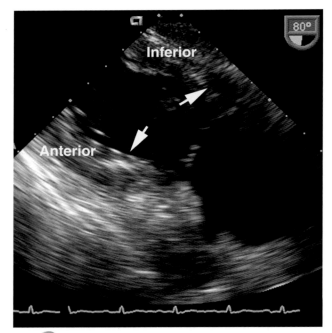

Fig 1-38. From the transgastric short-axis view, the image plane is rotated to 80 degrees to obtain a two-chamber view of the ventricle. As in the high TEE two-chamber view, this image plane shows the anterior and inferior walls, and 'hinge points' (**arrows**).

Comments

Assessment of coronary disease by echocardiography is most often based on the pattern of wall motion abnormalities, rather than by direct visualization of the coronary vessels. In order to fully evaluate all segments of the ventricular myocardium, multiple image planes are used, with the standard views being the four-chamber, two-chamber and long-axis views from a high transesophageal position and the midventricular short-axis view from a transgastric position, with each wall divided into thirds—basal, midventricular and apical. The lateral wall and inferior septum are seen in the four-chamber view, the inferior and anterior walls in the two-chamber view and the anterior septum and posterior (or inferior–lateral) wall in the long-axis view. The short-axis view provides an orthogonal view of these same segments. A transgastric two-chamber view can also be obtained by rotating 90 degrees from the short-axis view. In some patients, transgastric apical views can also be obtained. However, on both TEE and transgastric views, the true ventricular apex may be foreshortened so that apical wall motion abnormalities may be missed.

In patients undergoing cardiopulmonary bypass, regional wall motion is evaluated before and after the bypass run. In patients undergoing off-pump coronary bypass surgery, the majority of wall segments can be evaluated during the procedure, although cardiac displacement may limit visualization of some segments.

Suggested Reading

1. Comunale ME, Body SC, Ley C et al. The concordance of intraoperative left ventricular wall-motion abnormalities and electrocardiographic S-T segment changes: association with outcome after coronary revascularization-Multicenter Study of Perioperative Ischemia (McSPI) Research Group. Anesthesiology 1998; 88:945–54.

2. Shanewise JS, Cheung AT, Aronson S et al. ASE/SCA guidelines for performing a comprehensive intraoperative multiplane transesophageal echocardiography examination: recommendations of the American Society of Echocardiography Council for Intraoperative Echocardiography and the Society of Cardiovascular Anesthesiologists Task Force for Certification in Perioperative Transesophageal Echocardiography. Anesth Analg 1999; 89:870–84.

3. Wang J, Filipovic M, Rudzitis A et al. Transesophageal echocardiography for monitoring segmental wall motion during off-pump coronary artery bypass surgery. Anesth Analg 2004; 99(4):965–73.

Case 1-7
Myocardial Infarction Followed by Heart Transplantation

This 58-year-old woman suffered an acute aortic dissection complicated by a perioperative anterior myocardial infarction 18 months ago. Because of an episode of ventricular tachycardia, she was treated with amiodarone and an automatic implanted defibrillator was placed. Because of her arrhythmias and low left ventricular ejection fraction (about 35%), she was undergoing evaluation for heart transplantation. She was now admitted with recurrent ventricular tachycardia, resistant to medical therapy. A donor became available, and she was taken to the operating room for heart transplantation.

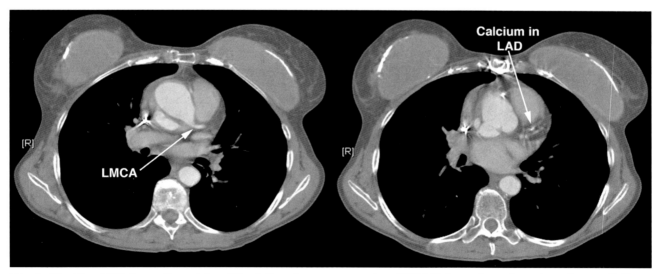

Fig 1-40. Chest CT shows the origin of the left main coronary artery (**LMCA**) from the enlarged aortic root (*left*). There is calcification of the left anterior descending (**LAD**) coronary artery (*right*).

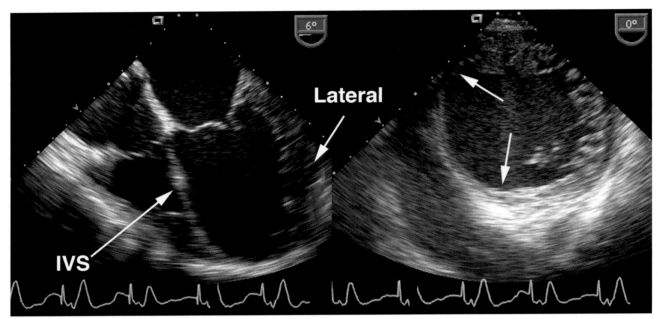

DVD **Fig 1-41.** In the TEE four-chamber view (*left*) the interventricular septum (**IVS**) is thin and akinetic, with relatively normal wall thickness and function of the lateral wall. The transgastric short-axis view (*right*) shows the thinned and akinetic anterior and inferior walls.

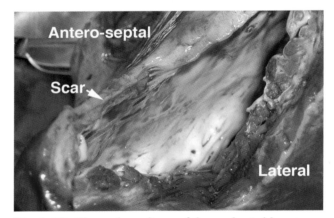

Fig 1-42. The endocardium of the explanted heart shows the area of scar along the septum.

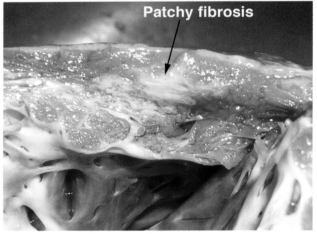

Fig 1-43. A transverse section of the lateral wall of the myocardium shows areas of patchy fibrosis.

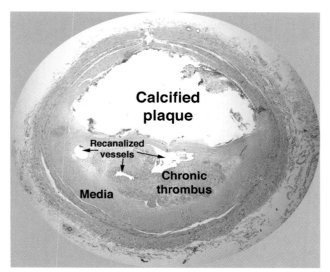

Fig 1-44. Microscopic section of the left anterior descending artery shows a calcified plaque, chronic thrombus and a small amount of recanalization.

Comments

In patients with coronary artery disease, myocardial wall thickness and systolic thickening is normal at rest if there has been no prior myocardial infarction, even when there is a significant degree of coronary stenosis. However, with ischemia there is a prompt decrease in endocardial motion and wall thickening in the myocardial segments supplied by the affected vessel. Wall motion returns to normal with relief of ischemia. This sequence of events is the basis of echocardiographic stress testing, with exercise or dobutamine. However, acute ischemia may also be seen in the operating room. With myocardial infarction, the irreversible changes in the myocardium correspond to a persistent wall motion. Wall thickness is normal early after infarction but, over time, scarring occurs, with decreased wall thickness and increased echogenicity. The degree of wall thinning corresponds to the transmural extent of the infarction. In this case, the echocardiographic findings were consistent with a large transmural anterior myocardial infarction with the thin akinetic segments on echocardiography corresponding to the area of scar on pathology. The lateral wall showed relatively normal function, even though patchy non-transmural infarction was found on pathology.

Suggested Reading

1. Marcovitz PA. Exercise echocardiography: stress testing in the initial diagnosis of coronary artery disease and in patients with prior revascularization or myocardial infarction. In: Otto CM, ed. The Practice of Clinical Echocardiography, 2nd edn. Philadelphia: WB Saunders, 2002: 275–300.

2. Marwick TH. Stress echocardiography with non exercise techniques: principles, protocols, interpretation and clinical applications. In: Otto CM, ed. The Practice of Clinical Echocardiography, 2nd edn. Philadelphia: WB Saunders, 2002: 301–41.

3. Savage RM, Lytle BW, Aronson S et al. Intraoperative echocardiography is indicated in high-risk coronary artery bypass grafting. Ann Thorac Surg 1997; 64(2):368–73.

Complications of Myocardial Infarction

Case 1-8
Post-myocardial Infarction Ventricular Septal Defect

This 75-year-old woman presented 3 weeks ago with an acute anterior myocardial infarction. Because she presented late after symptom onset, she did not receive reperfusion therapy and her postmyocardial infarction echocardiogram showed severely reduced left ventricular systolic function with an apical aneurysm. She was treated with warfarin for an apical thrombus.

Ten days ago, she presented with a large pericardial effusion and tamponade physiology. After removal of 600 ml of hemorrhagic pericardial fluid, hemodynamics improved but a new murmur was noted and echocardiography showed an apical ventricular septal defect (VSD). She was then transferred to our medical center for possible surgical intervention.

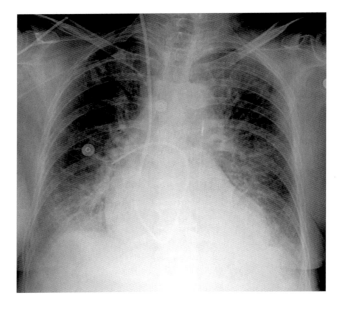

Fig 1-45. Chest radiography shows enlargement of the cardiac silhouette and pulmonary edema.

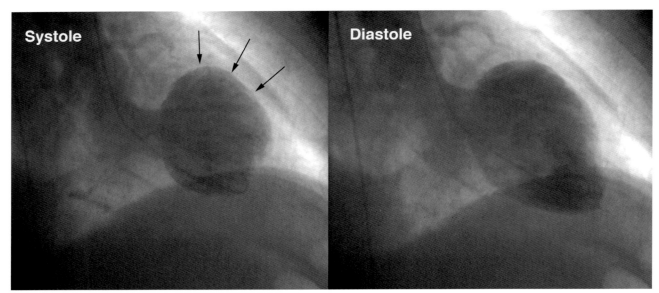

DVD ▶ **Fig 1-46.** Left ventricular angiography in a right anterior oblique projection shows the dilation of the anterior wall of the left ventricle in diastole and the akinetic segment in systole (**arrows**).

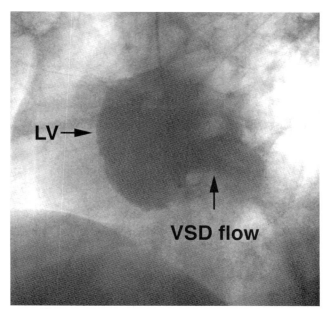

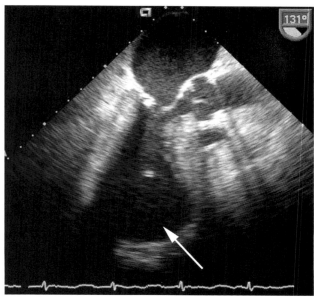

DVD **Fig 1-47.** Left ventricular angiography was also performed in the less traditional right posterior oblique projection to show contrast entering the right ventricle via the septal defect.

DVD **Fig 1-49.** In the transesophageal long-axis view, the diastolic contour abnormality and dyskinesis of the midventricular and apical segments of the anterior septum are seen. The arrow indicates the akinetic LV apex.

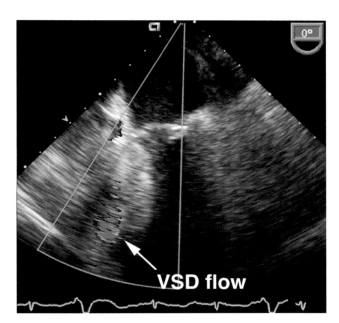

DVD **Fig 1-48.** In the transesophageal four-chamber view, color Doppler demonstrates turbulent systolic flow in the right ventricular apex.

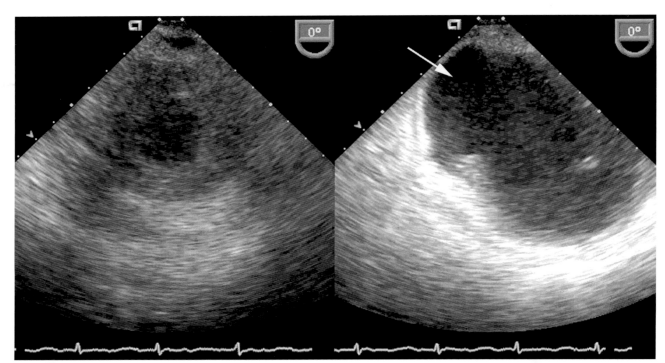

DVD **Fig 1-50.** In this transgastric short-axis view of the left ventricle, function at the midpapillary level is hyperdynamic (*left*), whereas the apex (*right*) is aneurysmal and akinetic. The arrow indicates the aneurysmal inferior

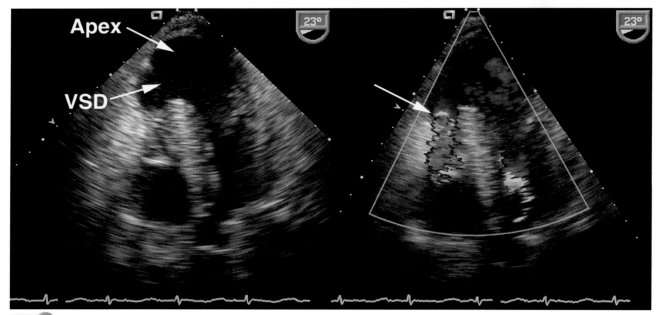

DVD **Fig 1-51.** In a transgastric apical view with anteflexion of the probe tip, the aneurysm of the apical septum is seen with an area of discontinuity in the septum. Color Doppler (**arrow**) confirms flow across the septum consistent with a post-myocardial infarction ventricular septal defect.

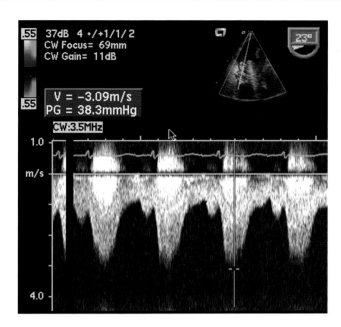

Fig 1-52. Continuous wave Doppler of the flow through the ventricular septal defects shows high-velocity flow in systole, consistent with the systolic pressure difference between the right and left ventricles. The velocity of 3.1 m/s (pressure difference of only 38 mmHg) is lower than expected with a chronic small ventricular septal defect, so might be an underestimate due to a non-parallel intercept angle. However, the patient's systolic blood pressure at the time of this recording was only 100 mmHg and pulmonary artery pressure was about 50 mmHg, indicating that velocity is only slightly underestimated. The persistent low-velocity flow in diastole is due to the slightly higher left than right ventricular diastolic pressure.

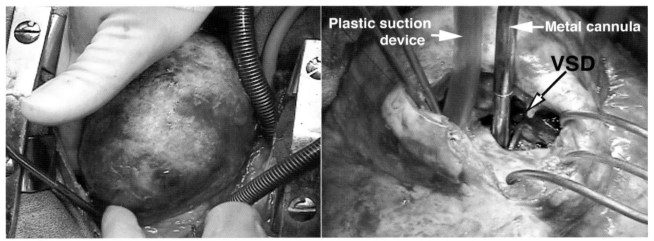

DVD **Fig 1-53.** On direct inspection at surgery, the anterior left ventricular wall is aneurysmal (*left*). The left ventricle has been opened through the apical scar with the metal suction cannula in the VSD (*right*).

Comments

Rupture of the myocardium is a rare but life-threatening complication of acute myocardial infarction (MI). Rupture of the left ventricular free wall leads to acute tamponade or a contained rupture with pseudoaneurysm formation (<1% of acute MI patients); rupture of the papillary muscle results in acute mitral regurgitation; and rupture of the septum leads to a VSD (2% of all MIs). Rupture occurs equally in the anterior and inferior septum and may be basal or apical. Risk factors for ventricular rupture include first myocardial infarction, transmural infarction (ST elevation or Q-wave formation) and a greater rise in cardiac enzymes. These factors suggest that the key parameters leading to rupture are the absence of collateral vessels and a larger infarction. Reperfusion therapy decreases the likelihood of rupture, although the clinical presentation may be earlier in those who do suffer this complication.

The clinical presentation in this patient is consistent with a post-myocardial infarction VSD, as clearly demonstrated on echocardiography. The history of pericardial tamponade is of concern, suggesting that she may also have had a contained free wall rupture. Outcome with a postmyocardial infarction VSD is poor, with a 30-day mortality as high as 74%.

Treatment includes medical stabilization followed by surgical repair, although the timing of surgery remains controversial.

Suggested Reading

1. Vargas-Barron J, Molina-Carrion M, Romero-Cardenas A et al. Risk factors, echocardiographic patterns, and outcomes in patients with acute ventricular septal rupture during myocardial infarction. Am J Cardiol 2005; 95(10):1153–8.

2. Crenshaw BS, Granger CB, Birnbaum Y et al. Risk factors, angiographic patterns, and outcomes in patients with ventricular septal defect complicating acute myocardial infarction. GUSTO-I (Global Utilization of Streptokinase and TPA for Occluded Coronary Arteries) Trial Investigators. Circulation 2000; 101(1):27–32.

Case 1-9
Dor Procedure (left ventricular apical exclusion)

This 65-year-old woman was referred for ventricular endoaneurysmorrhaphy, mitral valve repair and an atrial Maze procedure. Four months ago she suffered an anterior wall myocardial infarction. Despite thrombolytic therapy and emergency stent placement, she developed an akinetic anterior wall and apex. Over the ensuing 3 months of hospitalization, she had multiple complications, including intermittent congestive heart failure requiring several intubations, renal insufficiency, mitral regurgitation, pulmonary hypertension, anemia, a gastrointestinal bleed, pulmonary hypertension and paroxysmal atrial fibrillation. Serial echocardiograms demonstrated an akinetic anterior wall and apex with moderate to severe mitral regurgitation and pulmonary hypertension. A nuclear scan demonstrated no viability in the anterior wall. After an extensive discussion with the cardiology service, heart failure team, arrhythmia service and cardiac surgery service, the decision to proceed with surgical intervention was undertaken.

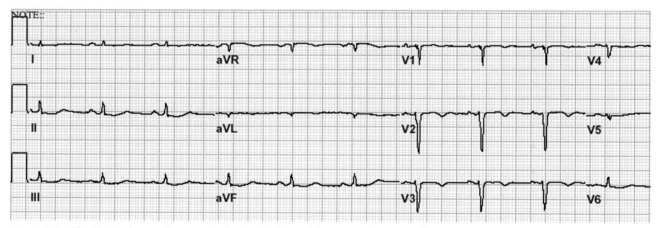

Fig 1-54. The ECG shows Q waves in leads V1–V5, with T-wave inversion but no acute ST changes, consistent with an old anterior myocardial infarction.

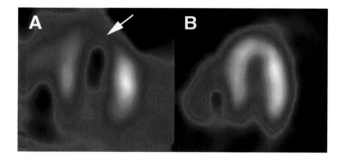

Fig 1-55. On the patient's resting radionuclide perfusion scan (A) in a four-chamber orientation, there is no uptake in the apical one-third of the ventricle (**arrow**), consistent with a large area of infarction. Late redistribution images showed no change in the pattern of perfusion, indicating that the apical region of the ventricle is not viable. A normal perfusion image from a different patient is shown (B) for comparison.

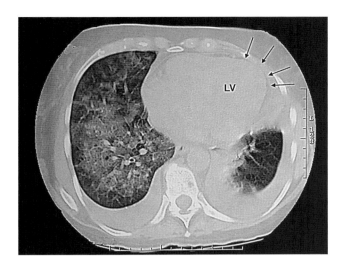

Fig 1-56. This chest computed tomographic (**CT**) scan at the level of the left ventricle (**LV**) shows the apical aneurysm (**arrows**).

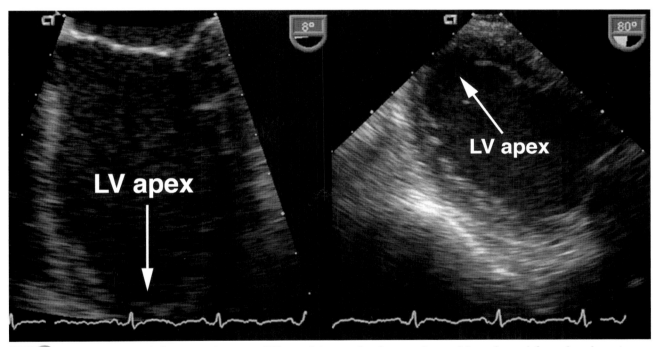

Fig 1-57. The left ventricular apex (**LV apex**) is seen in close up in a midesophageal four-chamber view (*left*) and a transgastric two-chamber view (*right*). In real time, the apex is seen to be dyskinetic.

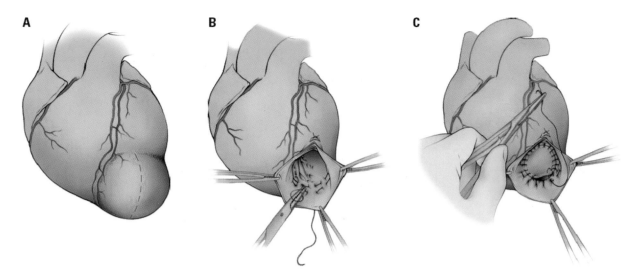

A   **B**   **C**

Fig 1-58. The Dor procedure is designed to exclude the akinetic scarred segment of the ventricle to restore normal left ventricular geometry and improve overall ventricular performance. The left ventricular cavity is opened in the middle of the aneurysm (*A*). One or more sutures of a 2-O Prolene monofilament are placed circumferentially approximately 1 cm above the border between the scarred and normal myocardium to restore the apex of the contracting ventricle (*B*). Then, a circular fabric (usually Dacron) patch, about 2 cm in diameter, is fixed inside the ventricle along this suture line to close the ventricular cavity (*C*). The scarred myocardium is closed over the patch. (Reproduced with permission from Franco KL, Verrier ED. Advanced Therapy in Cardiac Surgery 2e. Hamilton: BC Decker Inc. ©2003 BC Decker Inc.)

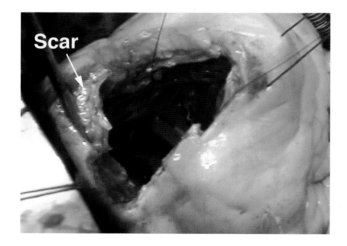

DVD **Fig 1-59.** At surgery the apical scar was opened, corresponding to step A in **Fig 1-58**. Normal trabeculations are seen in the ventricular chamber.

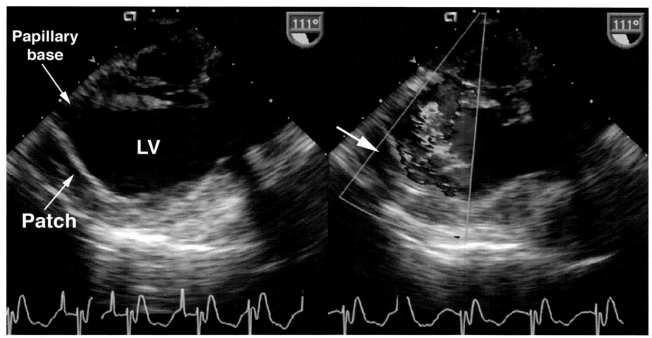

DVD **Fig 1-60.** The transgastric transesophageal image in a long-axis orientation, after completion of the procedure, shows the Dacron patch in the apical region. Color Doppler (*right*) demonstrates the patch to be intact, with no flow entering the excluded apex (**arrow**).

Comments

This patient developed a large apical aneurysm after anterior myocardial infarction. Ventricular performance can be improved by removal or exclusion of the scarred akinetic segment. The proposed mechanism of improvement is restoration of normal ventricular geometry, which leads to a decrease in wall stress because of the smaller ventricular diameter. With the Dor procedure, instead of excising the aneurysm, the aneurysmal area is excluded from the ventricular chamber with a patch closure of the residual opening between the normal part of the ventricle and the aneurysm, as detailed in the figures. Overall, operative mortality for this procedure is 8% with an average improvement in ejection fraction from 33% preoperatively to 50% 1 week after surgery, with sustained improvement in ventricular function at 1-year follow-up. The benefit of this procedure depends on the size of the myocardial scar. Thus, the echocardiographic examination focuses on defining the extent and location of wall thinning, akinesis and dyskinesis.

Suggested Reading

1. Dor V, Saab M, Coste P et al. Endoventricular patch plasties with septal exclusion for repair of ischemic left ventricle: technique, results and indications from a series of 781 cases. Jpn J Thorac Cardiovasc Surg 1998; 46(5):389–98.

2. Di Donato M, Sabatier M, Dor V et al. Akinetic versus dyskinetic postinfarction scar: relation to surgical outcome in patients undergoing endoventricular circular patch plasty repair. J Am Coll Cardiol 1997; 29(7):1569–75.

Case 1-10
Ventricular Rupture

This 68-year-old man presented with a 4-hour history of chest pain and ST elevation on ECG. He had no prior history of coronary disease but did have risk factors of hypertension, diabetes, smoking and hypercholesterolemia. He received thrombolytic therapy but had recurrent chest pain. He was transferred to our medical center and taken directly to the cardiac catheterization laboratory, where an occluded right coronary artery was successfully treated with two drug-eluting stents. An abnormal left ventriculogram prompted echocardiography and then surgical consultation.

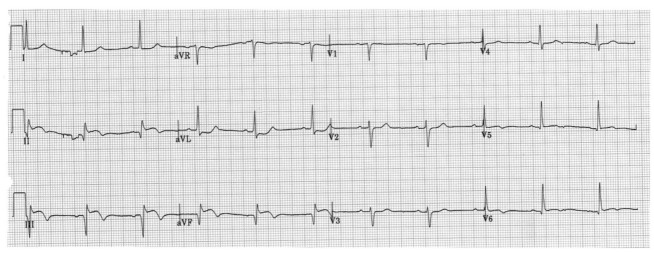

Fig 1-61. The ECG demonstrates an acute inferior myocardial infarction with Q waves, ST elevation and T-wave inversion in leads II, III and aVF.

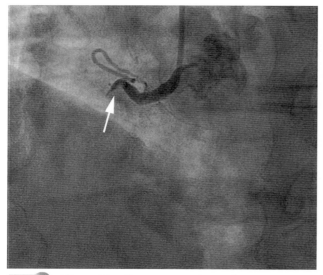

DVD **Fig 1-62.** Coronary angiography demonstrated only mild disease in the left anterior descending and circumflex coronary arteries. The right coronary artery was acutely occluded (**arrow**). The vessel was opened and a stent placed with restoration of normal blood flow.

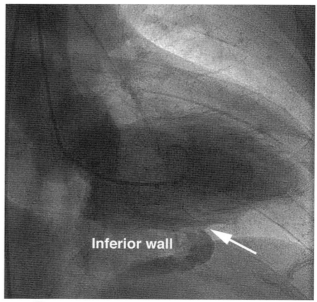

Inferior wall

DVD **Fig 1-63.** The left ventriculogram in a right anterior oblique projection shows an unusual extension of the contrast (**arrow**) out of the ventricular chamber in the mid-segment of the inferior wall.

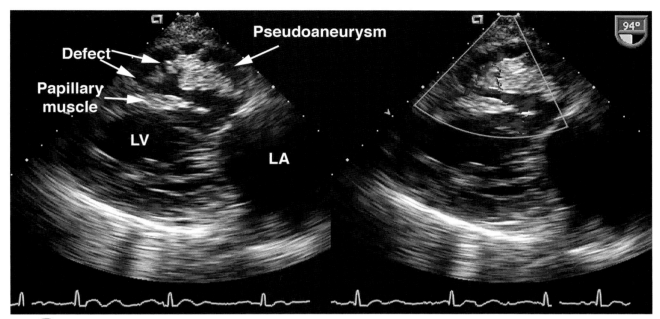

DVD **Fig 1-64.** Intraoperative transesophageal imaging in a two-chamber view from a transgastric position shows the defect in the inferior left ventricular wall, immediately adjacent to the papillary muscle. On color Doppler, flow into this region is seen.

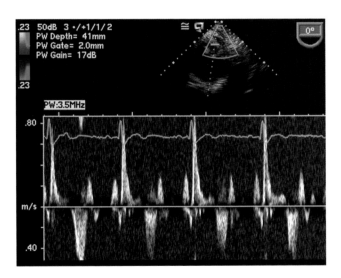

Fig 1-65. Pulsed Doppler confirms low-velocity flow into this space in early systole with reversed flow in late systole.

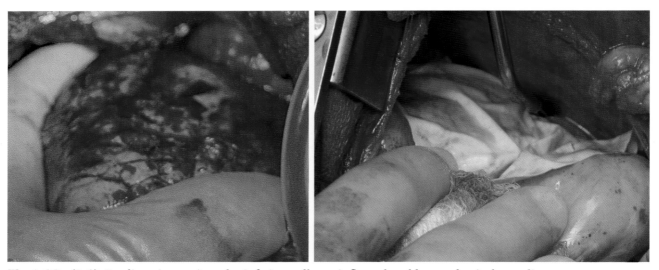

Fig 1-66. (*Left*) On direct inspection, the inferior wall was inflamed and hemorrhagic, but a discrete rupture was not identified. A patch was placed over the area of impending rupture. (*Right*) Two days later, the patient had recurrent chest pain. At that time, a transthoracic imaging showed that the LV rupture was contained by the surgical patch.

Comment

Ventricular rupture can occur up to 2 weeks after myocardial infarction and may result in pericardial tamponade with rapid hemodynamic collapse and death. However, in some patients, the rupture is "contained" by pericardial adhesions so that, after an initial episode of chest pain and hypotension, the patient transiently improves. Accurate diagnosis of ventricular rupture at this point, as in this case, can be lifesaving. The incidence of ventricular rupture is similar in patients treated by either thrombolytic therapy or direct angioplasty, with rupture presenting up to 2 weeks after infarction. Rupture typically occurs earlier (within 24 hours) after myocardial infarction in patients who received thrombolytic therapy.

With a contained ventricular rupture, over time the adhesed pericardium forms a saccular aneurysm around the rupture site. This pseudoaneurysm is identified on echocardiography as having a ratio of the neck of the aneurysm to the maximum diameter of <0.5. The pseudoaneurysm may be lined with thrombus, and there is often Doppler evidence for flow out and into the ventricle at the rupture site. Unlike a true ventricular aneurysm, the wall of a pseudoaneurysm does not contain myocardium and the abrupt transition from normal myocardium to the defect in the wall can often be appreciated on 2D imaging.

However, early in the course of ventricular rupture, the classic findings of a pseudoaneurysm may not be seen, with the echocardiogram simply showing discontinuity in the ventricular wall and Doppler evidence for flow outside the ventricular chamber, as in this case.

Suggested Reading

1. Vargas-Barron J, Molina-Carrion M, Romero-Cardenas A et al. Risk factors, echocardiographic patterns, and outcomes in patients with acute ventricular septal rupture during myocardial infarction. Am J Cardiol 2005; 95(10):1153–8.

2. McMullan MH, Maples MD, Kilgore TL Jr, Hindman SH. Surgical experience with left ventricular free wall rupture. Ann Thorac Surg 2001; 71(6):1894-8.

Transmyocardial Revascularization

Case 1-11
Transmyocardial Revascularization

This 43-year-old man with a history of smoking and hypercholesterolemia, and a family history of premature coronary disease, was referred for coronary bypass grafting for severe three-vessel coronary disease. At surgery, a left internal mammary graft (LIMA) graft was placed to the LAD and a saphenous vein graft was placed to the ramus intermedius. However, the distal vessels were diffused, diseased, the LIMA graft was small and there was concern that revascularization with these grafts was not adequate. No other suitable distal vessels were identified on careful evaluation. A decision was made to augment the myocardial perfusion with transmyocardial revascularization (TMR).

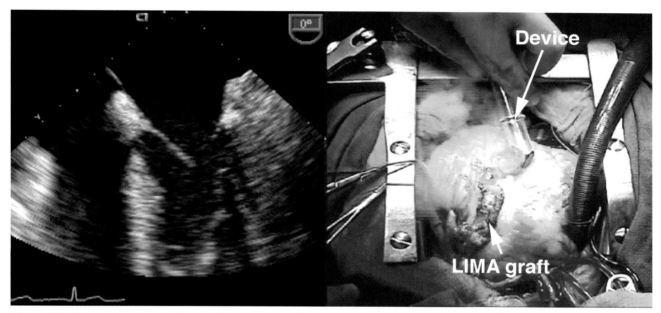

Fig 1-67. The transesophageal four-chamber view shows the ventricular septum at baseline (*left*). On the right, the intraoperative view shows the TMR device positioned over the anterior wall, adjacent to the left internal mammary artery (**LIMA**) graft to the left anterior descending coronary artery. The laser has been emitted, but has not yet come into contact with the myocardium.

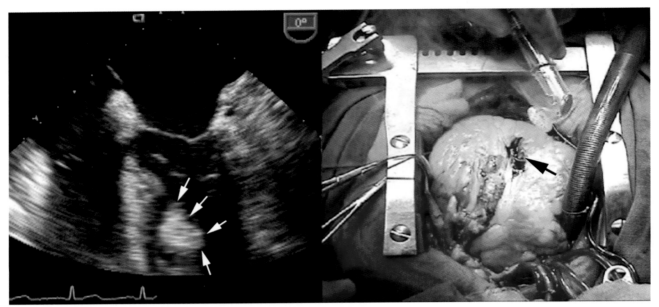

Fig 1-68. After completion of laser emission, contrast is seen in the left ventricle (*left*, **arrows**). This assures the surgeon that the channel created completely traverses all three layers of the left ventricle. The device has been removed from the heart, leaving a small area of epicardial injury. (*right*, **arrow**). Using this echocardiographic guidance, 10 TMR channels were placed on the antero-lateral wall surrounding the obtuse marginal and near the septum.

Comment

TMR is used for refractory anginal symptoms as an adjunct to revascularization in areas of myocardium that do not have suitable vessels for bypass grafting or percutaneous revascularization. TMR has been associated with clinical improvement in symptoms although the mechanism of this improvement is unclear. The small channels created by the device are closed within 24 hours and myocardial perfusion studies do not show improved myocardial blood flow. Proposed mechanisms of clinical improvement include stimulation of angiogenesis, myocardial fibrosis and sympathetic denervation.

In the operating room, TMR is monitored using TEE to detect the appearance of contrast in the ventricle with each channel. Potential complications of TMR that the echocardiographer should be alert to include atrial fibrillation, ventricular arrhythmias, myocardial infarction and left ventricular failure. The possible benefits of TMR remain controversial and it is unclear whether this approach will continue to be used in selected cases.

Suggested Reading

1. Szatkowski A, Ndubuka-Irobunda C, Oesterle SN, Burkhoff D. Transmyocardial laser revascularization: a review of basic and clinical aspects. Am J Cardiovasc Drugs 2002; 2(4):255–66.

Coronary Anomalies

Case 1-12
Anomalous Right Coronary Origin from Pulmonary Artery

This 37-year-old man was found to have a soft continuous murmur on physical examination. Transthoracic echocardiography showed an abnormal flow signal in the main pulmonary artery.

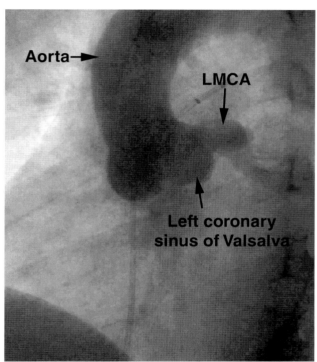

Fig 1-69. The aortogram demonstrates a large left main coronary artery (**LMCA**). The left-sided coronary arteries are enlarged because the flow in the right coronary artery is retrograde into the low-pressure pulmonary artery, creating a left-to-right shunt from the left coronary into the pulmonary artery. (Normal left main coronary diameter is 4.2 ± 0.7 mm.)

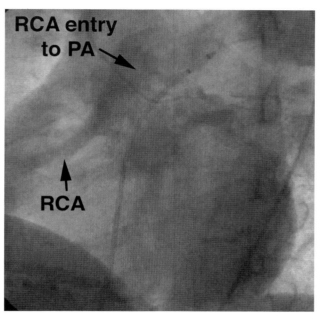

Fig 1-70. A late frame from the coronary angiogram shows contrast injected into the left coronary now traveling retrograde in the right coronary artery (**RCA**), with an entry into the pulmonary artery (**PA**).

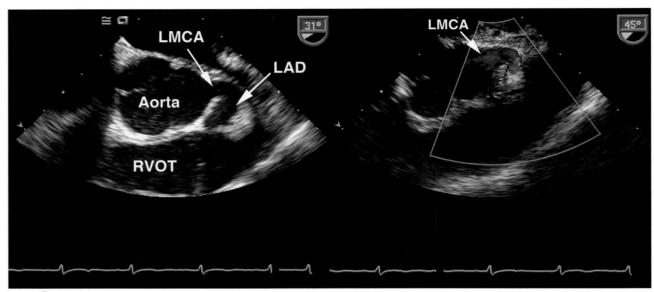

DVD **Fig 1-71.** On TEE, in a short-axis view just superior to the aortic valve, the enlarged left main coronary artery (**LMCA**) and the anteriorly directed left anterior descending coronary (**LAD**) are seen on 2D imaging (*left*) and with color Doppler (*right*). RVOT = right ventricular outflow tract.

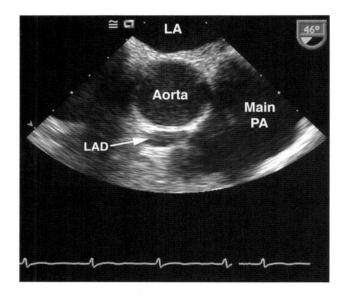

Fig 1-72. With slight adjustment of the image plane, the left anterior descending coronary, which is enlarged, is seen anterior to the aorta.

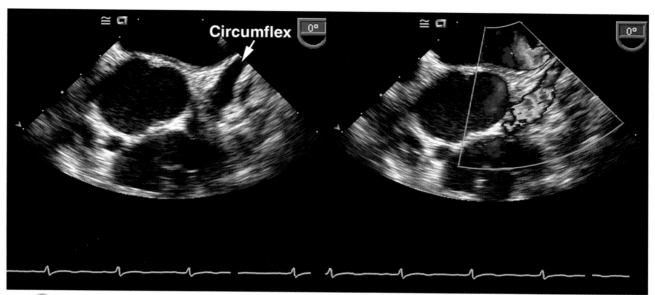

Fig 1-73. With the view rotated to 0 degrees, the enlarged circumflex artery is seen on 2D imaging (*left*) and with color Doppler (*right*).

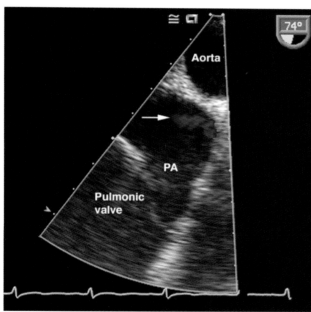

Fig 1-74. From a high esophageal probe position, subtle diastolic flow entering the pulmonary artery (**PA**) is seen (**arrow**).

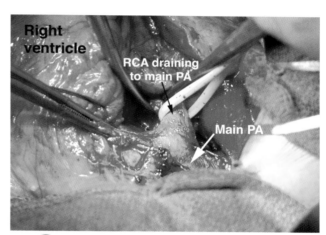

Fig 1-75. At surgery, the right coronary artery (**RCA**) origin from the main pulmonary artery (**PA**) was identified.

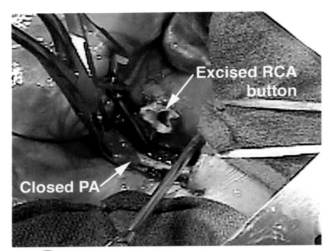

DVD ▶ **Fig 1-76.** The right coronary was excised with a small "button" of tissue and the defect in the pulmonary artery was repaired with a small pericardial patch.

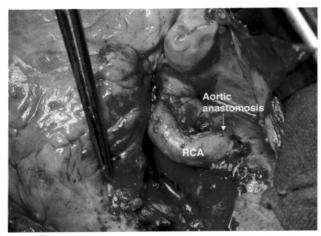

DVD ▶ **Fig 1-77.** The right coronary artery was then translocated to the aorta.

Comment

Abnormal origins of the coronary arteries are seen in about 0.4% of all congenital cardiac anomalies and usually involve an anomalous origin of a coronary artery from a different aortic sinus of Valsalva. The right or left coronary artery arising from the pulmonary artery, instead of the aorta, is rare and is usually an isolated finding. In patients with a coronary artery arising from the pulmonary artery, the clinical presentation depends on the hemodynamic consequences of the altered coronary blood flow patterns. In this patient, flow in the right coronary artery was retrograde into the low-pressure pulmonary artery. However, the patient did not have symptoms of ischemia, and left ventricular function was preserved because there was still adequate myocardial perfusion via the left coronary system. In effect, the myocardium supplied by the right coronary artery was perfused by left coronary to right coronary collateral flow.

Echocardiographic features that support the diagnosis of an anomalous coronary origin include the dilated left coronary arteries and the absence of diastolic flow reversal in the descending thoracic aorta (which is expected with a patent ductus arteriosus). On echocardiography, the diastolic flow signal is clearly not pulmonic regurgitation as it was detected distal to the pulmonic valve. Differentiation from a patent ductus arteriosus by echocardiography is more difficult. Direct visualization of the coronary origin would be the most definitive echocardiographic finding, but could not be obtained in this example.

Suggested Reading

1. Lerberg DB, Ogden JA, Zuberbuhler JR, Bahnson HT. Anomalous origin of the right coronary artery from the pulmonary artery. Ann Thorac Surg 1979; 27(1):87–94.
2. Veselka J, Widimsky P, Kautzner J. Reimplantation of anomalous right coronary artery arising from the pulmonary trunk leading to normal coronary flow reserve late after surgery. Ann Thorac Surg 2003; 76(4):1287–9.

Case 1-13
Anomalous Left Coronary Origin from the Pulmonary Artery

This 59-year-old man, with no prior medical problems, was admitted after a ventricular fibrillation arrest. Echocardiography showed moderate hypokinesis of the apical two-thirds of the anterior wall with an overall left ventricular ejection fraction of 42%. In addition, echocardiography suggested an anomalous left coronary artery, and he was taken to the cardiac catheterization laboratory where this diagnosis was confirmed.

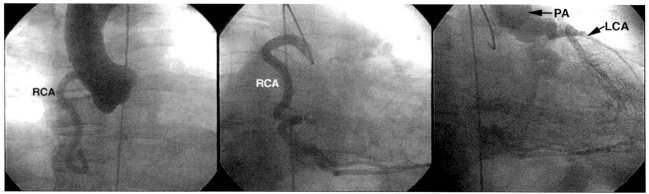

Fig 1-78. On aortography, dye injected into the aorta first fills the right coronary artery (**RCA**, *left*) and no left coronary is seen. With a selective injection of the RCA (center) after the right coronary fills, there is late opacification of the left coronary artery (**LCA**), which drains into the pulmonary artery (**PA**) (*right*).

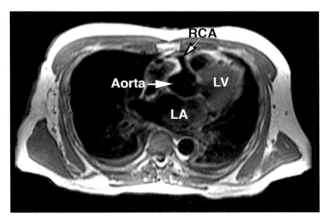

Fig 1-79. An MRI scan shows the right coronary artery (**RCA**) arising from the aorta in the normal position.

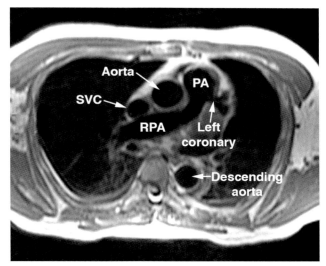

Fig 1-80. An MRI image slightly cephalad to **Fig 1-79** shows the left coronary artery arising from the pulmonary artery (**PA**). The bifurcation into the left anterior descending and circumflex coronaries can be seen.

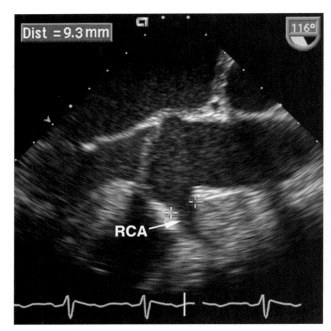

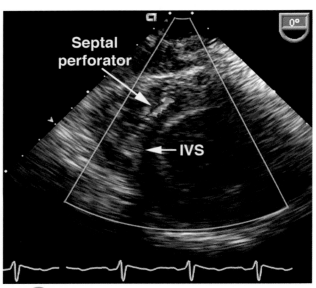

Fig 1-81. In a TEE long-axis view, the right coronary artery (**RCA**) origin from the aorta is in the normal position, but the vessel is larger than expected, at 9.3 mm. (Normal RCA diameter is 3.6± 0.8 mm.)

DVD **Fig 1-83.** An enlarged septal perforator branch is seen in a short-axis view of the ventricle due to the high volume of flow from the right coronary into the left coronary system.

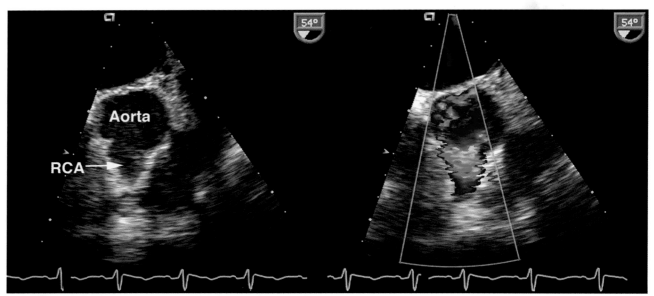

DVD **Fig 1-82.** In a short-axis view of the aorta at 30 degrees rotation, the enlarged right coronary ostium is seen on 2D imaging (*left*) and with color Doppler (*right*).

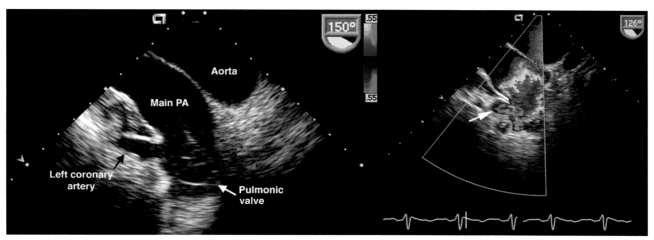

Fig 1-84. The left main coronary is identified originating from the main pulmonary artery (**PA**). Because pulmonary pressures are low, blood flow in the left coronary system is retrograde, with a left-to-right shunt from the aorta, via the right and then left coronary, with drainage into the PA (*right*, **arrow**).

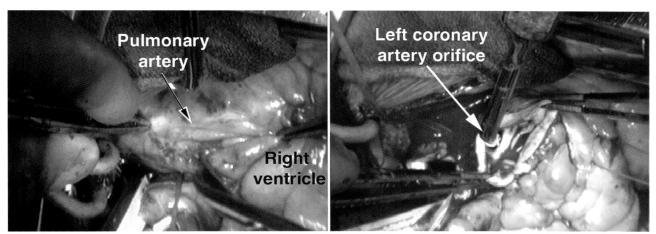

DVD ▶ **Fig 1-85.** At surgery the left coronary was identified arising from the pulmonary artery. The left main coronary was translocated to the aorta and the pulmonary artery was patched. In addition, a saphenous vein graft was placed to the mid-left anterior descending coronary artery. Postoperative ejection fraction was 58%.

Comment

Although the major adverse outcome in patients with an anomalous coronary artery is sudden cardiac death, as in this case, most patients with the left coronary artery arising from the pulmonary artery also have significant left ventricular dysfunction. An *anomalous left coronary artery from the pulmonary artery* is called the ALCAPA or Bland–White–Garland syndrome. The flow in the left coronary artery is retrograde into the low-pressure pulmonary artery. Thus, the entire myocardium is supplied by the right coronary artery, with right-to-left collaterals into the left coronary system. This often results in myocardial ischemia and subsequent left ventricular dysfunction. Most people with ALCAPA present in the first few months of life with myocardial ischemia and heart failure. Without surgical intervention, only 25% survive to adulthood; heart failure and ischemic mitral regurgitation are common in these survivors. Thus, the case presented here is quite unusual in that the patient was asymptomatic until his episode of sudden death and he had normal ventricular function after surgery.

Suggested reading

1. Angelini P. Coronary artery anomalies—current clinical issues: definitions, classification, incidence, clinical relevance, and treatment guidelines. Tex Heart Inst J 2002; 29:271–8.
2. Youn HJ, Foster E. Transesophageal echocardiography (TEE) in the evaluation of the coronary arteries. Cardiol Clin 2000; 18(4):833–48.

Case 1-14
Right Coronary to Left Ventricular Fistula

This 42-year-old woman had a known murmur for at least 25 years. Echocardiography showed a right coronary artery to left ventricular fistula. Left ventricular size was moderately increased (diastole 6.6 cm, systole 4.5 cm) with mild global hypokinesis and an ejection fraction of 52%. A stress nuclear perfusion study showed normal exercise tolerance for age, with a normal hemodynamic response to exercise. There was no evidence for inducible ischemia. Because serial echocardiograms had shown progressive left ventricular dilation with a reduction in ejection fraction, she was referred for surgical closure of the fistula.

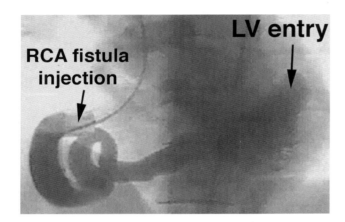

DVD **Fig 1-86.** Coronary angiography with selective injection into the right coronary artery (**RCA**) fistula demonstrates the dilated and tortuous course of the fistula, with contrast draining into the left ventricle (**LV**).

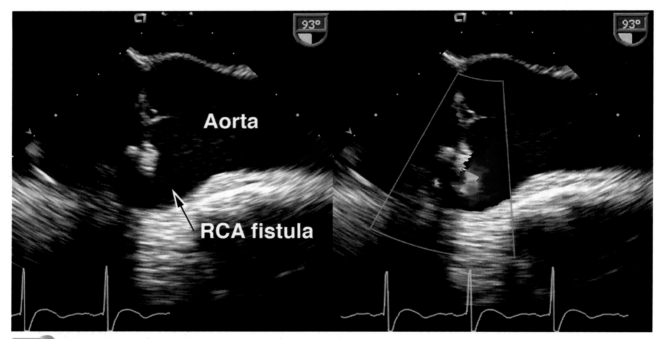

DVD **Fig 1-87.** In the TEE long-axis view of the ascending aorta, the enlarged right coronary artery fistula (**RCA**) is seen.

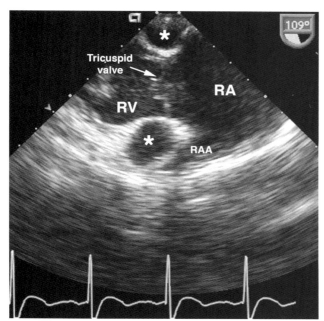

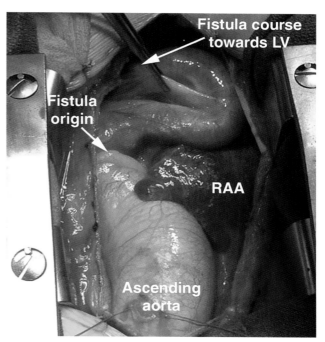

DVD **Fig 1-88.** In a right ventricular inflow view of the right atrium (**RA**) and right ventricle (**RV**), echolucent circular structures are seen in the atrioventricular groove on both sides of the tricuspid annulus (**asterisks**). Although the coronary sinus might be seen posteriorly in this location, it would not be seen anteriorly, and this structure is larger than the normal coronary sinus.

Fig 1-90. At surgery, looking from the patient's head toward his feet, the dilated fistula is seen originating from the ascending aorta proximal to the location of the right atrial appendage (**RAA**). The course of the fistula encircles the atrioventricular groove and courses towards the left ventricle (**LV**).

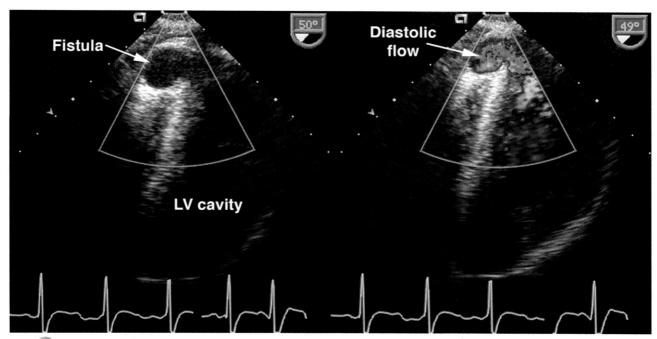

DVD **Fig 1-89.** The same structure seen in **Fig 1.88** is now seen entering the left ventricle in this two-chamber view. The echocardiographer can "follow" even a tortuous vessel, like this fistula, during the examination, by adjusting the angle of rotation and transducer position to sequentially image adjacent segments of the structure.

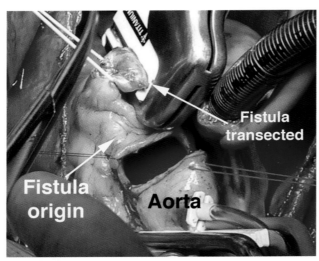

Fig 1-91. The fistula was transected just distal to its origin and the fistula orifice repaired from within the aorta with a patch. The fistula was also stapled close to its drainage into the left ventricle. A saphenous vein graft was placed to the posterior descending artery, just beyond a ligation that isolated the posterior descending artery from the remnants of the fistula. Echocardiography 2 years after surgery demonstrated a normal-sized left ventricle (dimensions 5.3 and 4.2 cm) with an ejection fraction of 56%.

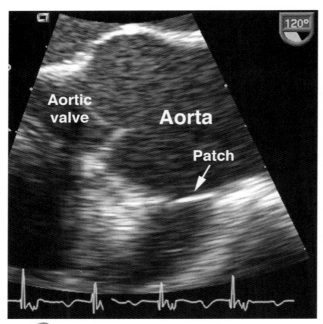

Fig 1-92. Postoperative TEE of the ascending aorta in a long-axis view shows the aortic patch covering the fistula orifice.

Comment

Most coronary fistulas from the coronary arteries into the cardiac chambers are congenital, although abnormal communications can also result from trauma or invasive procedures. Coronary fistulas are more common with the right coronary artery (55%) compared with the left coronary system and most often drain into the right ventricle (40%), right atrium (26%) or pulmonary artery (17%). Coronary fistulas that drain into the superior vena cava, coronary sinus or left ventricle, as in this case, are less common. The initial diagnosis is usually made based on the physical examination finding of a murmur, or on echocardiography requested for other reasons.

The echocardiographic findings depend on the origin and drainage of the fistula. The increased blood flow through the affected coronary artery leads to progressive dilation both of the coronary artery and the fistula. If the fistula drains into a right-sided chamber (in effect a left-to-right shunt), enlargement of the left-sided cardiac chambers, along with enlargement of the right ventricle (and right atrium if the fistula drains here) are expected. When the fistula drains into a left-sided chamber, creating increased flow from the aorta back into the left heart, progressive left ventricular dilation is expected, as in the case presented here. Transesophageal echocardiography is superior to transthoracic imaging for evaluation of the course of the fistula, drainage site and size of aneurysmal dilation. Other imaging modalities including coronary angiography and chest CT are also helpful.

In addition to progressive chamber enlargement and heart failure, complications of coronary fistulas include thrombosis and embolization with myocardial or systemic ischemic events, endocarditis, arrhythmias and pulmonary hypertension. Surgical or percutaneous closure is recommended to prevent these complications.

Suggested Reading

1. Vitarelli A, De Curtis G, Conde Y et al. Assessment of congenital coronary artery fistulas by transesophageal color Doppler echocardiography. Am J Med 2002; 113(2):127–33.

2. Armsby LR, Keane JF, Sherwood MC et al. Management of coronary artery fistulae. Patient selection and results of transcatheter closure. J Am Coll Cardiol 2002; 39(6):1026–32.

3. Frommelt PC, Frommelt MA. Congenital coronary artery anomalies. Pediatr Clin North Am 2004; 51(5):1273-88.

2

Mitral Valve Disease

Normal Mitral Valve

Case 2-1
Normal Mitral Valve Anatomy

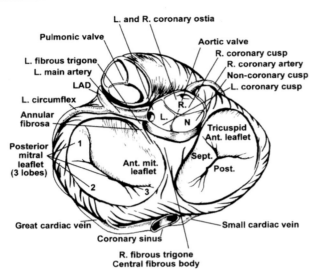

Fig 2-1. Anatomic view of the cardiac valves from the perspective of the base of the heart with the atria cut away and the great vessels transected. All four valves have a close anatomic relationship. In particular, the aortic valve is adjacent to the mitral valve along the midsegment of the anterior mitral leaflet. (Reproduced with permission from Otto CM. Valvular Heart Disease 2e. Philadelphia: WB Saunders. ©2004 Elsevier Inc.)

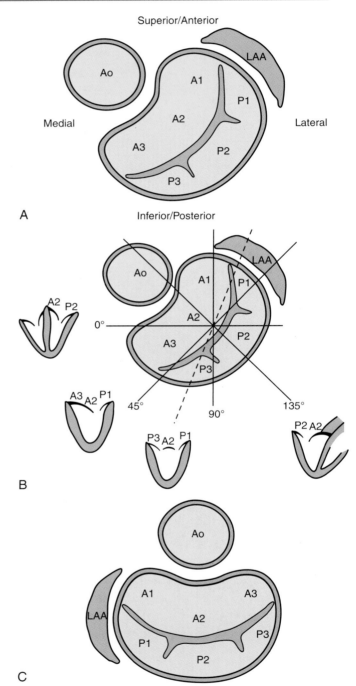

Fig 2-2. (A) Reference view displaying the mitral valve and its anatomic relationship to the aortic root (**Ao**) and the left atrial appendage (**LAA**) as seen from the left ventricular apex or TEE short axis view. (B) Reference view demonstrating the relationship of the TEE imaging planes to the mitral valve with the probe positioned in the standard midesophageal position. (C) Surgical view of the mitral valve as seen from left atrium with the heart rotated. (A1, A2, A3 = anterior leaflet sections; P1, P2, P3 = posterior leaflet sections.)(Reproduced with permission from Foster GP et al. Accurate localization of mitral regurgitant defects using multiplane transesophageal echocardiography. Ann Thoracic Surg 1998; 65:1025–1031. ©1998 Elsevier Inc.)

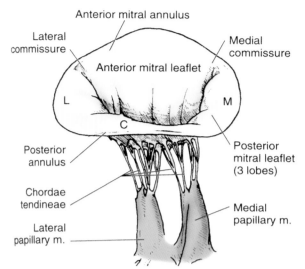

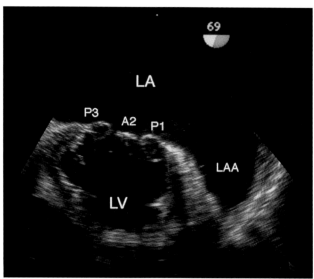

Fig 2-3. The mitral valve apparatus consists of the mitral annulus, anterior and posterior leaflets, chordae tendineae and the papillary muscles. **L** = lateral; **C** = central; **M** = medial. (Reproduced with permission from Otto CM. Valvular Heart Disease 2e. Philadelphia: WB Saunders. ©2004 Elsevier Inc.)

DVD **Fig 2-5.** TEE mitral commissural view, obtained here at 69 degrees by slight backward rotation from the two-chamber view, demonstrates the central segment of the anterior leaflet (**A2**) and the medial (**P3**) and lateral (**P1**) segments of the posterior leaflet.

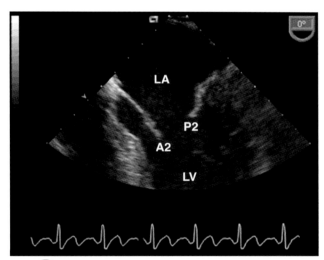

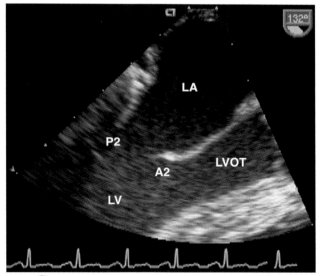

DVD **Fig 2-4.** TEE in a four-chamber view at 0 degrees demonstrating the central section of the anterior leaflet (**A2**) and the central scallop of the posterior leaflet (**P2**).

DVD **Fig 2-6.** Further rotation to 132 degrees results in a long-axis view, again showing the central section of the anterior leaflet (**A2**) and the central scallop of the posterior leaflet (**P2**).

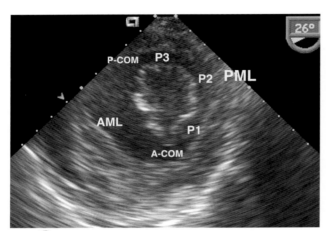

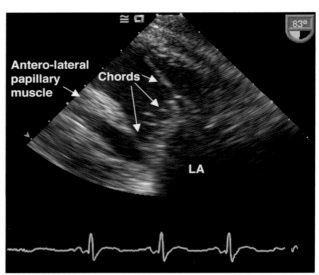

DVD **Fig 2-7.** The transgastric short-axis view at the level of the mitral valve demonstrates the anterior mitral leaflet (**AML**) and the three scallops of the posterior leaflet (**PML**), along with the posterior (**P-COM**) and anterior commissures (**A-COM**).

DVD **Fig 2-8.** Rotation to about 90 degrees (83 degrees in this case) from the transgastric short axis provides a two-chamber view with visualization of the mitral leaflets, chords and anterolateral papillary muscle.

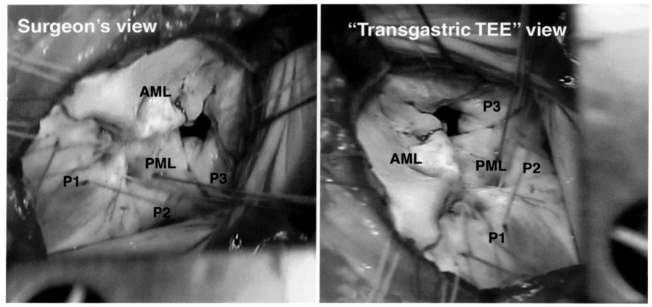

Fig 2-9. The normal mitral valve in vivo, as seen following incisions in the right atrium, and the inter-atrial septum. On the left is the surgeon's view from the right-hand side of the operating table. On the right is the valve as it would appear on a basal transgastric short axis TEE, as in **Figure 2-7**.

Comments

The mitral valve apparatus is a complex structure in three dimensions that includes the saddle-shaped mitral annulus, the leaflets, the chords and the papillary muscles. The anterior leaflet is longer than the posterior leaflet but extends only about one-third of the distance around the annulus circumference. The anterior leaflet does not have anatomically discrete segments but location can be described as the medial (A3), central (A2) and lateral (A1) aspects of the leaflet. The posterior leaflet is shorter but extends a greater distance around the mitral annulus. The posterior leaflet typically has three discrete scallops: medial (P3), central (P2) and lateral (P1).

Mitral regurgitant severity is best evaluated using multiple Doppler measures on a preoperative complete transthoracic echocardiogram (TTE). Decisions about timing of surgery are based not only on severity of regurgitation, but on serial changes in left ventricular dimensions and systolic function. When regurgitant severity is re-evaluated in the operating room (OR), regurgitant severity may be less than expected due to a lower afterload in the anesthetized versus awake patient. Useful measures of regurgitant severity in the OR include:

- Vena contracta width—the narrowest diameter of the regurgitant jet.
- Proximal isovelocity surface area (PISA)—the region of flow convergence on the ventricular side of the valve. The instantaneous regurgitant flow rate is the area of a hemisphere ($2\pi r^2$) times the aliasing velocity.
- Continuous wave (CW) Doppler—intensity and time course of the regurgitant velocity signal.
- Regurgitant orifice area (ROA)—calculated from PISA and CW Doppler velocity as discussed in Case 2.7 (see below).

The direction, size and shape of the regurgitant jet are less useful for quantitation of severity but often help identify the mechanism of regurgitation because the direction of the jet typically is opposite the affected leaflet, e.g. posterior leaflet prolapse results in an anteriorly directed jet.

Suggested Reading

1. Otto CM. Valvular regurgitation. In: Textbook of Clinical Echocardiography, 3rd edn. Philadelphia: Elsevier Saunders, 2004: 335–44.

2. Heinle SK. Quantitation of valvular regurgitation: Beyond color flow mapping. In: Otto CM, ed. The Practice of Clinical Echocardiography, 2nd edn. Philadelphia: WB Saunders, 2002: 367–88.

3. Zoghbi WA, Enriquez-Sarano M, Foster E, et al. Recommendations for evaluation of the severity of native valvular regurgitation with two-dimensional and Doppler echocardiography. J Am Soc Echocardiogr 2003; 16:777–802.

Myxomatous Mitral Valve Disease

Case 2-2
Posterior Leaflet Prolapse with Flail Central (P2) Scallop

A 46-year-old man with a 20-year history of a murmur was transferred from another hospital with increasing shortness of breath and hemoptysis of 1 month's duration. A loud holosystolic murmur at the apex was noted on physical examination. Because the patient also had a long history of intravenous drug use, blood cultures were obtained and the patient was started on empiric intravenous antibiotics for possible endocarditis.

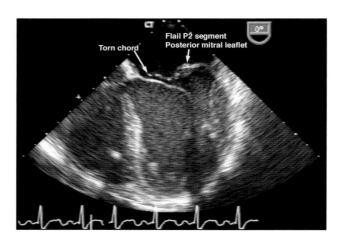

Transthoracic echocardiography showed severe mitral regurgitation with a posterior leaflet flail segment and an anteriorly directed regurgitant jet. Left ventricular size was at the upper limits of normal (end-systolic dimension 39 mm) with an ejection fraction of 60%. The left atrium was moderately enlarged and pulmonary pressures were severely elevated with an estimated systolic pressure of 70 mmHg. Transesophageal echocardiography was performed to evaluate for possible vegetations. This study demonstrated a flail central scallop of the posterior leaflet with severe mitral regurgitation. He was referred for mitral valve surgery.

Fig 2-10. Intraoperative 2D images of the mitral valve from a high esophageal position at 0 degrees rotation show the relatively thin anterior leaflet with normal motion and a thickened, redundant posterior leaflet. The flail segment of the posterior leaflet is seen on the atrial side of the annulus with the tip of the leaflet pointing away from the left ventricular apex. In contrast, with severe prolapse but intact chordae, there is bowing of the leaflet into the atrium, with the leaflet tip still pointing towards the ventricular apex.

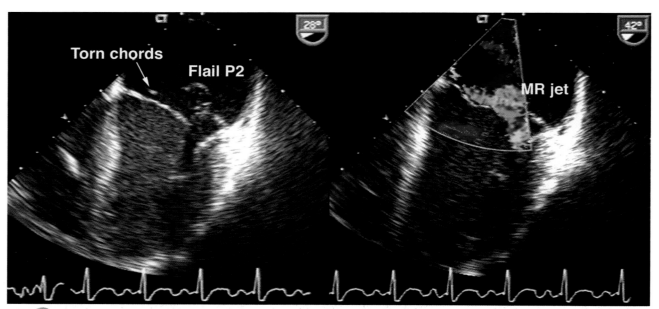

DVD **Fig 2-11.** Rotation of the 2D-image plane to 28 degrees (*left*) more clearly demonstrates the flail middle scallop of the posterior leaflet (**P2**) with a torn chord on the left atrial side of the valve in systole. Color flow Doppler at 42 degrees rotation (*right*) demonstrates a wide eccentric mitral regurgitant (**MR**) jet with flow acceleration on the ventricular side of the valve. The jet is directed away from the affected leaflet; e.g. an anteriorly directed jet with posterior leaflet disease.

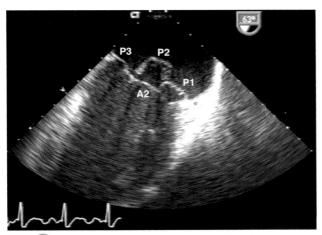

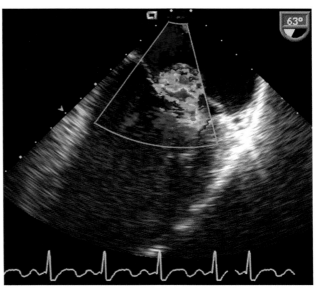

DVD **Fig 2-12.** Further rotation of the image plane to the mitral commissural view (63 degrees) shows the severe prolapse and partial flail of the central scallop of the posterior leaflet (**P2**).

DVD **Fig 2-14.** Color Doppler in the mitral commissural plane shows significant mitral regurgitation with a vena contracta width of 9 mm.

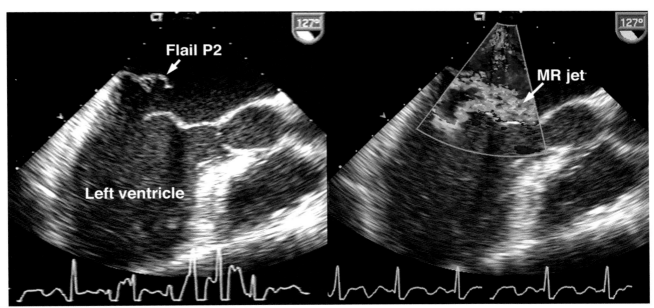

DVD **Fig 2-13.** Rotation of the 2D-image plane to 127 degrees (*left*) also demonstrates the flail middle scallop of the posterior leaflet (**P2**). Color flow Doppler at 127 degrees rotation (*right*) also demonstrates a wide eccentric mitral regurgitant (**MR**) jet with flow acceleration on the ventricular side of the valve. The jet is directed away from the affected leaflet; e.g. an anteriorly directed jet with posterior leaflet disease.

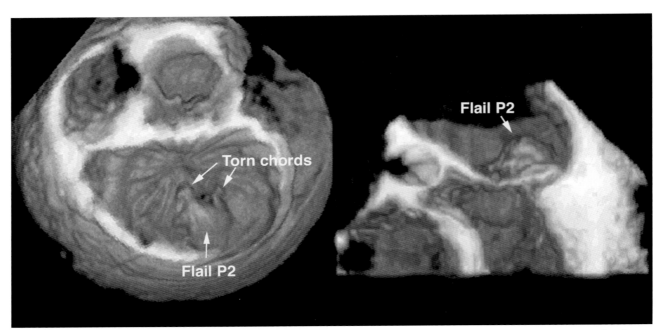

DVD **Fig 2-15.** 3D reconstructed images from a rotational TEE scan are oriented to show the mitral valve from the left atrial aspect (*left*) and in a long-axis orientation (*right*). The torn chords and the flail middle scallop of the posterior leaflet (**P2**) are clearly demonstrated. (Courtesy of Ed Gill, MD.)

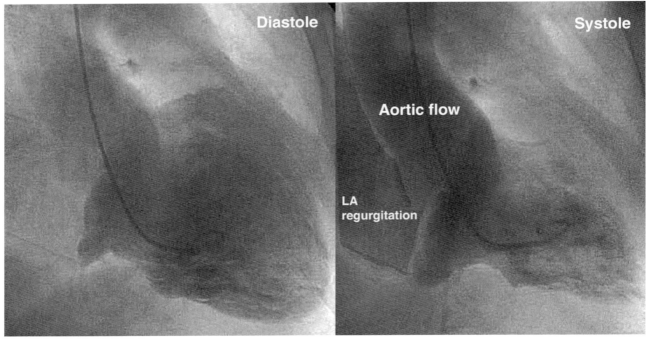

DVD **Fig 2-16.** Left ventricular angiography shows regurgitation across the mitral valve with opacification of the left atrium (**LA**) equal to the left ventricle after several beats consistent with moderate to severe mitral regurgitation.

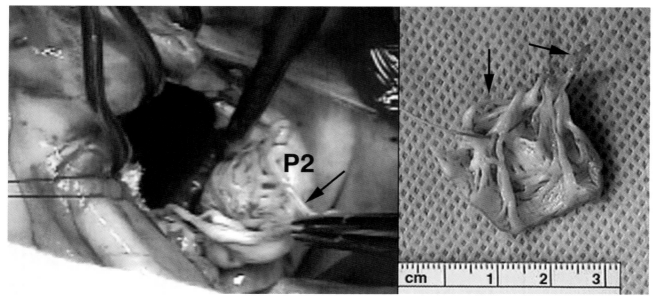

DVD **Fig 2-17.** Intraoperative visualization of the valve confirmed the flail middle scallop of the posterior leaflet with the surgical view shown on the left and the resected leaflet segment shown on the right. The anterior mitral leaflet was normal but there were three sets of ruptured chords to the central scallop of the posterior leaflet (**P2**) (**arrows**). There was no evidence for vegetation or abscess. The **DVD** shows that after resection of the flail leaflet segment and reapproximation of the leaflet edges, an annuloplasty ring was placed with the sutures positioned in the annulus and then the ring positioned.

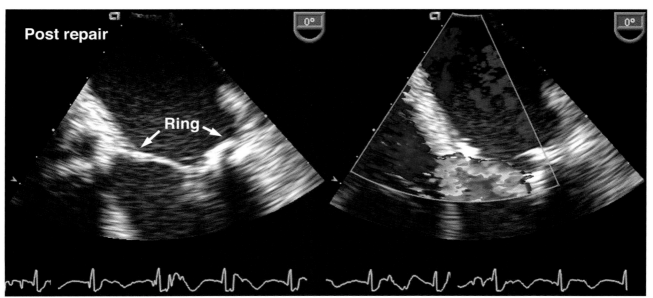

DVD **Fig 2-18.** Post-repair images at 0 degrees show increased echogenicity of the posterior leaflet and the annuloplasty ring, with normal leaflet closure in systole on 2D imaging (*left*) and the absence of mitral regurgitation on color flow imaging (*right*).

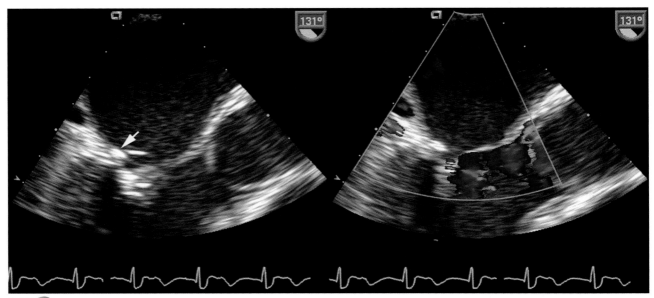

DVD ▶ **Fig 2-19.** Post-repair images in a long-axis view (131 degrees) show the annuloplasty ring (**arrow**) and the site of the posterior leaflet resection and repair (*left*). It is important to evaluate for regurgitation in multiple views; no regurgitation is seen with color flow imaging in this view (*right*).

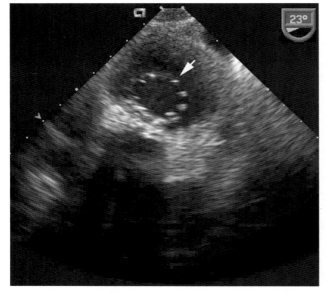

Fig 2-20. From the transgastric short-axis view, the annuloplasty ring is seen (**arrow**).

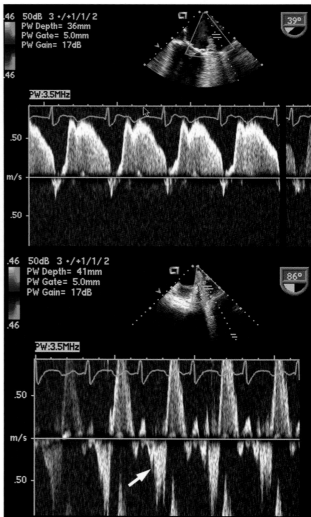

Fig 2-21. Pulsed Doppler evaluation of flow in the left upper pulmonary vein shows normal diastolic and systolic atrial inflow (*top*). In contrast, the pre-repair pulmonary venous flow (*bottom*) shows holosystolic reversal of flow (**arrow**) consistent with severe mitral regurgitation.

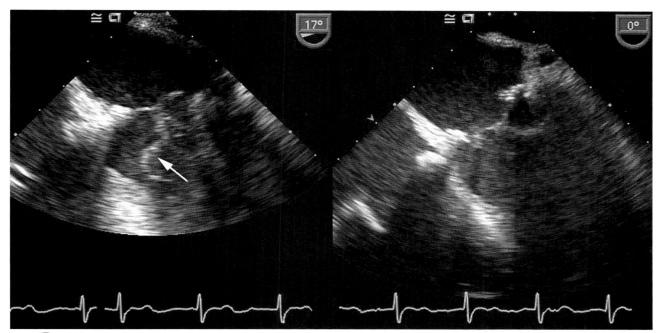

DVD **Fig 2-22.** In another patient with similar pathology and an identical procedure, postoperative TEE in the four-chamber view showed systolic anterior motion (**SAM**) of the anterior mitral leaflet (arrow) (*left*). After adjustment of loading conditions, the SAM resolved (*right*).

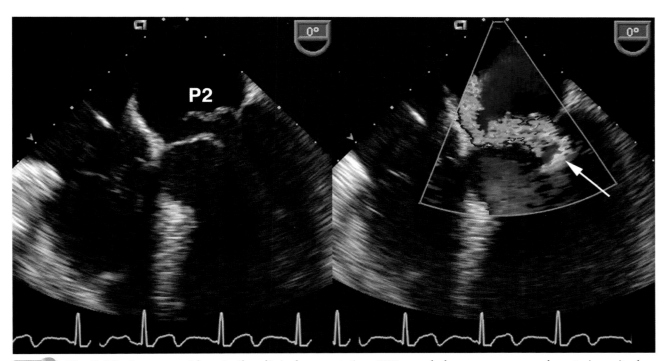

DVD **Fig 2-23.** In a case with a similar clinical presentation, TEE revealed more pronounced posterior mitral leaflet pathology. In the four-chamber view, P2 is seen to be flail, with an anteriorly directed jet of MR (**arrow**).

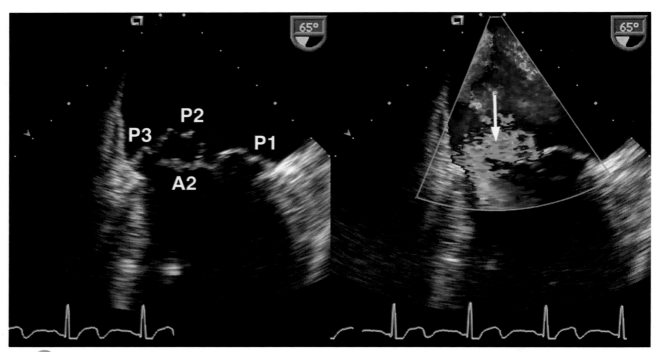

DVD ▶   **Fig 2-24.** In a bicommissural view, P2 is flail, and seen posteriorly to A2; in addition, excessive motion of P3 is also seen. The jet of MR (**arrow**) is seen between the anterior leaflet and both P2 and P3.

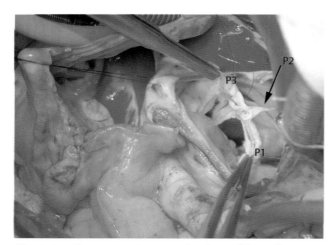

Fig 2-25. Intraoperative examination of the valve reveals redundancy in both P2 and P3, with a torn chord from P2 (**arrow**).

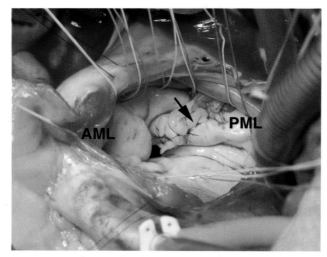

Fig 2-26. The involved posterior leaflet tissue has been resected and the defect closed (**arrow**).

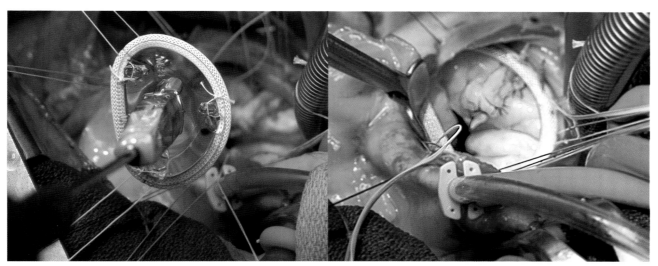

Fig 2-27. A complete annuloplasty ring is chosen, as opposed to the C-shaped ring used in the first case.

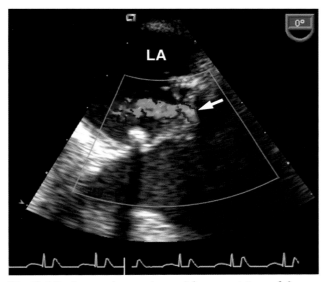

Fig 2-28. In another patient with an excision of the P2 scallop, postoperative imaging revealed a very eccentric jet (**arrow**) through the repaired posterior leaflet, suggesting that the posterior leaflet closure was not intact. This was confirmed on re-exploration, and re-repaired.

Comments

The first step in evaluation of a patient with mitral regurgitation is to establish the cause of valve dysfunction. Causes of mitral regurgitation are divided into primary anatomic abnormalities of the valve apparatus and secondary regurgitation due to left ventricular dilation and dysfunction with an anatomically normal valve. Common causes of primary mitral regurgitation include myxomatous mitral valve disease (e.g. mitral valve prolapse), rheumatic valve disease and endocarditis. In this patient, the etiology of valve dysfunction was myxomatous mitral valve disease. Although endocarditis was considered in the differential diagnosis of this patient's initial presentation, there was no evidence for valve infection on pathologic examination. However, differentiation of a valvular vegetation from a flail leaflet can be difficult, even with TEE imaging, as both have a similar echocardiographic appearance.

In patients with myxomatous mitral valve disease, attention is next focused on defining the exact anatomy of the valve leaflets and chords. The likelihood of a successful valve repair is highest with posterior leaflet involvement, particularly when the problem is isolated to the central (or P2) scallop. With severe prolapse, the leaflet bows into the left atrium in systole but the tip of the leaflet still points towards the LV apex because the chords are intact. In contrast, with chordal rupture and a flail leaflet segment, the leaflet tip points away from the LV apex, often with small mobile chords attached, as in this case. With the typical anatomy of regurgitation due to dysfunction of the central scallop of the posterior leaflet, quadrangular resection of the flail segment followed by placement of an annuloplasty ring usually results in a functional valve apparatus. The two broad categories of annuloplasty rings that have been used in the current era of mitral valve repair have been the C-shaped ring, and the complete ring. The former was used when it was assumed that there was no chance of dilation in the intertrigonal area, but some surgeons prefer a complete ring as distention in the intertrigonal area can occur.[1]

In patients with mitral valve repair, systolic anterior motion (SAM) of the anterior leaflet can result in significant dynamic left ventricular outflow tract obstruction. In many cases, SAM is transient as cardiopulmonary bypass is weaned and resolves with restoration of normal loading conditions. When significant outflow obstruction persists after normalization of loading conditions, a second pump run for correction of this abnormality should be considered. Systolic anterior motion can often be prevented by use of the "sliding-leaflet" technique where the posterior leaflet is separated from the mitral annulus at the time of posterior leaflet quadrangular resection and then reattached after reducing annular size with a flexible ring.

Suggested Reading

1. Hayek E, Gring CN, Griffin BP. Mitral valve prolapse. Lancet 2005; 365:507–18.
2. Pellerin D, Brecker S, Veyrat C. Degenerative mitral valve disease with emphasis on mitral valve prolapse. Heart 2002; 88(Suppl 4):20–28.
3. Omran AS, Woo A, David TE et al. Intraoperative transesophageal echocardiography accurately predicts mitral valve anatomy and suitability for repair. J Am Soc Echocardiogr 2002; 15:950–7.

Case 2-3
Posterior Leaflet Prolapse of Lateral (P1) Scallop

This 55-year-old woman was referred for mitral valve surgery for symptomatic severe mitral regurgitation. She had a long history of mitral valve prolapse. The four-chamber view showed no abnormalities of mitral leaflet motion.

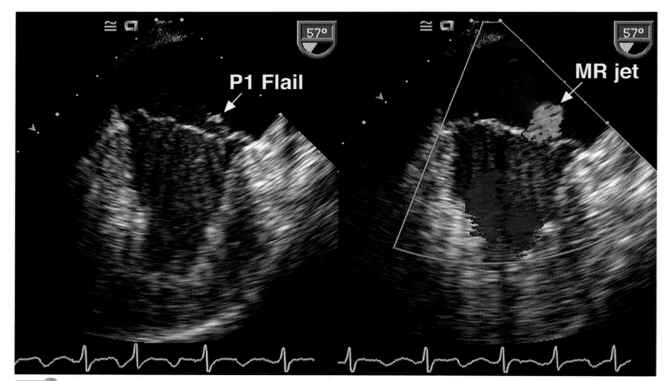

DVD **Fig 2-29.** The mitral commissural view, at about 60 degrees of rotation from a high TEE position, is helpful for defining which scallop of the posterior leaflet is abnormal. In this patient, the lateral segment or P1 scallop of the posterior leaflet is flail, with color Doppler showing the mitral regurgitant (**MR**) jet.

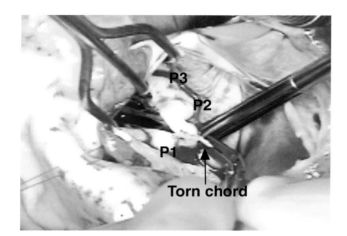

DVD **Fig 2-30.** At surgical inspection, the torn chord on the lateral scallop (**P1**) was identified.

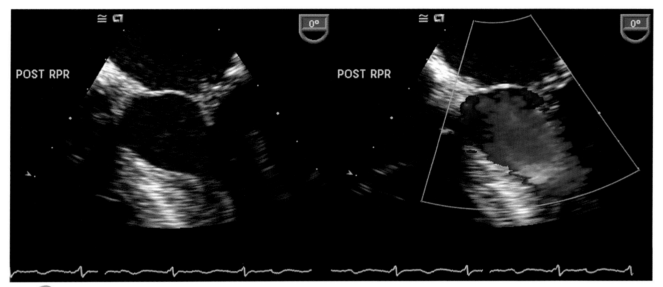

DVD **Fig 2-31.** After valve repair with resection of the flail segment and placement of an annuloplasty ring, the four-chamber view shows normal leaflet coaptation in systole with no detectable mitral regurgitation.

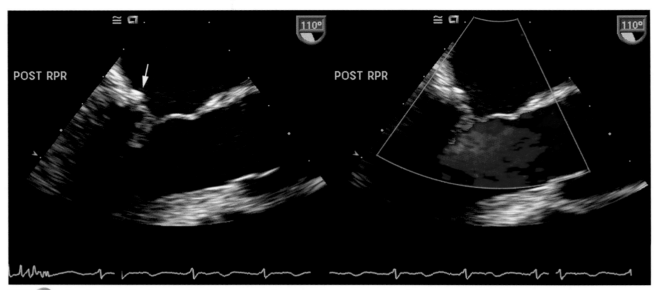

DVD **Fig 2-32.** The long-axis view, at 110 degrees of rotation, also shows normal leaflet coaptation, the annuloplasty ring (**arrow**) and no color Doppler evidence of regurgitation.

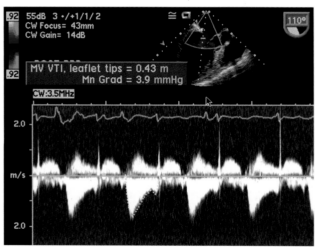

Fig 2-33. The continuous wave (**CW**) Doppler signal of transmitral flow shows a mildly increased antegrade velocity, with a steep deceleration slope, consistent with a small transmitral gradient but no significant obstruction to flow. There is no evidence for mitral regurgitation by CW Doppler.

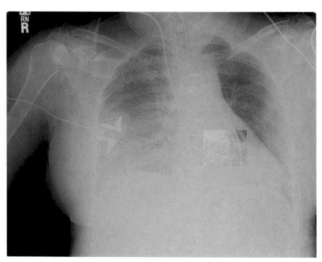

Fig 2-34. A postoperative digital chest radiograph, with processing in the region over the mitral valve to enhance prosthetic structures, shows the position of the mitral annuloplasty ring on the cardiac silhouette.

Case 2-4
Anterior Leaflet Prolapse

This 25-year-old man, with a known bicuspid aortic valve and history of aortic coarctation repair at age 2, presented with increasing dyspnea on exertion over the past several weeks. Physical examination showed a very hyperdynamic precordium with a loud, palpable P2. In addition, there was a grade 3/6 holosystolic murmur at the apex, radiating to the axilla, consistent with mitral regurgitation. Echocardiography showed a flail anterior mitral valve leaflet with severe mitral regurgitation. Aortic valve function was normal and there was no residual aortic coarctation. However, pulmonary systolic pressure was severely elevated at 90 mmHg. Because of severe symptomatic mitral regurgitation, he was referred for mitral valve surgery.

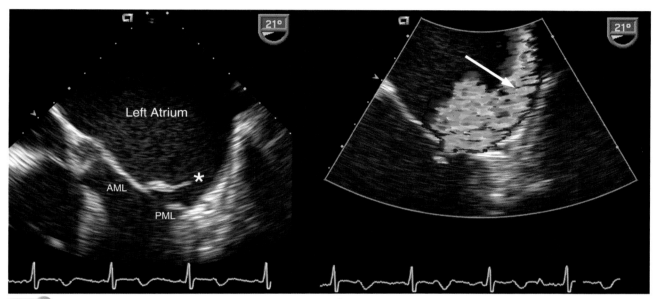

Fig 2-35. 2D imaging in an anteriorly angulated four-chamber view at 21 degrees rotation demonstrates a flail leaflet segment (**asterisk**) most consistent with anterior leaflet disease (*left*) with color flow imaging showing a posteriorly directed mitral regurgitant jet (*right*; **arrow**).

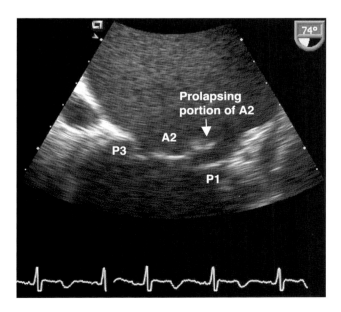

Fig 2-36. High TEE view at 74 degrees in a mitral commissural orientation shows a portion of the mitral leaflet in the left atrium in systole. In this view, the medial (**P3**) and lateral (**P1**) scallops of the posterior leaflet are typically seen with the central segment of the anterior leaflet (**A2**) seen in the center of the annular plane.

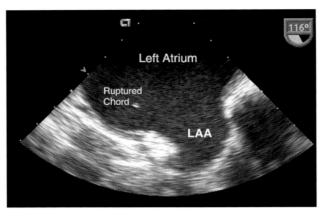

DVD **Fig 2-37.** In a view of the left atrium (**LA**) at the level of the atrial appendage (**LAA**), the tip of the ruptured mitral chord is seen intermittently in the image plane because the direction of the partial flail segment is superiorly into the left atrium.

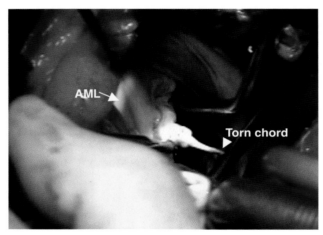

Fig 2-38. Visualization of the anterior leaflet at surgery demonstrated the torn chord at the mid-section of the anterior leaflet. Mitral valve repair was attempted. However, because of persistent significant mitral regurgitation after repair, the patient underwent mitral valve replacement.

Comments

Intraoperative TEE by an experienced echocardiographer for evaluation of the adequacy of mitral valve repair and for detection of any complications is indicated in all patients undergoing valve repair surgery. A second bypass pump run with revision of the repair or valve replacement is needed in about 5–10% of cases due to residual significant mitral regurgitation.

Baseline images provide a standard of reference for post-repair evaluation of valve function. However, it is important to ensure that the loading conditions, as measured by systemic blood pressure, heart rate and forward cardiac output, are similar on the pre- and post-valve repair studies. A lower blood pressure or cardiac output on the post-repair study may result in underestimation of regurgitant severity. The echocardiographic instrument settings also should be similar, including image depth, frame rate, 2D and color gain, wall filters and color map. The valve should be carefully evaluated in multiple image planes after the repair, and the direction and shape of any residual mitral regurgitation may be different than shown on the pre-repair images.

The surgeon may also assess the adequacy of repair by direct visual inspection of the amount of backflow across the valve when the ventricle is filled, as was done in this case.

Suggested Reading

1. Griffin BP, Stewart WJ. Echocardiography in patient selection, operative planning and intraoperative evaluation of mitral valve repair. In Otto CM, ed. The Practice of Clinical Echocardiography, 2nd edn. Philadelphia: WB Saunders, 2002: 417–34.

2. Agricola E, Oppizzi M, Maisano F et al. Detection of mechanisms of immediate failure by transesophageal echocardiography in quadrangular resection mitral valve repair technique for severe mitral regurgitation. Am J Cardiol 2003; 91:175–9.

3. Shah PM, Raney AA. Echocardiographic correlates of left ventricular outflow obstruction and systolic anterior motion following mitral valve repair. J Heart Valve Dis 2001; 10:302–6.

Rheumatic Mitral Valve Disease

Case 2-5
Rheumatic Mitral Stenosis

This 56-year-old man presented with severe symptomatic mitral stenosis and atrial fibrillation and was initially considered for percutaneous balloon valvotomy. The preoperative TEE showed typical rheumatic mitral valve disease with superimposed calcification and an immobile posterior leaflet with overall mitral valve morphology that was suboptimal for a percutaneous procedure. In addition, there was a large laminated left atrial thrombus. Thus, he was referred for surgical intervention.

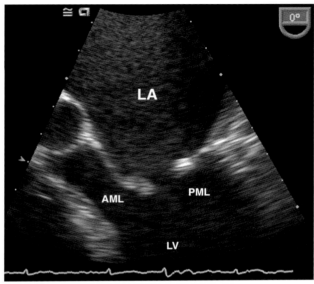

Fig 2-39. In a high TEE view, a mid-diastolic frame shows the mitral leaflets with thickening and tethering of the leaflet tips, resulting in the "doming" of the valve in diastole that is typical of rheumatic valve disease. This appearance is due to commisural fusion, along with chordal thickening and shortening.

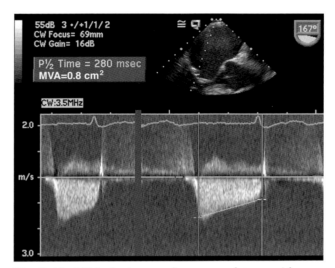

Fig 2-40. With the image plane rotated to provide a long-axis view of the mitral valve with the direction of the CW Doppler beam parallel to the jet through the narrowed mitral valve, the diastolic flow signal is recorded. The patient is in atrial fibrillation with variation in R-R interval and no a-velocity. The line shows the diastolic slope of the velocity curve with calculation of the pressure half-time. The pressure half-time is the time interval from the peak transmitral gradient to the point where the gradient is half the peak gradient. Mitral valve area is the pressure half-time divided by the empiric constant 220.

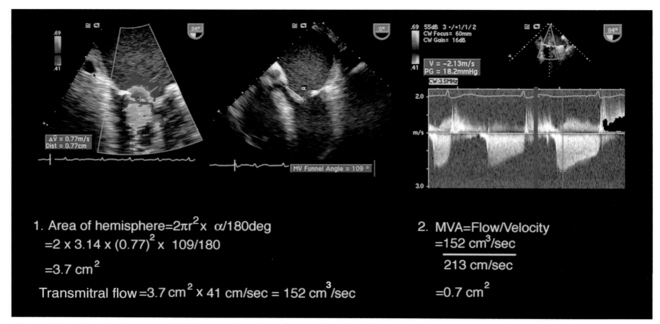

1. Area of hemisphere=$2\pi r^2 \times \alpha/180\deg$
   $= 2 \times 3.14 \times (0.77)^2 \times 109/180$
   $= 3.7\ cm^2$
   Transmitral flow $= 3.7\ cm^2 \times 41\ cm/sec = 152\ cm^3/sec$

2. MVA=Flow/Velocity
   $= \dfrac{152\ cm^3/sec}{213\ cm/sec}$
   $= 0.7\ cm^2$

Fig 2-41. Mitral valve area (**MVA**) can also be calculated using the continuity principle. The maximal transmitral volume flow rate is calculated from a color flow image of the proximal acceleration of flow as shown (Equation 1), analogous to the PISA calculation of regurgitation flow rate. The maximum flow rate is then divided by maximum velocity to estimate MVA (Equation 2). This method assumes that maximal velocity and maximal flow rate occur at the same point in time.

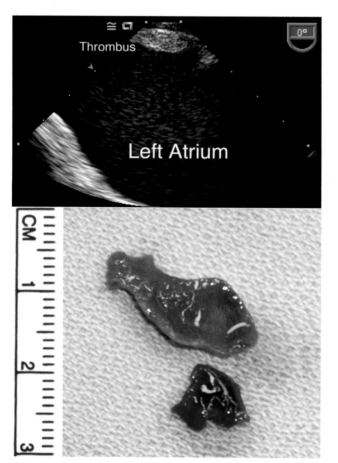

Fig 2-42. (*Top*) A mass in the dome of the left atrium. (*Bottom*) Fragments of the mass that pathologically was identified as platelets and fibrin, consistent with recent thrombus.

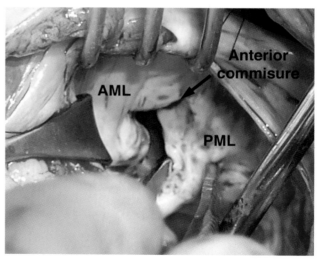

Fig 2-43. Intraoperative visualization of the valve shows leaflet thickening that is characteristic of rheumatic disease. There was dense fusion of the anterior and posterior leaflets at the commissures, with retraction and calcification of the central scallop of the posterior leaflet. A repair was performed with a commissurotomy and placement of an annuloplasty ring. Although initial postoperative TEE images showed only mild regurgitation, when loading conditions returned to the preoperative baseline, moderate-to-severe regurgitation was seen. The patient then underwent a second pump run with mitral valve replacement.

Case 2-6
Rheumatic Mitral Stenosis and Regurgitation

This 52-year-old man with congestive heart failure was referred to cardiac surgery for severe rheumatic mitral valve disease with both stenosis and regurgitation.

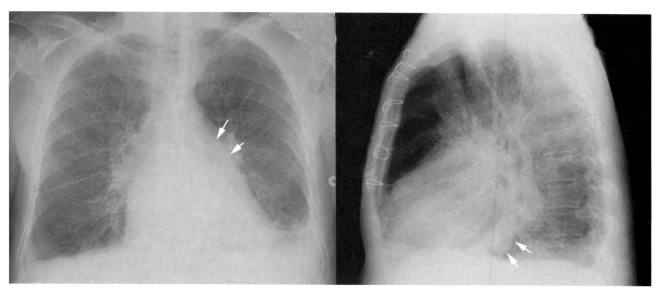

Fig 2-44. The AP (*left*) chest radiograph shows cardiomegaly and increased pulmonary vascularity. The left atrium is enlarged, as evidenced by the abnormal left heart contour. The lateral chest radiograph also shows left atrial enlargement (**arrows**).

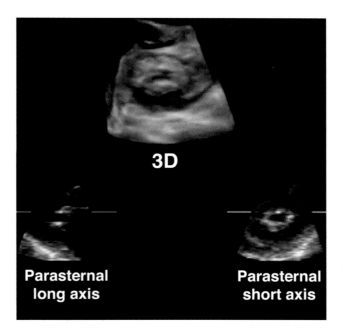

3D

Parasternal long axis

Parasternal short axis

DVD **Fig 2-45.** Selected images from his preoperative real-time 3D transthoracic echocardiogram show simultaneous parasternal long- and short-axis views of the rheumatic mitral valve (*bottom left and right*) and a 3D reconstruction of the valve orifice in a short-axis orientation "looking" from the LV apex towards the valve. Note the commissural fusion resulting in a small symmetric elliptical orifice at the leaflet tip level.

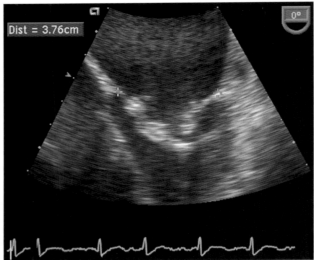

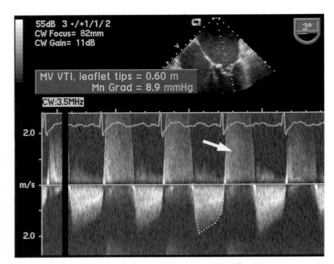

Fig 2-46. Intraoperative TEE in a four-chamber view demonstrates several features: left atrial enlargement with spontaneous contrast; diffuse thickening of the mitral leaflets with evidence of chordal thickening and shortening; and an enlarged mitral annulus.

Fig 2-48. CW Doppler of the mitral inflow pattern shows an increased velocity with a mean pressure gradient of 9 mmHg. Mitral regurgitation is evident above the baseline (**arrow**).

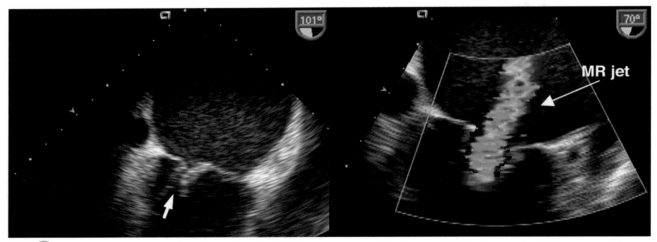

Fig 2-47. In a two-chamber view, the leaflets appear to close incompletely in systole (**left arrow**) with a broad central jet of mitral regurgitation (**MR**).

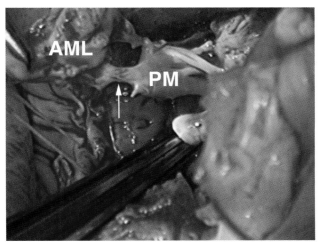

Fig 2-49. At surgical examination, the mitral chords (**arrow**) were severely thickened and shortened. The mitral valve was replaced with preservation of both anterior and posterior chords to preserve annular–papillary muscle continuity. AML = anterior mitral leaflet; PM = papillary muscle.

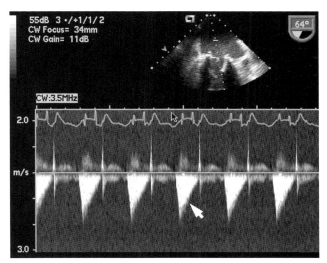

Fig 2-51. CW Doppler flow across the mitral prosthesis shows a normal antegrade velocity with a steep deceleration slope, indicating the absence of stenosis (**arrow**). No mitral regurgitation is detected.

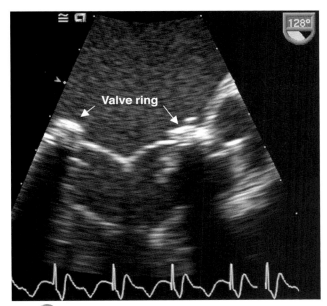

Fig 2-50. Immediate postoperative images in a long-axis view show the valve ring and the thin leaflets of the tissue prosthesis closed in systole.

Comments (for Cases 2-5 and 2-6)

The hallmark of rheumatic valve disease is commissural fusion of the mitral leaflets with the typical echocardiographic appearance of diastolic doming of the leaflets. The standard approach to measurement of mitral valve area on transthoracic imaging is 2D planimetry of the orifice. However, this view can rarely be obtained on transesophageal imaging, as it is difficult to obtain a short-axis view at the leaflet tips.

The mitral pressures half-time method, based on the Doppler velocity curve, is useful in the OR because the mitral jet is directed away from the transducer and it is relatively easy to obtain a parallel intercept angle between the ultrasound bean and mitral stenosis jet.

The continuity equation valve area can be estimated from maximal flow rate and velocity as shown. Alternatively, the total flow in diastole can be calculated by measurement of flow in the pulmonary artery and valve area, calculated by dividing by the velocity time integral of the CW Doppler signal. As in this case, these alternate methods for evaluation of mitral stenosis severity should show reasonable agreement. However, stenosis severity has usually been evaluated in detail preoperatively so that confirmation by pressure half-time is adequate.

References

1. Otto CM. Valvular stenosis. In: Textbook of Clinical Echocardiography, 3rd edn. Philadelphia: Elsevier Saunders, 2004: 295–303.

2. Longo M, Previti A, Morello M et al. Usefulness of transesophageal echocardiography during open heart surgery of mitral stenosis. J Cardiovasc Surg (Torino) 2000; 41:381–5.

3. Lee TY, Tseng CJ, Chiao CD et al. Clinical applicability for the assessment of the valvular mitral stenosis severity with Doppler echocardiography and the proximal isovelocity surface area (PISA) method. Echocardiography 2004; 21:1–6.

Mitral Regurgitation Due to Coronary Artery Disease

Case 2-7
Ischemic Mitral Regurgitation

This 83-year-old man with severe aortic stenosis and a left ventricular ejection of 7% was also found to have severe mitral regurgitation. Coronary angiography showed a 60% stenosis of the left anterior descending coronary artery and an 80% stenosis of a large first obtuse marginal branch of the circumflex coronary artery. Mitral leaflet anatomy was normal but there was thinning and akinesis of the posterior–lateral left ventricular wall, suggesting that the etiology of mitral regurgitation was ischemic. After aggressive medical management and placement of an intra-aortic balloon pump, he was referred for aortic valve replacement, coronary bypass grafting and mitral valve repair.

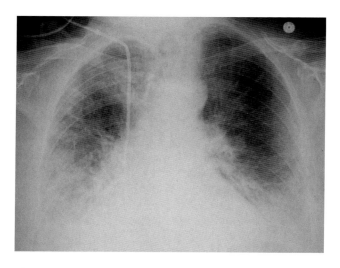

Fig 2-52. The portable PA chest radiograph shows cardiomegaly with increased pulmonary vascularity and pulmonary edema.

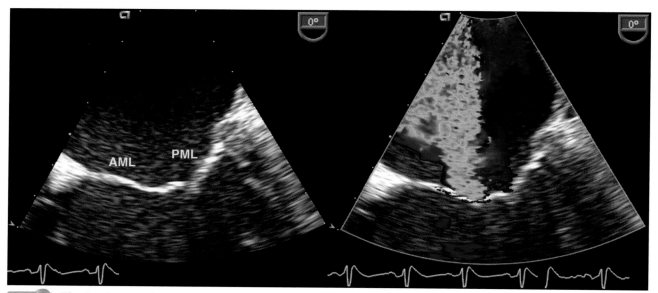

DVD ▶ **Fig 2-53.** In a four-chamber TEE view, the mitral leaflets and chords appear anatomically normal but the annulus is dilated and the anterior leaflet appears to "slide" behind the posterior leaflet due to tethering (or inadequate closure) of the posterior leaflet. Color Doppler demonstrates a central jet of regurgitation. AML = anterior mitral leaflet, PML = posterior mitral leaflet.

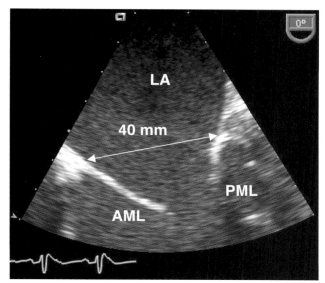

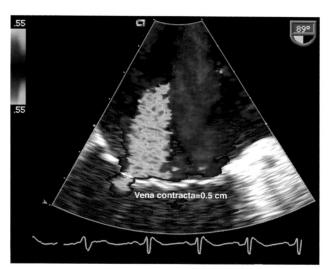

Fig 2-54. Because an annular ring is often used in the surgical approach to ischemic mitral regurgitation, it is helpful to obtain an annulus dimension for surgical planning. Typically, this measurement is made in mid-diastole using a view that clearly shows the attachment of the leaflets to the annulus. AML = anterior mitral leaflet, PML = posterior mitral leaflet, LA = left atrium.

Fig 2-55. Quantitation of mitral regurgitant severity begins with measurement of vena contracta width. The vena contracta is measured at the narrowest jet width with a clearly defined 'waist' between the proximal flow acceleration and distal jet expansion. The width of 0.5 cm is consistent with moderate mitral regurgitation and indicates that further quantitation is needed.

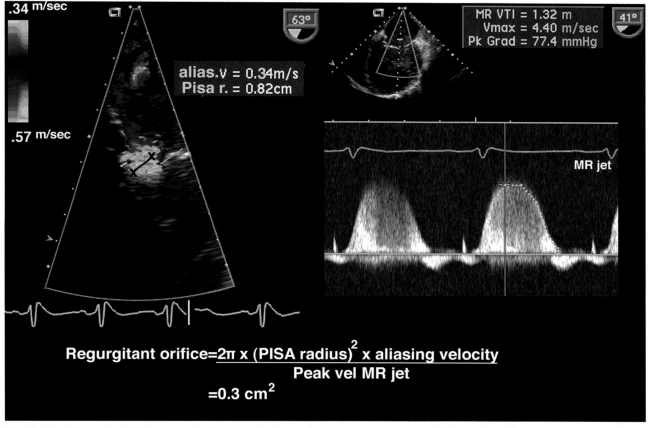

Fig 2-56. Using the PISA approach for quantitation of regurgitant severity, a PISA radius of 0.8 cm is measured at an aliasing velocity of 0.34 m/s. Multiplying the surface area of a hemisphere with a radius of 0.8 cm times the aliasing velocity yields a maximum regurgitant flow rate of 137 ml/s. Maximum regurgitant orifice area (**ROA**) is then determined by dividing by the CW Doppler MR jet velocity. An ROA of 0.3 cm^2 is consistent with moderate mitral regurgitation.

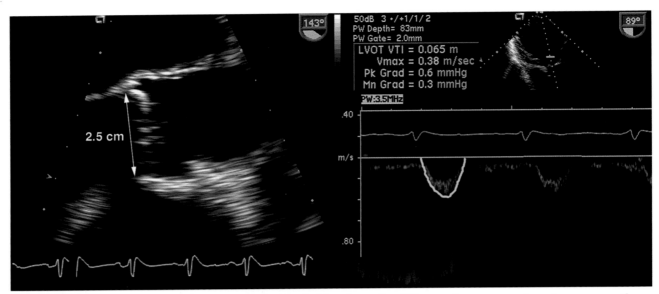

Fig 2-57. Regurgitant volume can then be calculated either from the difference between stroke volume across the mitral versus aortic valve or by multiplying the velocity time integral (**VTI**) by the ROA, as shown here. The regurgitant fraction is then the ratio of regurgitant stroke volume to total stroke volume (**RSV** + antegrade flow in the **LVOT**). Both the regurgitant volume of 40 ml and the regurgitant fraction of 56% are consistent with moderate mitral regurgitation. It is likely that regurgitation is more severe when the patient is not under general anesthesia.

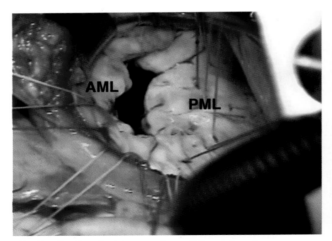

Fig 2-58. Surgical inspection of the valve shows incomplete valve closure with relatively normal valve leaflets. Sutures have been placed in the mitral annulus for securing the annuloplasty ring. AML = anterior mitral leaflet, PML = posterior mitral leaflet.

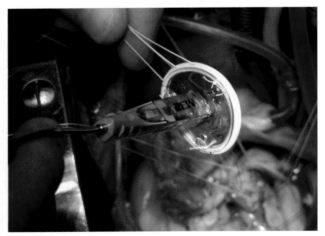

Fig 2-59. The annuloplasty ring being prepared for placement.

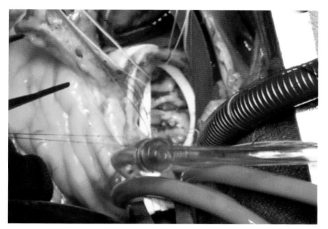

Fig 2-60. The annuloplasty ring in position.

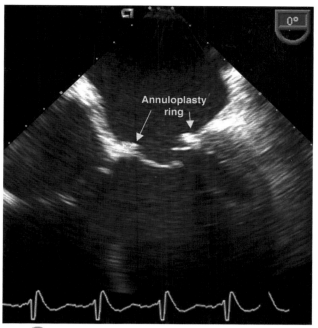

DVD **Fig 2-61.** Immediate postoperative images show the annuloplasty ring in position and the normal coaptation of the mitral leaflets in systole. There was no detectable mitral regurgitation on color Doppler examination.

Comments

Ischemic mitral regurgitation can be due to several different mechanisms. Wall motion abnormalities localized to the regions underlying the papillary muscles result in mitral regurgitation at rest, when the myocardium is infarcted, or only with stress, when there is intermittent ischemia. In patients with left ventricular dilation and systolic dysfunction due to coronary artery disease, regurgitation has a mechanism similar to that seen in patients with dilated cardiomyopathy (Case 2-11). The most catastrophic form of ischemic mitral regurgitation is papillary muscle rupture (Cases 2-8 and 2-9).

With ischemic mitral regurgitation due to a regional wall motion abnormality, "tethering" of the posterior leaflet is typical, as seen in this case. The posterior leaflet appears relatively immobile and fails to move completely towards the mitral annulus in systole, so that the normal motion of the anterior leaflet results in the appearance that it is "sliding" behind the coaptation point with the posterior leaflet. Revascularization alone has variable effects on the severity of ischemic mitral regurgitation, so that many surgeons will place an annuloplasty ring to reduce the size of the posterior aspect of the annulus, resulting in more complete leaflet coaptation in systole.

Suggested Reading

1. Levine RA, Hung J, Otsuji Y et al. Mechanistic insights into functional mitral regurgitation. Curr Cardiol Rep 2002; 4:125–9.

2. Hung J, Papakostas L, Tahta SA et al. Mechanism of recurrent ischemic mitral regurgitation after annuloplasty: continued LV remodeling as a moving target. Circulation 2004; 110:II85–90.

3. Grigioni F, Enriquez-Sarano M, Zehr KJ et al. Ischemic mitral regurgitation: long-term outcome and prognostic implications with quantitative Doppler assessment. Circulation 2001; 103(13):1759–64.

Case 2-8
Papillary Muscle Rupture

This 64-year-old man presented with chest pain and an abnormal ECG. His past medical history was remarkable for hypertension, hypercholesterolemia and smoking. Coronary angiography showed diffuse disease in the left anterior descending artery, a chronically occluded right coronary artery and a 95% stenosis in the first obtuse marginal branch, which was considered to be the "culprit" lesion. The left ven-

tricular angiogram showed an ejection fraction of 45% with akinesis of the inferior and lateral walls.

He underwent percutaneous angioplasty of the obtuse marginal vessel with only a small residual stenosis. However, due to progressive hypotension and pulmonary congestion, an intra-aortic balloon pump was inserted and an echocardiogram was requested.

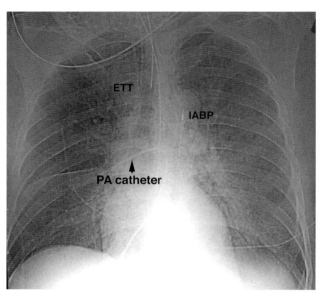

Fig 2-62. The portable bedside chest radiograph shows a normal size heart with mild pulmonary congestion. The endotracheal tube (**ETT**), intra-aortic balloon pump (**IABP**) and pulmonary artery (**PA**) catheter are seen.

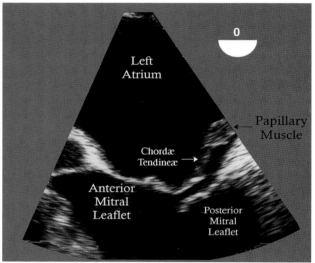

DVD **Fig 2-64.** The four-chamber view shows a ruptured papillary muscle attached to the anterior leaflet, with the entire papillary muscle prolapsing into the left atrium in systole, with corresponding severe mitral regurgitation.

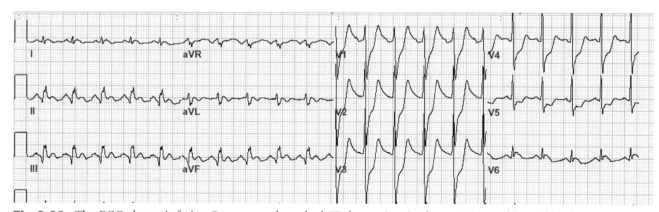

Fig 2-63. The ECG shows inferior Q waves and marked ST depression in the anterior and lateral leads.

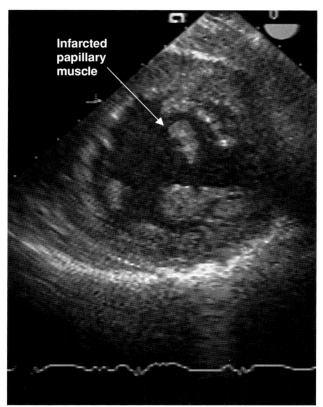

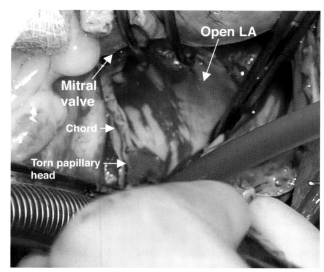

Fig 2-66. Operative findings showed papillary muscle rupture with disruption of chordal attachments to the anterior mitral leaflet resulting in a partial flail leaflet. The anatomy was not amenable to repair so that mitral valve replacement was performed.

DVD **Fig 2-65.** The transgastric short-axis view demonstrates the chaotic motion and smaller size of the ruptured posterior–medial papillary muscle.

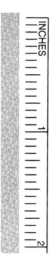 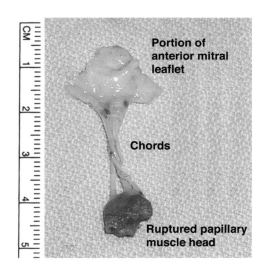

Fig 2-67. The excised leaflet and papillary muscle head.

Case 2-9
Another Case of Papillary Muscle Rupture

This 72-year-old female presented to the hospital with acute chest pain, and rapidly deteriorated with evidence of cardiogenic shock and pulmonary edema. Surface echocardiography revealed severe mitral regurgitation. The patient was taken to the cardiac catheterization laboratory and was found to have an acutely occluded circumflex artery, which was opened with stent/angio-

plasty. Her hemodynamic status improved, but did not normalize, over the next several days. Echocardiography showed normal left ventricular systolic function but persistent severe mitral regurgitation. She was taken to the OR, where TEE demonstrated a ruptured papillary muscle. This was successfully treated with bioprosthetic mitral valve replacement.

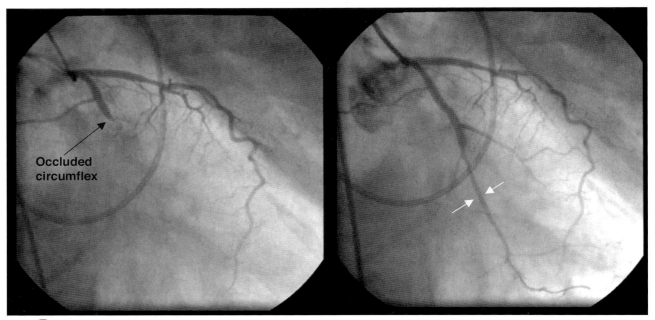

DVD **Fig 2-68.** Selective coronary angiography demonstrates an occluded circumflex artery (*left*) (see DVD), which was successfully stented (**arrows**, *right*).

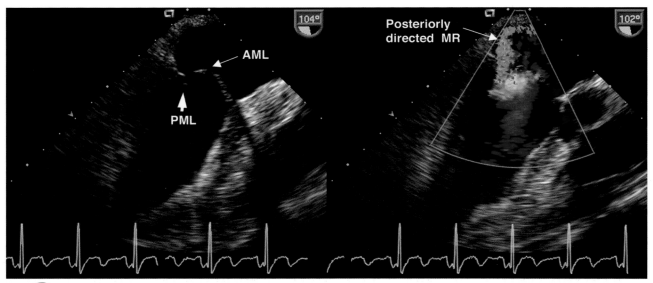

DVD **Fig 2-69.** TEE at approximately 100 degrees rotation reveals a severely prolapsing anterior mitral leaflet (**AML**), and a posteriorly directed jet of mitral regurgitation (**MR**). PML = posterior mitral leaflet.

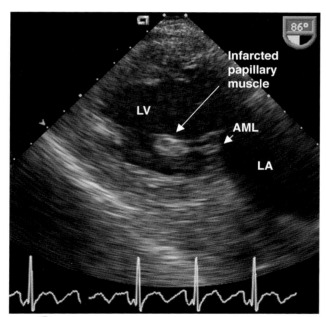

Fig 2-70. Transgastric long-axis view of the left ventricle (**LV**), reveals the ruptured head of the anterior papillary muscle. LA = left atrium; AML = anterior mitral leaflet.

Comments (for Cases 2-8 and 2-9)

Papillary muscle rupture is a rare (<0.1%) but often fatal (95% mortality within 2 weeks) complication of acute myocardial infarction. The onset of papillary muscle rupture is usually several days after the infarction and typically occurs with small, localized trans-mural myocardial damage, rather than with a large infarction. The patient presents with heart failure symptoms ranging from acute pulmonary edema to frank cardiogenic shock, depending on how much of the papillary muscle has ruptured, and consequent mitral regurgitant severity.

Although echocardiography is the optimal approach to diagnosis, care is needed in the examination as overall left ventricular systolic function may appear relatively normal and the rupture of papillary muscle is often not visualized on transthoracic examination. TEE is diagnostic with demonstration of the flail leaflet, with the detached papillary muscle head prolapsing into the left atrium in systole. In the first example, rupture of the posterior–medial papillary muscle was obvious on the first images. However, in the second case, the ruptured papillary muscle did not prolapse into the left atrium, and could only be visualized by transgastric imaging. The normality of the woman's left ventricular systolic function suggested a discrete rupture of the anterior–lateral papillary muscle.

Suggested Reading

1. Chevalier P, Burri H, Fahrat F et al. Perioperative outcome and long-term survival of surgery for acute post-infarction mitral regurgitation. Eur J Cardiothorac Surg 2004; 26:330–5.

2. Minami H, Mukohara N, Obo H et al. Papillary muscle rupture following acute myocardial infarction. Jpn J Thorac Cardiovasc Surg 2004; 52:367–71.

3. Tavakoli R, Weber A, Vogt P et al. Surgical management of acute mitral valve regurgitation due to post-infarction papillary muscle rupture. J Heart Valve Dis 2002; 11:20–5.

Other Causes of Mitral Regurgitation

Case 2-10
Radiation-induced Mitral Valve Disease

This 45-year-old man, who had undergone radiation therapy for Hodgkin's disease 24 years ago, presented with increasing fatigue and dyspnea on exertion. TTE showed severe mitral annular calcification with moderate functional mitral stenosis and mild regurgitation but moderate pulmonary hypertension with an estimated pulmonary systolic pressure of 55 mmHg. He was referred for mitral valve repair or replacement.

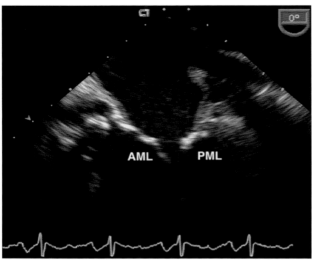

DVD **Fig 2-71.** On TEE imaging in a four-chamber view, the mitral leaflets are irregularly thickened with increased echogenicity and reduced systolic motion. In contrast to rheumatic disease, the leaflet tips are not restricted and diastolic doming is not seen. AML = anterior mitral leaflet, PML = posterior mitral leaflet.

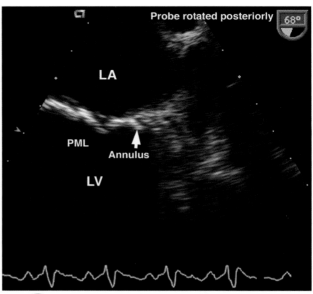

DVD **Fig 2-72.** Rotation of the probe posteriorly from the two-chamber view shows that the increased echogenicity extends from the leaflet base into the adjacent mitral annulus.

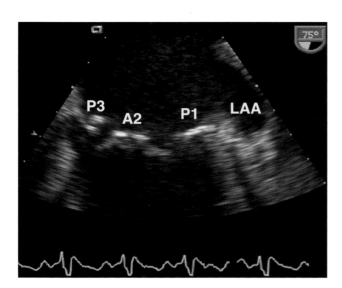

DVD **Fig 2-73.** The mitral commissural view shows calcification of P1, P3, and A2. LAA = left atrial appendage.

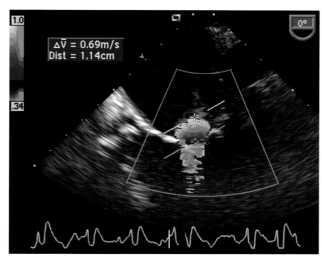

Fig 2-74. Color Doppler demonstrates the PISA proximal to the mitral orifice as blood accelerates into the narrowed mitral orifice.

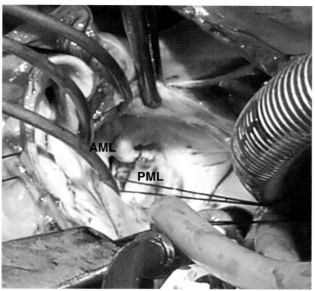

Fig 2-76. Surgical inspection of the valve showed thickened rigid leaflets. AML = anterior mitral leaflet, PML = posterior mitral leaflet.

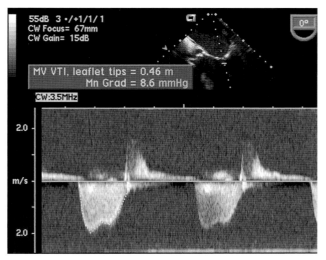

Fig 2-75. CW Doppler recording of the antegrade mitral flow shows an increased velocity consistent with a mean gradient of about 9 mmHg. Although the deceleration slope appears prolonged, measurement of the pressure half-time is limited by the short diastolic period prior to the a-velocity, making it difficult to accurately define the mid-diastolic slope.

Comments

About 6% of patients with prior mediastinal radiation therapy (20–25 years ago) present with clinical evidence of valve dysfunction. The mitral and tricuspid valves are involved most often, with pathologic changes including fibrosis and thickening of the leaflets. By echocardiography, the valve leaflets appear thickened and retracted with decreased motion. Unlike rheumatic disease, commissural fusion is not seen. These patients are at high risk for valve surgery because the radiation therapy also results in pericardial fibrous thickening (making surgical access to the valve problematic), perivascular myocardial fibrosis (often with left ventricular diastolic dysfunction) and accelerated coronary atherosclerosis.

Suggested Reading

1. Hull MC, Morris CG, Pepine CJ, Mendenhall NP. Valvular dysfunction and carotid, subclavian, and coronary artery disease in survivors of Hodgkin lymphoma treated with radiation therapy. JAMA 2003; 290:2831–7.

2. Heidenreich PA, Hancock SL, Lee BK et al. Asymptomatic cardiac disease following mediastinal irradiation. J Am Coll Cardiol 2003; 42:743–9.

3. Hering D, Faber L, Horstkotte D. Echocardiographic features of radiation-associated valvular disease. Am J Cardiol 2003; 92:226–30.

Case 2-11
Mitral Regurgitation Associated with Dilated Cardiomyopathy

This 35-year-old woman with heart failure due to dilated cardiomyopathy was referred for surgical intervention for severe mitral regurgitation. Her TTE showed mild left ventricular dilation, with an end-diastolic dimension of 59 mm, but with moderate global hypokinesis, with an end-systolic dimension of 52 mm and an ejection fraction of 44%. The left atrium was severely dilated at 58 mm and pulmonary systolic pressure was mildly elevated at 35 mmHg. Severe mitral regurgitation was present, with a vena contracta width of 10 mm and a regurgitant fraction of 78%.

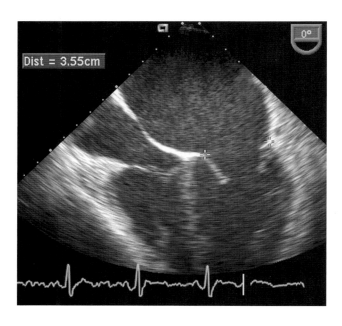

Fig 2-77. In a four-chamber view, the severely dilated left atrium and left ventricle are seen. The mitral annulus is dilated at 3.6 cm. The mitral leaflets and chords appear anatomically normal. In real time, left ventricular systolic function is severely reduced.

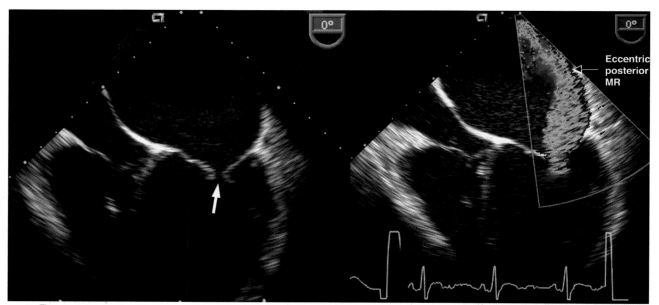

DVD **Fig 2-78.** During systole, the mitral leaflets fail to coapt (*left*, **arrow**). Color Doppler shows a large eccentric posteriorly directed mitral regurgitant (**MR**) jet in the left atrium (*right*).

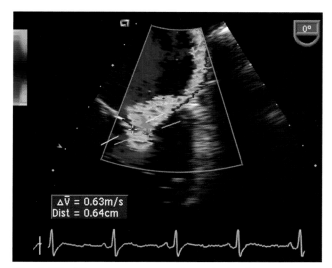

Fig 2-79. The vena contracta is optimized by decreasing the interrogation depth and enlarging the area of interest to minimize error in measurement. The vena contracta is seen as the narrow waist between the PISA and the expansion of the jet in the atrium. This vena contracta width of 0.6 cm is consistent with moderate regurgitation.

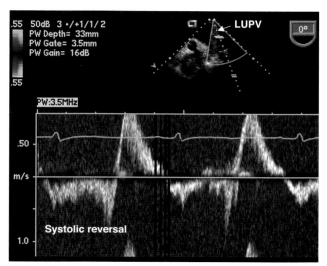

Fig 2-80. Pulsed Doppler evaluation of pulmonary vein flow provides an additional approach to evaluation of regurgitant severity. This image shows holosystolic flow reversal in the left upper pulmonary vein (**LUPV**) as expected, given the direction of the regurgitant jet.

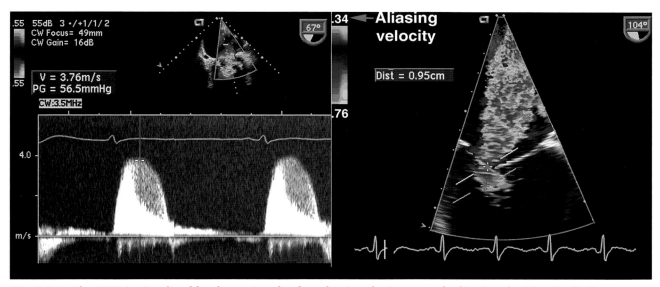

Fig 2-81. The PISA is visualized by decreasing depth, enlarging the image and adjusting the Nyquist limit to optimize the image. The maximum regurgitant flow rate (cm^3/s) is calculated by multiplying the PISA ($2\pi(0.95\ cm)^2$) by the aliasing velocity (34 cm/s). Maximal regurgitant orifice area (**ROA**) is then estimated by dividing by the peak regurgitant jet velocity (376 cm/s). The ROA of 0.5 cm^2 is consistent with severe regurgitation.

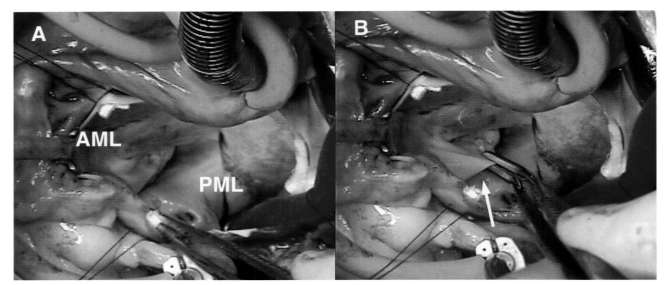

Fig 2-82. At surgery, the mitral annulus was enlarged with normal mitral leaflets and chordae (*A*). The thinness of the anterior leaflet (**arrow**) is demonstrated during retraction (*B*).

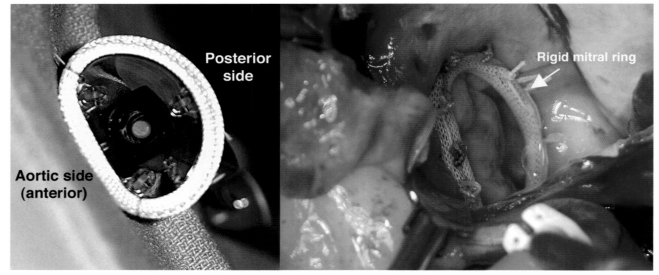

Fig 2-83. An annuloplasty was performed, with this image showing the positioning of the mitral annuloplasty ring (*right*). On the left, the ring is shown prior to implantation.

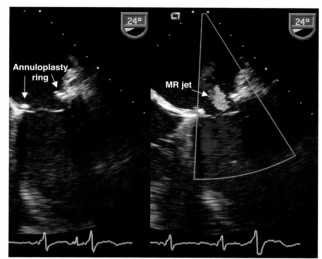

Fig 2-84. Post-annuloplasty images show the ring on the left atrial side of the valve at the junction of the leaflets with the annulus (*left*), with color Doppler showing only mild residual regurgitation.

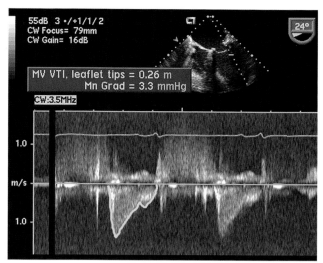

Fig 2-86. The antegrade velocity across the mitral valve is rechecked after the procedure to ensure there is no significant functional stenosis by measurement of the mean gradient (now 3 mmHg) and visual examination of the deceleration slope (note the steep slope on the first beat).

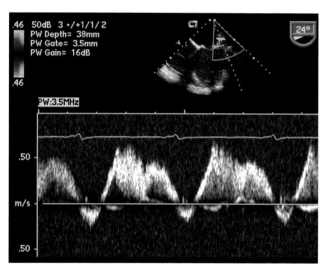

Fig 2-85. Post-annuloplasty, the left upper pulmonary vein flow pattern now shows normal antegrade flow in systole (compare with **Fig 2-80**).

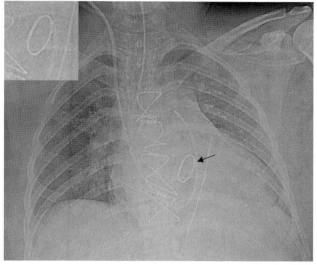

Fig 2-87. The postoperative chest radiography shows the sternotomy wires, the pulmonary artery catheter, the endotracheal tube, a chest tube, and the semi-circular annuloplasty ring (**arrow**), also seen in the inset.

Comments

Mitral regurgitation often accompanies dilated cardiomyopathy and contributes to heart failure symptoms. The exact mechanism of mitral regurgitation remains controversial with proposed alterations in the 3D anatomy of the mitral apparatus, including an altered angle between the papillary muscles and mitral annulus, altered left ventricular curvature and strain patterns, and mitral annular dilation. Mitral regurgitation due to dilated cardiomyopathy often responds to medical therapy for the underlying left ventricular systolic dysfunction. However, some patients with refractory regurgitation are referred for surgical intervention. Because the surgical approach usually includes placement of a mitral annuloplasty ring, measurement of mitral annular dimensions is helpful; most often measurements are made in the four-chamber and long-axis planes. It is important to identify the point where the anterior mitral leaflet joins the annulus (or aortic root) for each leaflet for an accurate measurement.

Suggested Reading

1. Aikawa K, Sheehan FH, Otto CM et al. The severity of functional mitral regurgitation depends on the shape of the mitral apparatus: a three-dimensional echo analysis. J Heart Valve Dis. 2002; 11:627–36.

2. Kwan J, Shiota T, Agler DA et al. Geometric differences of the mitral apparatus between ischemic and dilated cardiomyopathy with significant mitral regurgitation: real-time three-dimensional echocardiography study. Circulation 2003; 107:1135–40.

3. Tibayan FA, Lai DT, Timek TA et al. Alterations in left ventricular curvature and principal strains in dilated cardiomyopathy with functional mitral regurgitation. J Heart Valve Dis 2003; 12:292–9.

3

Aortic Valve Disease

Normal aortic valve

Aortic stenosis

Aortic regurgitation

The bicuspid aortic valve

Normal Aortic Valve

Case 3-1
Normal Aortic Valve

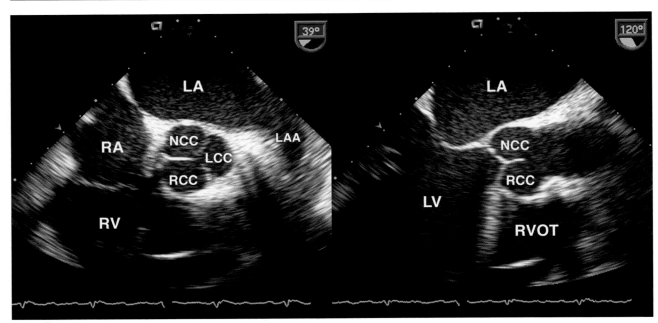

Fig 3-1. Intraoperative transesophageal echocardiography in a short-axis view (*left*) shows the closed aortic valve and the orientation of the three cusps: non-coronary cusp (**NCC**), left coronary cusp (**LCC**) and right coronary cusp (**RCC**). The long-axis view (*right*) shows the RCC and NCC; these are the cusps most often seen in the long-axis orientation, although occasionally the LCC is seen instead of the NCC. LA = left atrium, LAA = left atrial appendage, RA = right atrium, RV = right ventricle, RVOT = right ventricular outflow tract.

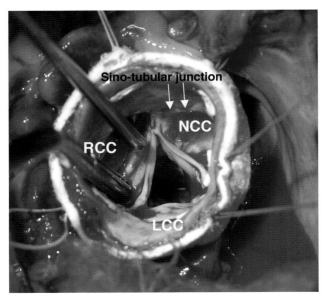

Fig 3-2. At surgery, in an image taken from the head of the operating table, a normal aortic valve is seen. The leaflets are thin and non-calcified. The commissural attachments to the sino-tubular junction are seen.

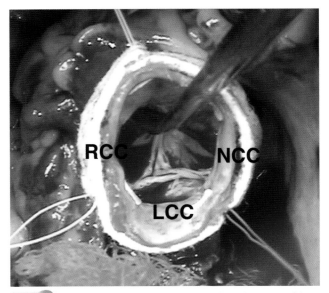

Fig 3-3. The valve is now closed, as would be the case in diastole.

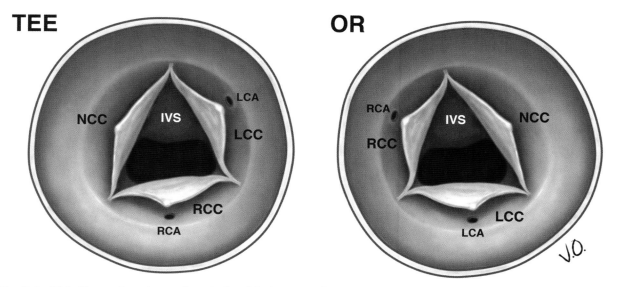

Fig 3-4. This illustration shows the relationship between the normal aortic valve and associated structures as seen on TEE, and as seen in the OR from the patient's head.

Aortic Stenosis

Case 3-2
Severe Calcific Aortic Stenosis

This 89-year-old woman presented with a 1-month history of near-syncope and increasing dyspnea on exertion. She was otherwise healthy and lived independently. Echocardiography showed calcific aortic stenosis with a maximum aortic velocity of 4.9 m/s recorded from the apical window, a mean gradient of 58 mmHg and a continuity equation valve area of 0.7 cm². There was moderate concentric left ventricular hypertrophy with a normal ejection fraction. Coronary angiography showed no significant coronary artery disease.

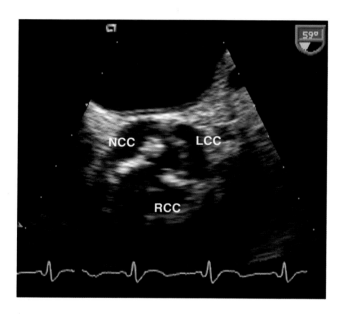

DVD **Fig 3-5.** Intraoperative transesophageal echocardiography in a short-axis view, obtained with rotation of the image plane to 59 degrees and slight flexion of the probe, shows a heavily calcified trileaflet aortic valve with reduced systolic opening. Although this short-axis image is correctly aligned, planimetry of the valve area is not possible due to shadowing and reverberations from the valve calcium and the irregular shape of the orifice. In addition, the stenotic valve often has a complex 3D shape with a non-planar orifice that may not be visualized in a single 2D-image plane. **LCC** = Left coronary cusp; **NCC** = non-coronary cusp; **RCC** = right coronary cusp.

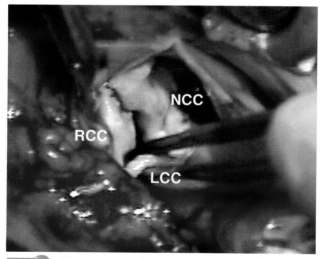

Fig 3-6. With rotation of the image plane to 148 degrees and leftward turning of the probe, a long-axis view of the aortic valve, aortic root and left ventricular outflow tract is obtained. This long-axis view shows severe leaflet calcification with reduced systolic motion. **DVD** of combined views from **Figs 3-5** and **3-6**.

DVD **Fig 3-7.** On direct visualization, the trileaflet aortic valve was heavily calcified with increased stiffness of the leaflets, as shown by the surgeon prior to valve removal. The stenotic aortic valve was replaced with a 21 mm tissue valve and she had an uneventful hospital course.

Comments

In current clinical practice, aortic stenosis is best evaluated by transthoracic echocardiography. The standard evaluation of stenosis severity is based on:

1. 2D imaging of valve anatomy, the extent of calcification and leaflet motion.
2. Continuous wave Doppler measurement of the antegrade velocity across the valve (the aortic "jet") with calculation of maximum and mean pressure gradients.
3. Calculation of valve area using the continuity equation.

On 2D imaging the number of valve leaflets is identified, although severe calcification of a bicuspid valve may be indistinguishable from a severely calcified trileaflet valve. When the leaflets are thin with a systolic separation >1.5 cm, severe stenosis is not present. However, when leaflet separation is reduced, Doppler data are needed for evaluation of stenosis severity.

The aortic jet velocity is recorded from the acoustic window that shows the highest velocity signal. This is especially important, as accurate velocity data (and calculated pressure gradients) depend on a parallel intercept angle between the ultrasound beam and the high-velocity jet. Because the 3D direction of the jet is unpredictable, in practice the jet velocity is recorded from multiple windows with careful patient positioning to ensure a parallel intercept angle is obtained. The most useful windows are apical and suprasternal, but in some cases the highest velocity is recorded from a subcostal or high right parasternal position. The most common error in assessment of aortic stenosis severity is failure to obtain a parallel intercept angle, which results in underestimation of stenosis severity.

Transaortic pressure gradients (ΔP in mmHg) are calculated with the simplified Bernoulli equation using the aortic jet velocity (V_{AS}) as:

$$\Delta P = 4(V_{AS})^2$$

The maximum instantaneous gradient is calculated from the maximum velocity; the mean gradient is calculated by averaging the instantaneous gradients over the ejection period, or can be approximated by the formula:

$$\Delta P_{mean} = 2.4(V_{AS})^2$$

The physiologic cross-sectional area of flow across the stenotic valve is calculated using the continuity equation, based on the principle that the stroke volume (SV) proximal to and in the orifice must be equal. Volume flow rate at any site equals the 2D cross-sectional area × the velocity time integral of flow (mean velocity × ejection period) through that site.

Stroke volume in the left ventricular outflow tract (LVOT) and in the narrowed aortic stenotic (AS) orifice are equal:

$$SV_{LVOT} = SV_{AS}$$

So that:

$$CSA_{LVOT} \times VTI_{LVOT} = AVA \times VTI_{AS}$$

Solving for aortic valve area (AVA):

$$AVA = (CSA_{LVOT} \times VTI_{LVOT})/VTI_{AS}$$

In clinical practice, this equation is often simplified by using maximum velocities, instead of velocity time integrals:

$$AVA = (CSA_{LVOT} \times VTI_{LVOT})/V_{AS}$$

Clinical decision making is primarily based on the patient's symptoms, and there are no absolute values for stenosis severity that define symptom onset. However, stenosis severity is classified in general terms as severe when jet velocity is >4 m/s and valve area <1.0 cm^2, moderate when jet velocity is 3–4 m/s and valve area 1.0–1.5 cm^2, and mild when jet velocity is <3.0 m/s and valve area >1.5 cm^2.

This case illustrates the use of transthoracic echocardiography for evaluation of aortic stenosis severity. When Doppler data are diagnostic, invasive evaluation of stenosis severity is not indicated, although coronary angiography may be needed to evaluate for possible coronary disease. Intraoperative echocardiography provided visual confirmation of the diagnosis and was useful in monitoring ventricular function.

Suggested Reading

1. Otto CM. Valve stenosis. In: Textbook of Clinical Echocardiography, 3rd edn. Philadelphia: Elsevier Saunders, 2004: 277–314.
2. Otto CM. Valvular aortic stenosis: disease severity and timing of intervention. J Am Coll Cardiol 2006; 47(11):2141–51.

Case 3-3
Aortic Stenosis with Epiaortic Scanning

This 41-year-old woman with multiple sclerosis had a history of a bicuspid aortic valve. She presented with increasing dyspnea on exertion, presyncope and chest pain. Transthoracic echocardiography showed a bicuspid aortic valve with secondary calcification. The antegrade velocity was 4.9 m/s and continuity equation valve area was 0.8 cm^2. Left ventricular systolic function was normal, with an ejection fraction of 75% measured by the apical biplane method.

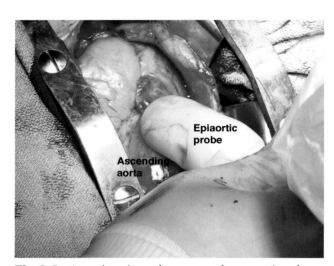

Fig 3-8. An epiaortic probe was used to examine the aortic valve at the time of surgery, which illustrates the use of alternate transducer positions in the operating room for evaluation of aortic stenosis severity. The probe (in a sterile sleeve) is positioned by the surgeon or echocardiographer directly on the ascending aorta, as shown here. The probe position is then adjusted, with rotation and angulation as needed, to obtain standard image planes of the aortic valve. In some cases, improved images are obtained by using a stand-off (such as a fluid-filled glove) or repositioning the transducer so that the area of interest is in the focal zone of the ultrasound beam instead of in the near field of the image.

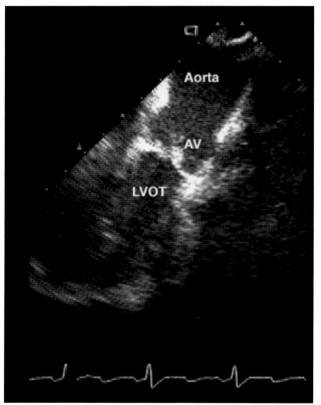

DVD **Fig 3-9.** The epiaortic long-axis images of the aortic valve show the ascending aorta with the sinotubular junction. The aortic valve leaflets are severely calcified with reduced mobility. AV = aortic valve; LVOT = left ventricular outflow tract.

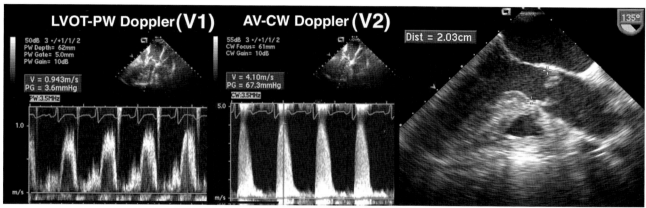

Fig 3-10. This composite image shows calculation of the continuity equation valve area using epiaortic scanning to obtain Doppler flows and a transesophageal long-axis view of the left ventricular outflow tract (**LVOT**) for measurement of outflow tract diameter (2.0 cm). The pulsed wave (**PW**) Doppler sample volume was positioned just on the ventricular side of the aortic valve to obtain a smooth velocity curve with a narrow band of velocities and a well-defined peak at 0.9 m/s. Continuous wave (**CW**) Doppler of the aortic valve (**AV**) showed an aortic jet velocity of 4.1 m/s. The aortic valve area (**AVA**) calculated with the continuity equation is 0.7 cm^2. The Doppler aortic jet velocity is lower than the 4.9 m/s jet obtained on transthoracic examination, most likely due to a lower cardiac output during anesthesia, although a non-parallel intercept angle between the ultrasound beam and aortic jet is also a possibility. However, LVOT velocity is similarly lower, so that the continuity equation valve area of 0.7 is similar to the value obtained preoperatively.

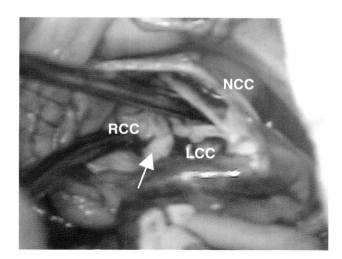

Fig 3-11. Direct inspection of the valve through the aortotomy shows a bicuspid aortic valve with severe calcification of the leaflets. The arrow indicates the raphe in the congenitally fused right and left coronary cusps (**RCC, LCC**). She underwent valve replacement with a 21 mm bioprosthetic valve. Her postoperative course was uneventful and she was discharged 6 days after surgery.

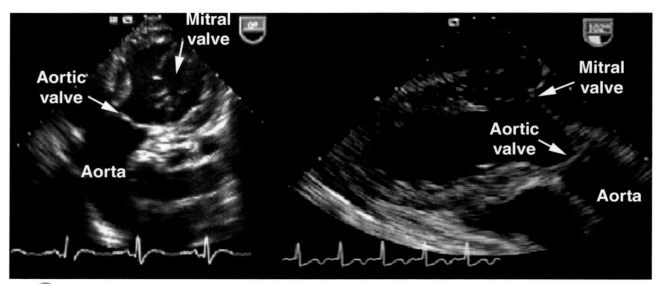

DVD ▶ **Fig 3-12.** From a transesophageal probe position, the ultrasound beam is relatively perpendicular to left ventricular outflow, precluding quantitative Doppler data. However, even from the transgastric view, it is rarely possible to obtain a view where the ultrasound beam is parallel to the flow direction. As this example from another patient shows, although the LVOT can be visualized in a transgastric long-axis view at 90 degrees rotation from the transgastric short-axis view, the angle between the ultrasound beam and aortic flow is not parallel. From a transgastric apical view, although the alignment looks better in this 2D plane, this view is foreshortened and an optimal angle in the elevational plane has not been obtained.

Comments

Evaluation of the severity of aortic stenosis on TEE is problematic. Some centers have found that planimetry of valve area from short-axis views is accurate, but this approach remains controversial due to shadowing and reverberations from valve calcification. In our experience, 2D planimetry is most useful in patients with mild-to-moderate stenosis when valve opening can be clearly visualized. With more severe stenosis, valve area may be overestimated by 2D imaging if areas of calcification in the body of the leaflet are mistaken for the leaflet edge or if the image plane is not at the level of the narrowest valve orifice.

Doppler evaluation of stenosis severity is suboptimal due to the limited acoustic windows available from the transesophageal approach. Unlike transthoracic imaging, transducer positioning is constrained to the narrow window provided by the esophagus and stomach. It is rarely possible to align the Doppler beam parallel to ventricular outflow from either a trans-esophageal or transgastric probe position. Occasionally, the aortic jet can be accurately recorded from a transgastric apical view, although alignment in the elevational plan cannot be evaluated. Deviations from a parallel intercept angle result in substantial errors: for example, with an actual jet velocity of 5 m/s, the measured velocity is only 4.3 m/s at an intercept angle of 30 degrees and 2.5 m/s at a 60 degree intercept angle. This corresponds to an actual maximum pressure gradient of 100 mmHg being underestimated at 75 or even 25 mmHg.

Thus, we recommend that all patients with suspected aortic stenosis undergo a careful and complete TTE examination as part of the preoperative evaluation. If an unsuspected abnormal aortic valve is noted during the intraoperative echocardiogram and no prior evaluation is available, the possibility that stenosis severity may be underestimated by intraoperative Doppler should be taken into consideration.

Suggested Reading

1. Cormier B, Iung B, Porte JM et al. Value of multiplane transesophageal echocardiography in determining aortic valve area in aortic stenosis. Am J Cardiol 1996; 77:882–5.
2. Kim KS, Maxted W, Nanda NC et al. Comparison of multiplane and biplane transesophageal echocardiography in the assessment of aortic stenosis. Am J Cardiol 1997; 79:436–41.

Case 3-4
Moderate Aortic Stenosis in a Patient Undergoing Coronary Bypass Surgery

A 70-year-old man with coronary artery disease is noted to have a systolic murmur on preoperative examination. Transthoracic echocardiography shows an aortic jet velocity of 3.4 m/s, a mean transaortic gradient of 26 mmHg and a continuity equation valve area of 1.3 cm².

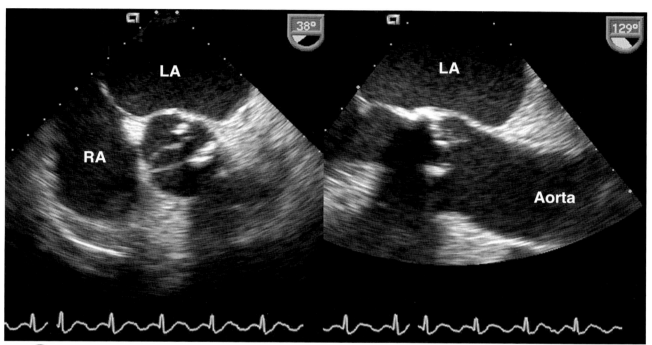

Fig 3-13. Intraoperative imaging in a long-axis (*right*) and short-axis (*left*) view of the aortic valve shows a bicuspid valve with moderate leaflet calcification and moderately reduced systolic motion.

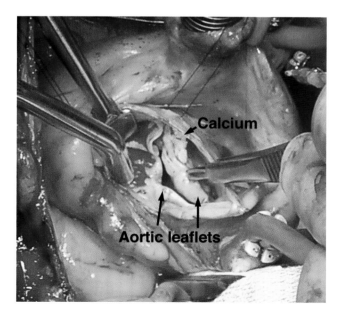

Fig 3-14. Direct visualization of the valve by the surgeon confirms the moderately calcified bicuspid aortic valve with increased leaflet stiffness. The leaflets were resected in preparation for valve replacement.

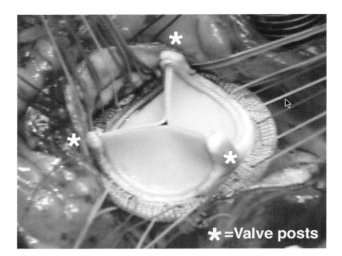

DVD **Fig 3-15.** This intraoperative photograph shows the implantation of the stented tissue valve.

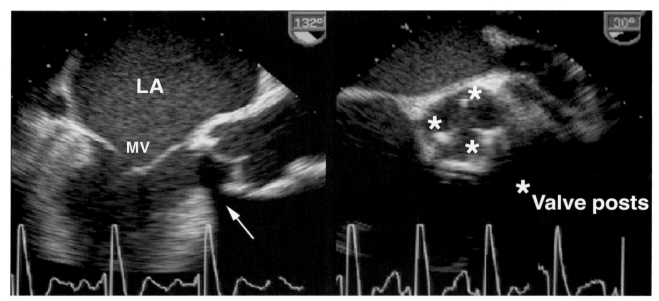

Fig 3-16. After weaning from cardiopulmonary bypass, short-axis (*left*) and long-axis (*right*) images of the aortic valve in diastole show the prosthetic valve posts and the thin leaflets. Note the shadowing by the prosthetic valve (**arrow**). LA = left atrium, MV = mitral valve.

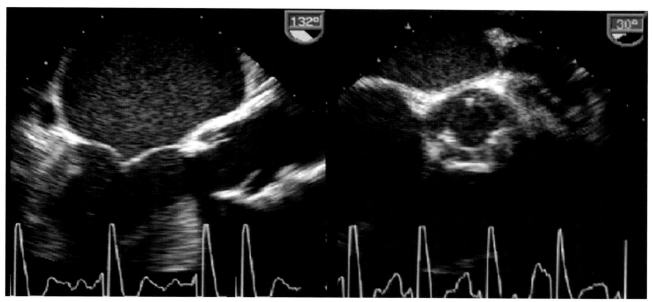

Fig 3-17. Systolic images of the stented tissue prosthesis show the open leaflets in a short-axis (*left*) and long-axis (*right*) view. In real time [DVD ▶] the normal motion of the thin prosthetic leaflets is seen.

Comments

In patients with asymptomatic aortic valve stenosis who are undergoing surgery for coronary artery, aortic root or mitral valve disease, the option of concurrent aortic valve replacement should be considered. The rationale for aortic valve replacement in these patients is that progression of aortic stenosis leading to symptoms is predictable and inevitable and the risk of repeat surgery is high. Balanced against these potential benefits are the additional surgical time and risk for the current procedure and the durability, suboptimal hemodynamics and potential complications of a prosthetic valve.

Recent prospective Doppler echocardiographic studies have improved our understanding of the natural history of asymptomatic aortic stenosis. In patients with mild stenosis (jet velocity <3.0 m/s) progression to severe symptomatic aortic stenosis occurs in only 10–15 % by 2–3 years, compared with 80% in those with severe stenosis (jet velocity >4.0 m/s). Thus, there now is general agreement that valve surgery for asymptomatic disease may not be needed when stenosis is mild but is appropriate when stenosis is severe. Decision making is more difficult in patients with moderate stenosis, as in this case, with a progression to severe symptomatic disease in about 30% at 3 years.

In patients with moderate stenosis, other factors that are taken into account include patient age, preferences and comorbidities; the expected hemodynamics and durability of available prosthetic valves; and the degree of valve calcification. Significant valve calcification is associated with rapid disease progression. In this case example, the decision to proceed with valve replacement was based on the finding of significant calcification of a bicuspid valve with moderate obstruction to outflow. As our choices for valve replacement improve, with durable valves that have favorable hemodynamics and do not require anticoagulation, the balance may shift towards valve replacement at the time of other cardiac surgery in more patients with aortic valve disease.

Suggested Reading

1. Bonow RO, Carabello BA, Chatterjee K et al. ACC/AHA 2006 guidelines for the management of patients with valvular heart disease: a report of the American College of Cardiology/American Heart Association Task Force on Practice Guidelines (Writing Committee to Develop Guidelines for the Management of Patients with Valvular Heart Disease). American College of Cardiology Web Site. Available at: http://www.acc.org/clinical/guidelines/valvular/index.pdf.

2. Otto CM, Burwash IG, Legget ME et al. A prospective study of asymptomatic valvular aortic stenosis: clinical, echocardiographic, and exercise predictors of outcome. Circulation 1997; 95:2262–70.

3. Rosenhek R, Klaar U, Scholten C et al. Mild and moderate aortic stenosis: natural history and risk stratification by echocardiography. Eur Heart J 2004; 25:199–205.

Case 3-5
Rheumatic Aortic Stenosis

This 56-year-old man presented 3 months ago with shortness of breath and atrial fibrillation. Physical examination showed a grade IV/VI systolic murmur at the base and he was referred for echocardiography. The transthoracic examination showed severe aortic stenosis with a jet velocity of 4.3 m/s, a mean gradient of 40 mmHg and a valve area of 0.9 cm^2. There was moderate aortic regurgitation. In addition, the mitral valve had changes consistent with rheumatic disease, with mild mitral stenosis.

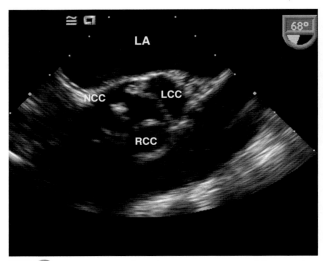

Fig 3-18. This short-axis image of the aortic valve in systole shows a trileaflet valve with a triangular orifice due to commissural fusion, as is typical with rheumatic valve disease. The DVD loop shows the reduced systolic opening of the leaflets on 2D imaging (*left*) and with color Doppler (*right*) showing only mild aortic regurgitation.

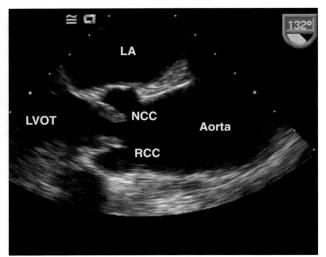

Fig 3-19. The long-axis view of the aortic valve and ascending aorta shows doming of the leaflets in systole, again typical for rheumatic disease. The anterior cusp of the aortic valve in this view is the RCC. The posterior cusp is usually the NCC, although the LCC may be seen, depending on the exact position of the valve relative to the transducer in the esophagus (see the short-axis view for reference).

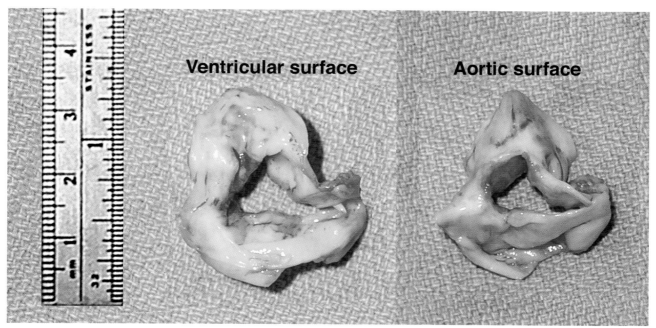

Fig 3-20. The explanted valve shows dramatic commissural fusion with a triangular orifice at the leaflet tips, seen both from the ventricular and aortic aspects. The leaflets are diffusely thickened, including the leaflet edges, with a smooth surface and only mild superimposed calcification, in contrast to the irregular calcific masses seen in the central part of the leaflets with calcific valve disease.

Comments

Although calcific valve disease is the most common cause of aortic stenosis in Europe and North America, rheumatic valve disease is highly prevalent in Asia, Africa and the Pacific Islands and sporadic cases are seen in every country. Rheumatic valve disease is the long-term sequela of acute rheumatic fever. The pathognomonic features of rheumatic valve disease are primary involvement of the mitral valve, with characteristic commissural fusion and chordal fusion and shortening. The aortic valve is affected in about 40% of cases, with involvement of the tricuspid valve in only 6% of those patients with rheumatic mitral valve disease. Rheumatic aortic valve disease can be recognized by the characteristic mitral valve changes and evidence for commissural fusion and diffuse leaflet thickening, particularly along the leaflet edges, of the aortic valve. In systole, a central triangular orifice is seen, in contrast to the complex stellate orifice of calcific aortic stenosis. Aortic valve by planimetry may be difficult in the latter instance, as shadowing may obscure the margins of the stenotic orifice (see Fig 3.4—arrow)

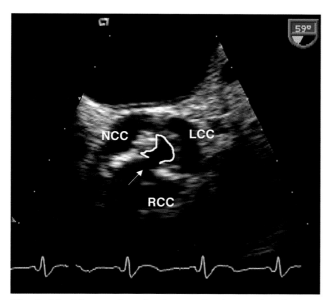

Fig 3-21. The aortic valve is seen in short axis. The arrow indicates the dropout that results in difficulty in measuring the aortic valve area by planimetry.

Suggested Reading

1. Faggiano P, Aurigemma GP, Rusconi C et al. Progression of valvular aortic stenosis in adults: literature review and clinical implications. Am Heart J 1996; 132 (2 Pt 1): 408–17.

Aortic Regurgitation

Case 3-6
Chronic Aortic Regurgitation

This 56-year-old man was noted to have a murmur on routine physical examination for 4 years. He was asymptomatic and had no history of endocarditis. The transthoracic examination showed normal aortic root dimensions and anatomy with a trileaflet aortic valve. Small mobile echos were seen on the ventricular side of the valve, thought to be an old vegetation versus a partial flail leaflet, and Doppler studies were consistent with moderate-to-severe aortic regurgitation. Blood cultures were negative. He was treated with an angiotensin-converting enzyme inhibitor and followed with annual echocardiography.

Date	LVESD	LVEDD	EF	Symptoms
3/01	37	57	65%	None
7/02	43	62	56%	None
12/02	38	63	64%	None
5/03	40	63	63%	None
1/04	47	60	51%	Decreased exercise tolerance

EF, ejection fraction; LVESD, left ventricular end-systolic diameter; LVEDD, left ventricular end-diastolic diameter.

Four years after diagnosis of aortic regurgitation, he reported decreased exercise tolerance and his echocardiogram showed a decline in ejection fraction, prompting referral for aortic valve replacement.

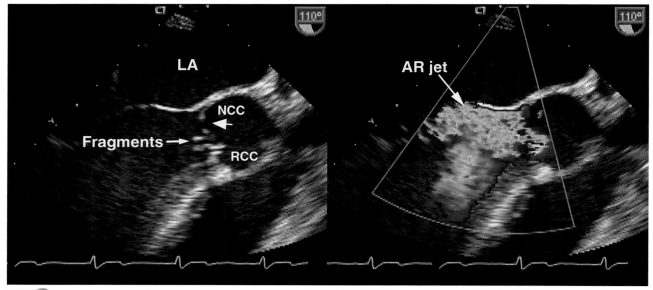

DVD **Fig 3-22.** Intraoperative 2D echocardiographic imaging (*left*) in a long-axis view of the aortic valve shows thin leaflets but with some small mobile leaflet fragments on the ventricular side of the valve. The arrow points to an apparent defect in the NCC. In real time, the RCC appears to prolapse. Color flow imaging (*right*) shows severe aortic regurgitation with a wide vena contracta width and a color jet that fills most of the left ventricular outflow tract in diastole. As on the transthoracic study, aortic root dimension is normal and root anatomy is normal with normal contours of the sinuses of Valsalva, a well-defined sinotubular junction and a normal dimension of the ascending aorta.

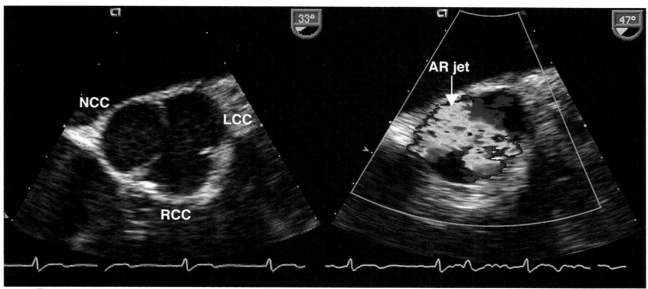

DVD Fig 3-23. Short-axis views at the aortic valve level (*left*) demonstrate a trileaflet aortic valve. Color flow imaging shows the aortic regurgitant (**AR**) jet (**arrow**) filling the region of the NCC, consistent with a hole in this leaflet.

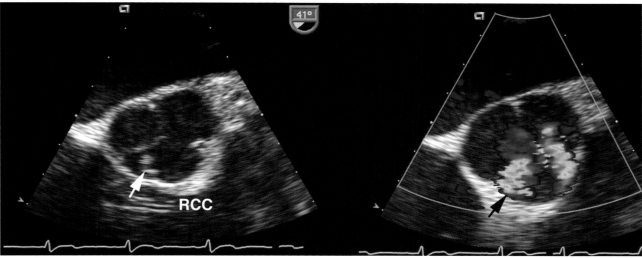

DVD Fig 3-24. Still in the short axis, but with the transducer further rotated, the RCC does not coapt properly (**arrow**) (*left*). On the right, color flow shows aortic regurgitation in this area (**arrow**).

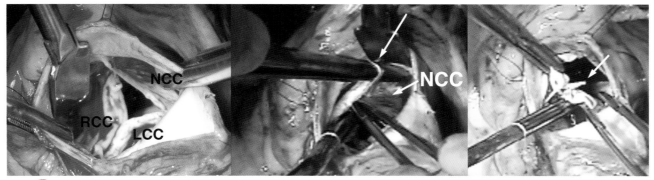

DVD Fig 3-25. Intraoperative examination of the trileaflet valve in situ shows thin leaflets with a fenestration along the free edges of the NCC shown by the probe through this region of the leaflet (**arrows**) (*center*). On the right, a small subvalvular fragment is seen (**arrow**).

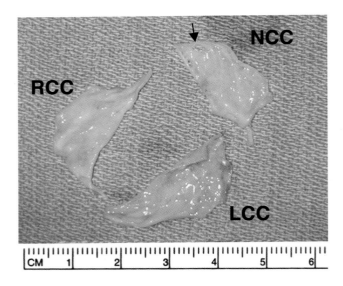

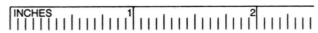

Fig 3-26. Pathologic examination of the explanted valve showed thin, floppy leaflets with fenestrations along the free edges of two leaflets. Microscopic examination was consistent with myxomatous degeneration.

Comments

Chronic aortic regurgitation may be due to disease of the valve leaflets or the aortic root. Examples of aortic root disease include Marfan syndrome and cystic medial necrosis. The most common primary diseases of the valve leaflets are a congenitally bicuspid aortic valve and rheumatic disease. Congenital valve fenestrations, as seen in this case, are unusual but there are several case reports of similar cases. It has been proposed that when congenital fenestrations are in the overlapping part of the valve closure plane, valve function is normal. With an increase in aortic size, possibly related to aging, these overlap regions become load-bearing, resulting in stretching of the fenestration and aortic regurgitation. Myxomatous valve disease usually primarily involves the mitral valve, with involvement of the aortic valve leaflets seen in only 2% of patients with mitral valve prolapse. Isolated myxomatous changes of the aortic valve, as in this case with a normal mitral valve on echocardiography, are unusual.

The timing of surgery in chronic aortic regurgitation is based on the response of the left ventricle to chronic volume overload and clinical symptoms. Surgery is recommended for patients with severe aortic regurgitation at symptom onset, with the initial symptom typically dyspnea on exertion, as in this case. Patients who remain asymptomatic are at risk of developing irreversible left ventricular systolic function so that annual echocardiography is recommended for monitoring. The parameters that are most useful for predicting a decline in left ventricular contractility are left ventricular size and systolic performance. The most useful echocardiographic parameters are left ventricular end-systolic and end-diastolic dimension and the 2D apical biplane ejection fraction. Although some clinicians prefer left ventricular volume calculations, dimension measurements are more widely used due to their simplicity and reproducibility.

The ACC/AHA Guidelines for Valvular Heart Disease recommend aortic valve surgery for chronic aortic regurgitation when symptoms are present or, in asymptomatic patients, when ejection fraction is <50%, end-systolic dimension is >55 mm, or end-diastolic dimension is >75 mm. The indication for surgery in the case presented here was symptom onset, although the change in ejection fraction was also worrisome.

Treatment with afterload reducing agents to delay the rate of left ventricular dilation in patients with chronic aortic regurgitation is controversial, with conflicting results in two small randomized studies.

Suggested Reading

1. Borer JS, Bonow RO. Contemporary approach to aortic and mitral regurgitation. Circulation 2003; 108:2432–8.

2. Akiyama K, Ohsawa S, Hirota J, Takiguchi M. Massive aortic regurgitation by spontaneous rupture of a fibrous strand in a fenestrated aortic valve. J Heart Valve Dis 1998; 7:521–3.

3. Evangelista A, Tornos P, Sambola A et al. Long-term vasodilator therapy in patients with severe aortic regurgitation. N Engl J Med 2005; 353:1342–9.

4. Zoghbi WA, Enriquez-Sarano M, Foster E et al. Recommendations for evaluation of the severity of native valvular regurgitation with two-dimensional and Doppler echocardiography. J Am Soc Echocardiogr 2003; 16(7):777–802.

Case 3-7
Rheumatic Aortic Regurgitation

This 44-year-old man had a long history of rheumatic valvular heart disease. Four years ago he had an episode of endocarditis due to *Streptococcus viridans* and was treated with 6 weeks of intravenous antibiotics. Four months ago he had another episode of endocarditis with blood cultures positive for *Haemophilus segnis* and was again treated with 6 weeks of intravenous antibiotics. However, he had the onset of congestive heart failure symptoms, due to increasing aortic regurgitation. Echocardiography showed a left ventricular end-systolic dimension of 59 mm, an end-diastolic dimension of 72 mm and an ejection fraction of 44%. Coronary angiography was normal.

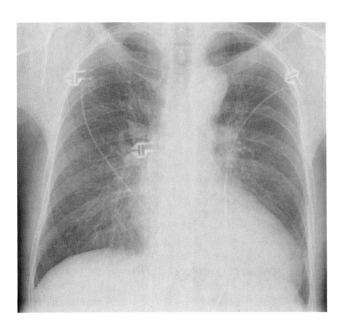

Fig 3-27. Chest radiography shows severe left ventricular enlargement with clear lung fields.

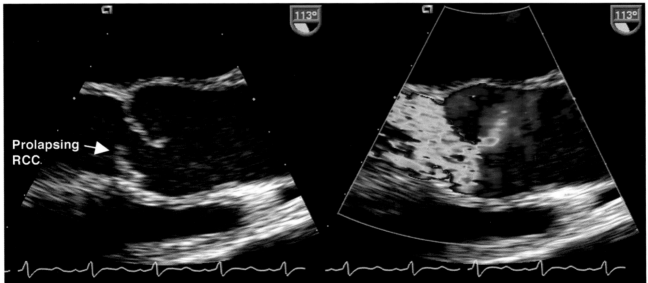

Fig 3-28. Long-axis images (*left*) of the aortic valve were obtained by rotating the image plane to 113 degrees. The aortic leaflets are thickened with slight systolic doming and with partial prolapse of the more anterior leaflet (probably the **RCC**) into the outflow tract in diastole. Color flow images (*right*) show severe aortic regurgitation with a wide (vena contracta width = 8 mm) eccentric jet through the area on non-coaptation of the leaflets.

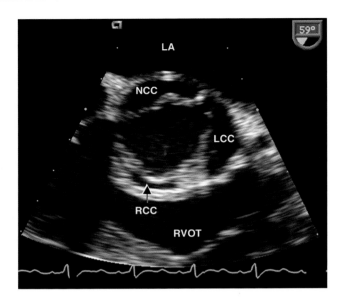

Fig 3-29. Short-axis images of the aortic valve obtained at 59 degrees rotation of the image plane show a trileaflet valve with thickening and fusion at the commissure typical for rheumatic disease.

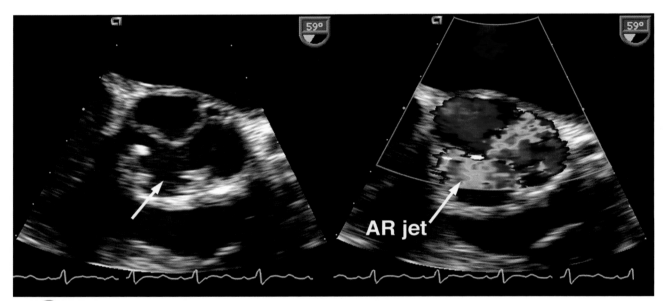

DVD **Fig 3-30.** Short-axis images of the aortic valve in diastole demonstrate partial destruction of the right coronary cusp due to endocarditis (**arrow**)(*left*) with color Doppler (*right*) demonstrating the aortic regurgitant (**AR**) jet in cross section.

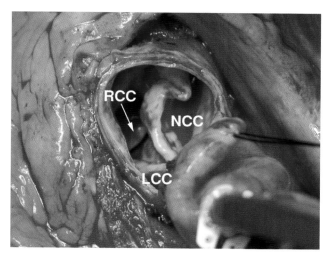

Fig 3-31. At surgery, the valve was trileaflet with commissural fusion typical of rheumatic valve disease and with evidence of destruction of the RCC, due to previous endocarditis, but no evidence of active infection.

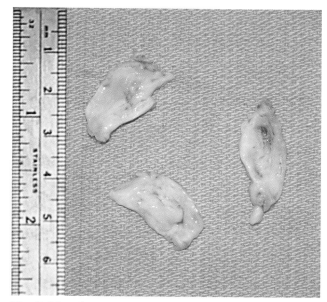

Fig 3-32. The explanted valve shows thickened and deformed valve leaflets, especially along the leaflet edges. Microscopic examination of the valve leaflets demonstrated diffuse leaflet thickening with focal neovascularization consistent with a post-inflammatory process, which is typical for rheumatic valve disease.

Comments

This patient, with valve destruction due to endocarditis superimposed on chronic rheumatic valve disease, illustrates the issues in establishing the etiology of aortic regurgitation by echocardiography. Evaluation of aortic root anatomy is essential, as surgical intervention for aortic regurgitation due to root disease differs from the management of primary valve disease. The long-axis image of the ascending aorta demonstrates the sites needed for aortic measurements in patients undergoing aortic valve and/or root surgery:

1. Diameter measurements just proximal to the valve (e.g. the left ventricular outflow tract) are used for continuity equation valve area calculations and correspond to the sewing ring size of stented tissue and mechanical valves.
2. Aortic root enlargement is often most severe at the sinuses of Valsalva.
3. The normal contour of the sinotubular junction is absent in patients with Marfan syndrome and this measurement site is especially important when a stentless valve is implanted.
4. It is important to visualize and measure ascending aortic diameter in patients with aortic valve disease as the aorta is often abnormal as well.

The physiology in this patient is consistent with a combination of chronic and acute regurgitation. Chronic regurgitation due to rheumatic disease led to significant left ventricular dilation, with preserved systolic function. However, the additional volume of aortic regurgitation due to valve destruction with endocarditis, led to clinical decompensation with symptoms of heart failure and a decline in ejection performance.

Case 3-8
Traumatic Acute Aortic Regurgitation

This previously healthy 73-year-old woman was transferred directly from the emergency department to the operating room with a diagnosis of acute severe aortic regurgitation. She had been kicked by a horse on her left upper chest and fell backwards, hitting a metal pole, with loss of consciousness. She was intubated in the field and then underwent emergency transthoracic and transesophageal echocardiography that showed severe aortic regurgitation and a pericardial effusion.

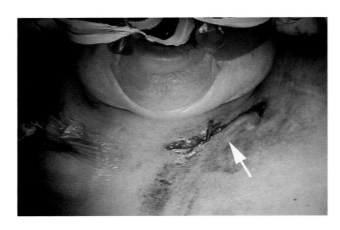

Fig 3-33. Photograph of the patient's chest wall shows trauma from the horse's kick (**arrow**).

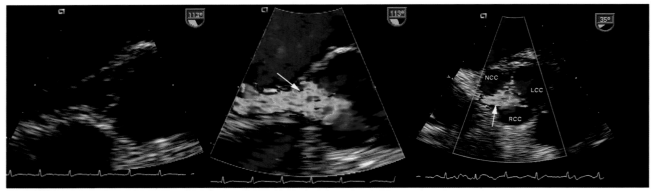

DVD ▶ **Fig 3-34.** Transesophageal echocardiography in a long-axis view of the aortic valve shows apparent thickening and prolapse of the aortic valve leaflets. On real-time imaging the flail trileaflet valve is seen. On color Doppler, the regurgitant jet (**arrows**) nearly fills the outflow tract in both long- and short-axis views with a vena contracta diameter >15 mm.

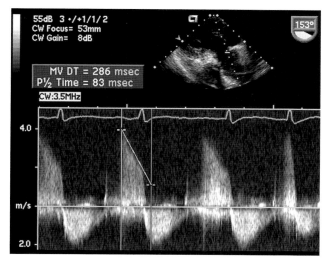

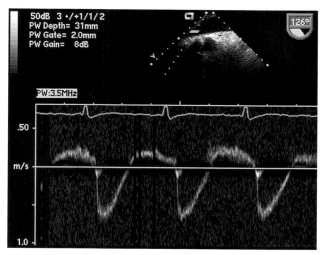

Fig 3-35. Continuous wave Doppler was recorded from a transgastric long-axis view. Although the intercept angle between the ultrasound beam and aortic regurgitant jet may result in underestimation of velocity, the intensity of the velocity curve relative to antegrade flow indicates severe regurgitation. In addition, the steep deceleration slope indicates rapid equilibration of aortic and ventricular diastolic pressures consistent with acute regurgitation.

Fig 3-36. Pulsed Doppler recording of flow in the descending thoracic aorta shows holodiastolic flow reversal confirming the presence of severe aortic regurgitation. This signal is best recorded starting from a short-axis view of the descending thoracic aorta, rotating the image plane to a long-axis view and then placing the pulsed Doppler sample volume as distal as possible in the aorta, to obtain a relatively parallel intercept angle. If the Doppler beam is perpendicular to the direction of flow, there will be no Doppler signal, because the cosine of 90 degrees (in the Doppler equation) is zero.

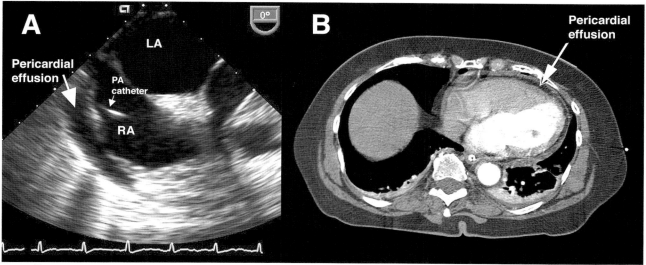

DVD **Fig 3-37.** A small pericardial effusion is present adjacent to the right atrium in this high transesophageal view, and on CT scanning. The pulmonary artery catheter is seen in the right atrium. On opening of the pericardium at surgery, there was evidence of high pericardial pressures with a moderate amount of pericardial fluid.

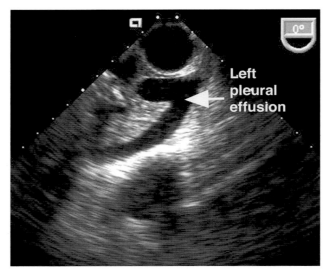

Fig 3-38. A left pleural effusion is noted when the image plane is oriented towards the descending thoracic aorta.

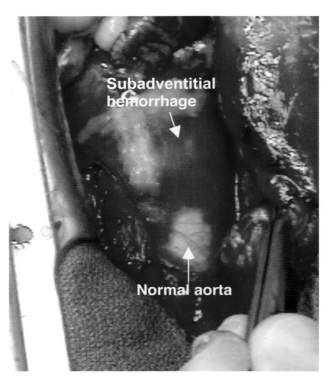

Fig 3-39. After sternotomy, aortic subadventitial hemorrhage was noted.

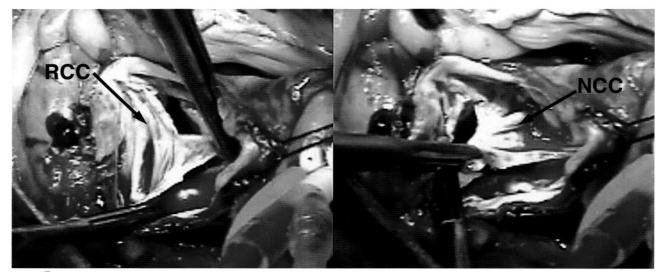

DVD **Fig 3-40.** On direct inspection of the aortic valve at surgery, there was disruption of the commissure between the right and non-coronary cusps, resulting in flail motion of both leaflets.

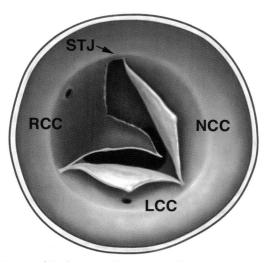

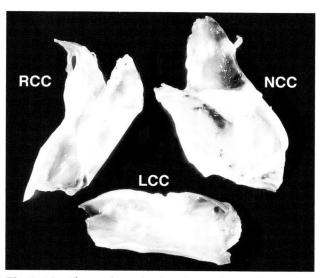

Fig 3-41. This drawing shows how disruption of the attachment of the RCC to the sinotubular junction (**STJ**) and tearing of the body of the leaflet would result in valvular incompetence. The torn NCC is not illustrated here.

Fig 3-42. The explanted valve shows the tearing and disruption of the right and non-coronary cusps. The aortic valve was replaced with a tissue prosthesis and the patient had a successful recovery.

Comments

Blunt trauma to the chest can cause a range of cardiac disorders, including myocardial contusion and disruption of the thoracic aorta, related to deceleration and traction. Valve injury is less common, with most cases involving the anteriorly located tricuspid valve. However, some valve damage is postulated to be related to sudden changes in ventricular or aortic pressure and may affect the left-sided valves. For example, in early diastole the closed aortic valve may be damaged by a sudden increase in aortic pressure, resulting in increased mechanical force on the valve leaflets. The acute onset in this case is consistent with either direct compression of the heart by the horse kick or a sudden rise in aortic pressure resulting in a flail aortic leaflet.

There are several approaches to quantitation of aortic regurgitation severity by echocardiography. A simple and useful approach is to measure the narrowest diameter of the regurgitant jet, or the vena contracta. Ideally, both the proximal flow convergence region and distal expansion of the jet are seen, with the vena contracta being the narrow segment just beyond the valve orifice. A vena contracta width >6 mm indicates severe regurgitation, 3–6 mm indicates moderate and <3 mm is consistent with mild aortic regurgitation. Another simple measure is evidence for holodiastolic flow reversal in the descending thoracic aorta. A small amount of early diastolic flow reversal is normal, but retrograde flow in the aorta throughout diastole is consistent with severe regurgitation. The signal strength of the continuous wave Doppler aortic regurgitation jet, relative to antegrade flow, provides a qualitative evaluation of regurgitant severity. In addition, the diastolic slope of the aortic regurgitation jet can be measured with a pressure half-time <200 (i.e. a steeper slope) consistent with severe regurgitation. This patient met all these criteria for severe aortic regurgitation with a wide vena contracta width, a dense continuous wave signal with a steep deceleration slope and dramatic holodiastolic flow reversal in the aorta. When the severity of regurgitation is less clear, regurgitant volume, fraction and orifice area can be calculated based on measurement of volume flow at two intracardiac sites.

Suggested Reading

1. Otto CM. Emergent valve disorders. In: Fink MP, Abraham E, Vincent JL, Kochanek P eds. Textbook of Critical Care, 5th edn. Philadelphia: Elsevier, 2005: 861–70.

2. Pretre R, Chilcott M. Blunt trauma to the heart and great vessels. N Engl J Med 1997; 336:626–32.

3. Zoghbi WA, Enriquez-Sarano M, Foster E et al. Recommendations for evaluation of the severity of native valvular regurgitation with two-dimensional and Doppler echocardiography. J Am Soc Echocardiogr 2003; 16(7):777–802.

Case 3-9
Perforated Aortic Valve with Regurgitation

This 49-year-old man presented with new-onset heart failure and a diastolic murmur on examination. Six months ago he suffered an inferior myocardial infarction that was treated with a percutaneous coronary intervention. Transthoracic echocardiography showed severe left ventricular dilation with a large area of inferior akinesis and an ejection fraction of 29%. There was moderate central mitral regurgitation due to abnormal left ventricular geometry resulting in tethering of the posterior leaflet. The estimated pulmonary systolic pressure was 75 mmHg. In addition, severe aortic regurgitation was present on Doppler examination, although the etiology of valve dysfunction was uncertain.

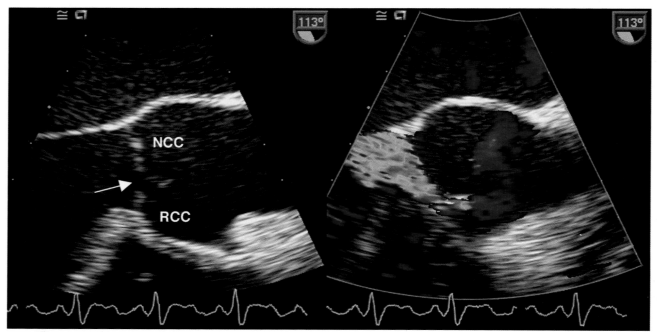

DVD **Fig 3-43.** The 2D long-axis view (*left*) shows the normal aortic root size and anatomy with the NCC and RCC of the aortic valve. Discontinuity is noted in the RCC (**arrow**) with an eccentric jet of aortic regurgitation through this region on color flow imaging (*right*).

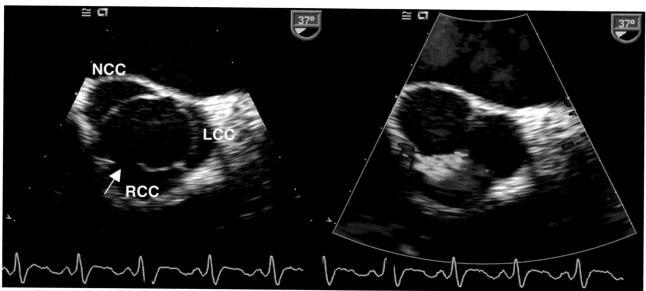

DVD **Fig 3-44.** The short-axis view of the aortic valve shows a trileaflet valve with normal systolic motion. Color flow imaging (*right*) shows a wide jet of aortic regurgitation in the region of the RCC. These findings are consistent with a perforation of the RCC (**arrow**, *left*).

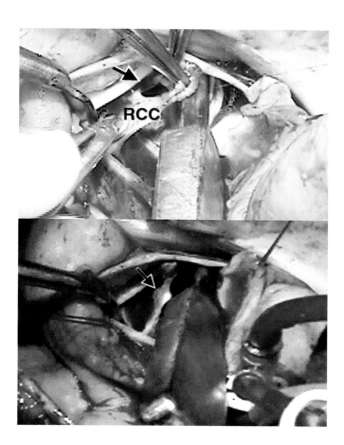

DVD **Fig 3-45.** (*Top*) Inspection of the valve at surgery showed a perforation in the RCC, as shown by the arrow. (*Bottom*) The valve was repaired with a pericardial patch on the RCC, as shown by the arrow.

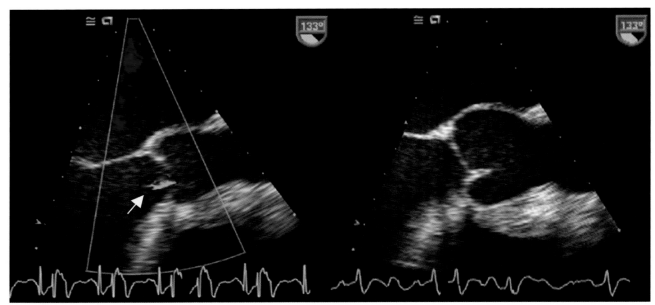

DVD **Fig 3-46.** After weaning from cardiopulmonary bypass, long-axis images of the repaired valve show normal motion and only trace aortic regurgitation (**arrow**).

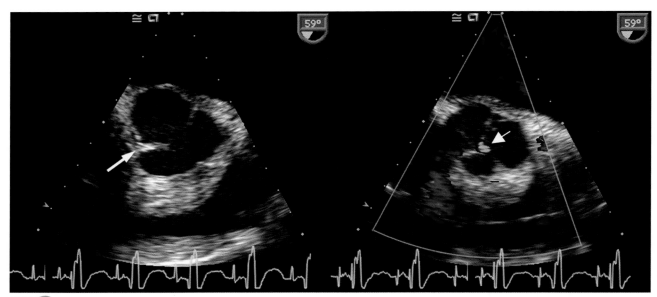

DVD **Fig 3-47.** Short-axis views of the aortic valve after RCC repair (*left*, **arrow**) show only a small jet of central aortic regurgitation (*right*, **arrow**).

Comments

Traumatic injury of the aortic valve due to a percutaneous coronary intervention is rare but is the most likely cause of aortic regurgitation in this patient given the perforation in the right coronary cusp and the normal tissue characteristics of the other valve leaflets. This patient tolerated the aortic regurgitation for several months before presenting with congestive heart failure symptoms, which suggests that an initial small tear in the leaflet may have gradually increased in size, resulting in subacute aortic regurgitation with time for ventricular compensation. The severe ventricular enlargement, which had improved by 6 months after surgery, is consistent with chronic volume overload of the left ventricle.

The Bicuspid Aortic Valve

Case 3-10
Severe Stenosis

A 55-year-old man with aortic stenosis was referred for valve replacement for severe symptomatic aortic stenosis.

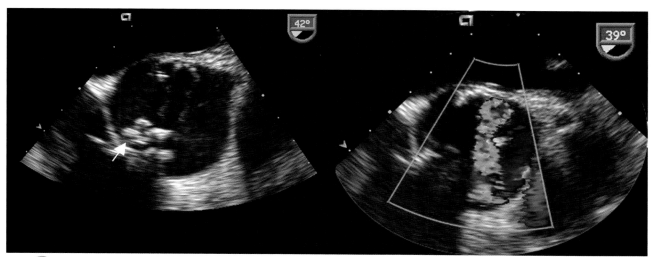

DVD **Fig 3-48.** Intraoperative TEE in a short-axis view shows a bicuspid aortic valve with two relatively equal-sized leaflets but with extensive calcification at the anterior aspect of the valve (*left,* **arrow**) and limited motion of the valve leaflets.

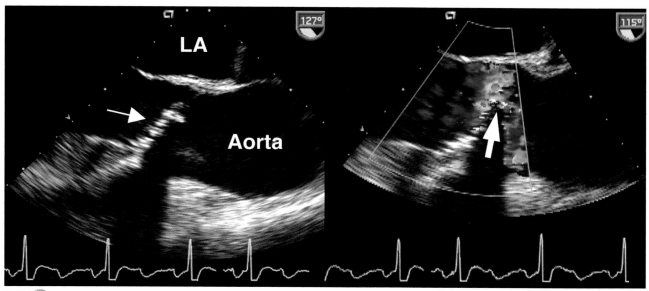

DVD **Fig 3-49.** Long-axis imaging of the aortic valve and ascending aorta shows the heavily calcified valve (*left,* **arrow**), and dilated ascending aorta (4.5 cm) and a narrow jet of aortic outflow (*right,* **arrow**). Note the shadowing from the valve calcification.

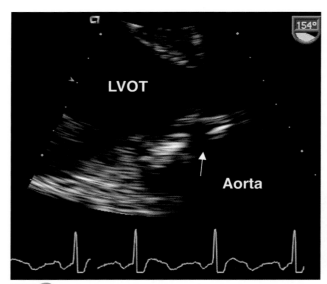

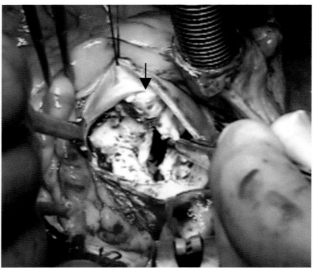

DVD **Fig 3-50.** Transgastric imaging of the aortic valve shows heavy calcification, a small orifice (**arrow**) and shadowing of the ascending aorta.

DVD **Fig 3-51.** Visualization of the valve at surgery shows the heavily calcified valve with an area of nodular calcification corresponding to the echocardiographic findings (**arrow**) (the anterior aspect of the valve is at the top of the screen). The stiffness of the calcified valve leaflets can be appreciated on the DVD.

Comments

This is a classic clinical presentation and typical appearance of a calcified bicuspid aortic valve resulting in significant aortic stenosis. Complete evaluation of valve anatomy and hemodynamics should be performed by preoperative transthoracic echocardiography. The intraoperative TEE provides confirmation of the diagnosis and can identify associated abnormalities, such as a dilated aortic root, that may not have been appreciated preoperatively.

Suggested Reading

1. Pachulski RT, Chan KL. Progression of aortic valve dysfunction in 51 adult patients with congenital bicuspid aortic valve: assessment and follow up by Doppler echocardiography. Br Heart J 1993; 69:237–40.

2. Chan KL, Ghani M, Woodend K et al. Case-controlled study to assess risk factors for aortic stenosis in congenitally bicuspid aortic valve. Am J Cardiol 2001; 88:690–3.

Case 3-11
Combined Stenosis and Regurgitation

A 52-year-old woman with a bicuspid aortic valve was referred for valve replacement. Fourteen years ago she underwent resection of a benign cardiac tumor that was located in the LVOT just proximal to the aortic valve. At that time, direct inspection of the aortic valve showed a bicuspid valve with thin leaflets and echocardiography showed normal valve function. Over the past 3 months she noted increasing dyspnea on exertion, with physical examination showing a 3/6 aortic stenosis murmur, a 2/6 aortic regurgitant murmur and diminished carotid upstrokes.

Transthoracic echocardiography results are as follows:

	Aortic jet velocity	Mean gradient	Valve area
6 years ago	4.1 m/s	40 mmHg	1.6 cm^2
1 year ago	4.8 m/s	54 mmHg	1.0 cm^2
Now	6.0 m/s	81 mmHg	0.9 cm^2

There is moderate coexisting aortic regurgitation with mild left ventricular dilation, moderate concentric hypertrophy and an ejection fraction of 61%. Dilation of the ascending aorta is present with a maximum diameter on chest CT of 5.0 cm.

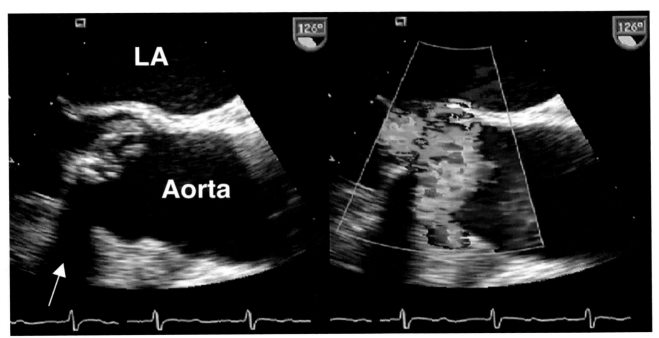

Fig 3-52. Intraoperative TEE in a long-axis view of the aortic valve in diastole with 2D images (*left*) and color flow Doppler (*right*). Note the thickening and calcification of the aortic valve with prominent shadowing (**arrow**). A broad jet of aortic regurgitation is seen, filling about 60% of the diameter of the outflow tract, with a vena contracta width >12 mm. On this frame, which best demonstrates the maximum width of the vena contracta of the aortic regurgitant jet, a flow disturbance (in green mosaic) is seen on the aortic side of the valve due to flow acceleration into the regurgitant orifice. The flow dynamics of the aortic regurgitation are better appreciated on the DVD.

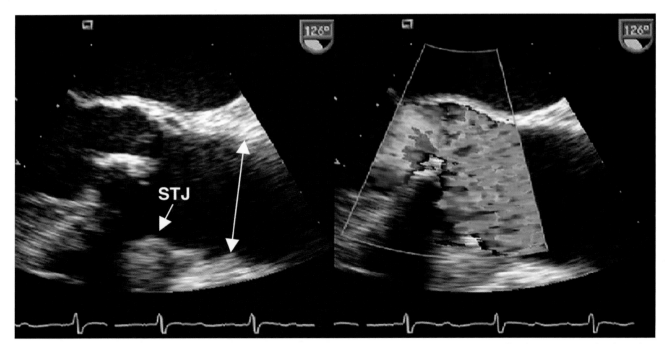

Fig 3-53. Long-axis view of the aortic valve in systole, with 2D images showing restricted valve opening (*left*) with an eccentric antegrade jet of flow on color Doppler (*right*). The bicuspid valve shows systolic "doming" with the smallest valve orifice at the leaflet tips. Also note the dilated ascending aorta (**arrows**) but with a normal contour of the sinotubular junction (**STJ**).

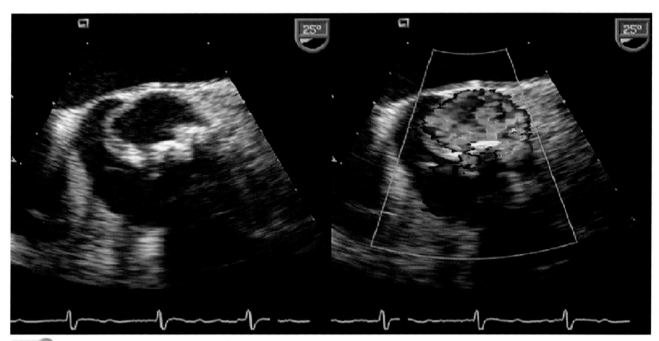

DVD **Fig 3-54.** Short-axis views of the aortic valve in mid-systole showing eccentric valve opening with only one commissure evident on 2D imaging (*left*). Color Doppler confirms that antegrade flow is confined to this eccentric orifice (*right*). With the doming of this bicuspid congenitally abnormal aortic valve, planimetry of valve area in short-axis views is problematic as the tomographic plane may be through the base of the doming leaflets, rather than at the leaflet tips. Thus, the apparent large opening seen on this image does not represent the smallest valve area and should not be measured. The continuity equation valve area is a more accurate descriptor of functional valve area in this situation.

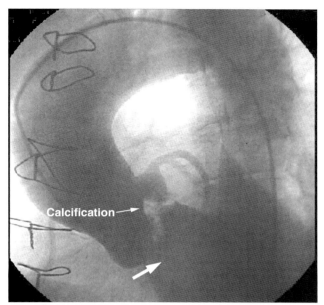

Fig 3-55. Aortogram with contrast injected into the ascending aorta shows severe valve calcification and dilation of the ascending aorta. Moderate aortic regurgitation is evident with contrast refluxing into the left ventricle, with an equal density of contrast in the left ventricle (**arrow**) and aorta after several beats.

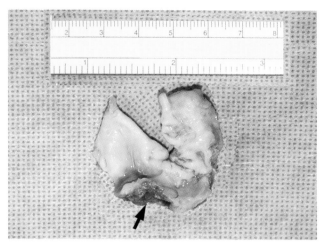

Fig 3-57. The excised valve appears unicuspid with severe calcification. The valve has been oriented to match the short-axis view in **Fig 3-54**. Note how the shape and size of the valve opening and the appearance of calcification on the pathology specimen correspond to the echocardiographic image. The arrow indicates the chronic inflammation beneath the right coronary cusp.

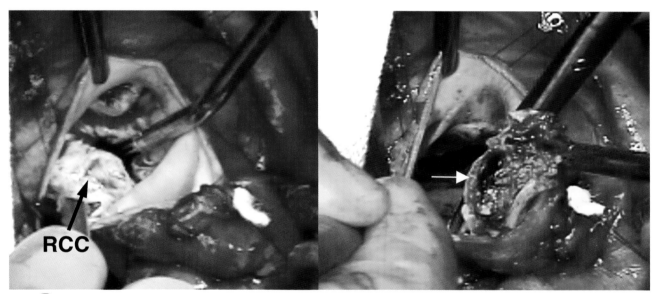

Fig 3-56. Inspection of the valve at surgery showed a bicuspid valve with severe fusion of 2 cusps resulting in a functional unicuspid valve (*left*). The valve was heavily calcified with evidence of chronic inflammation beneath the right coronary cusp (*right*, **arrow**), possibly due to a jet lesion related to her previous outflow tract tumor. The aortic valve was resected and replaced with a 27 mm Carpentier–Edwards pericardial valve and the dilated ascending was replaced with a woven polyester aortic graft.

Comments

Some patients with a congenital bicuspid aortic valve develop severe aortic regurgitation with left ventricular dilation, requiring valve surgery in young adulthood. However, most patients have normal valve function until the 5th–6th decade of life when progressive valve calcification results in outflow obstruction, often with some degree of coexisting aortic regurgitation. When severe stenosis results in symptoms, aortic valve replacement is needed. In this case, the extent of valve deformity may have been affected by abnormal subvalvular hemodynamics related to the woman's outflow tract tumor.

Aortic stenosis presents with symptoms at a younger age in patients with a bicuspid valve rather than a trileaflet valve, presumably related to earlier calcification secondary to the abnormal shear and tensile stresses of the bicuspid valve leaflets. However, once mild stenosis is present, the rate of hemodynamic progression is similar, regardless of underlying valve anatomy. Over the past 6 years, this woman's progression was typical, with an increase in jet velocity of 0.3 m/s per year and a decrease in valve area of 0.1 cm^2 per year.

Suggested Reading

1. Otto CM, Burwash IG, Legget ME et al. A prospective study of asymptomatic valvular aortic stenosis: clinical, echocardiographic, and exercise predictors of outcome. Circulation 1997; 95:2262–70.

2. Carabello BA. Clinical practice. Aortic stenosis. N Engl J Med 2002; 346(9):677–82.

Case 3-12
Bicuspid Valve with an Aortic Aneurysm

An asymptomatic 47-year-old man was referred for repair of an ascending aortic aneurysm. Chest CT showed dilation of the ascending aorta, extending into the proximal arch, with a maximum dimension of 58 mm. On transthoracic echocardiography, a bicuspid aortic valve with mild-to-moderate aortic regurgitation was seen with normal left ventricular size and systolic function. Cardiac catheterization showed normal coronary arteries, mild–moderate aortic regurgitation and a dilated ascending aorta.

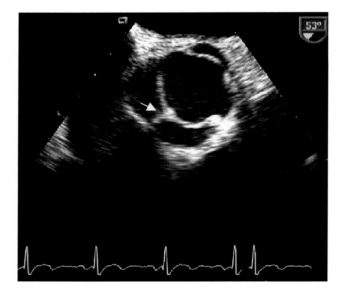

DVD **Fig 3-58.** The intraoperative TEE short-axis view of the aortic valve shows two leaflets open in systole with a raphe in the larger, anterior cusp (arrow).

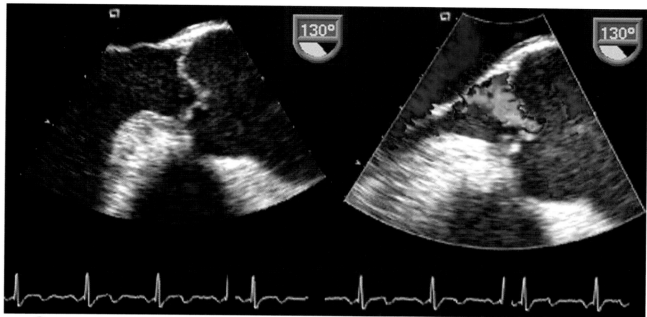

Fig 3-59. Long-axis view of the aortic valve in diastole with 2D imaging showing the slight thickening of the closed leaflets (*left*) and color Doppler (*right*) showing mild aortic regurgitation with a vena contracta width of 3 mm. The aortic regurgitation originates centrally, which is consistent with stretched leaflets resulting in inadequate central coaptation due to aortic root dilation.

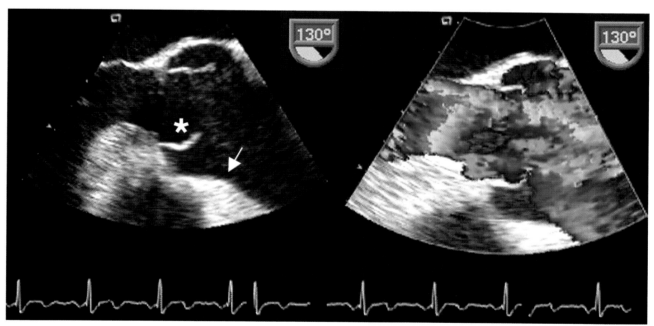

Fig 3-60. Long-axis view in systole with 2D imaging showing the open aortic leaflets (*left*) and color Doppler showing no outflow obstruction (*right*). The more anterior right coronary cusp is "domed" (**asterisk**). Note that the sinotubular junction (**arrow**) and contour of the sinuses of Valsalva appear normal despite the ascending aortic aneurysm.

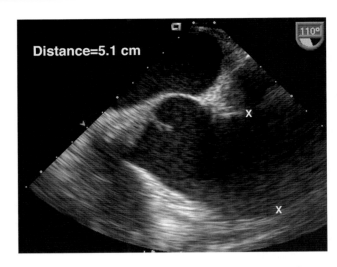

Distance=5.1 cm

Fig 3-61. Long-axis view of the ascending aorta reveals the aneurysmal dilation.

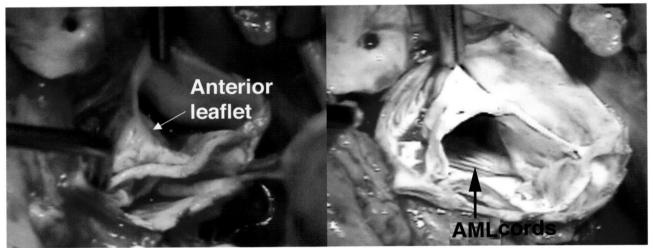

Fig 3-62. Surgical view of the bicuspid aortic valve (*left*). The larger anterior leaflet is excessively redundant and thinned (*right*). Chords of the anterior mitral leaflet (**AML**) are seen through the aortic valve orifice.

Comments

Although this patient presented primarily with an ascending aortic aneurysm, some degree of aortic dilation is common in patients with a bicuspid aortic valve. Even when the dilation is not as severe as in this case, the presence of a bicuspid aortic valve is associated with an increased risk of aortic dissection, even after valve replacement. Thus, evaluation of the ascending aorta and consideration of the surgical approach is essential in patients with a bicuspid aortic valve.

In this patient, the clinical presentation was similar to Marfan syndrome but can be differentiated based on the lack of associated clinical findings (e.g. ocular, musculoskeletal) and the preservation of the sino-tubular junction seen on echocardiography.

Suggested Reading

1. Fedak PW, Verma S, David TE et al. Clinical and pathophysiological implications of a bicuspid aortic valve. Circulation 2002; 106:900–4.
2. Ferencik M, Pape LA. Changes in size of ascending aorta and aortic valve function with time in patients with congenitally bicuspid aortic valves. Am J Cardiol 2003; 92:43–6.

Case 3-13
Chronic Aortic Regurgitation

This asymptomatic 49-year-old man, who had a 20-year history of a heart murmur followed with periodic echocardiography, was referred for aortic valve replacement for severe aortic regurgitation.

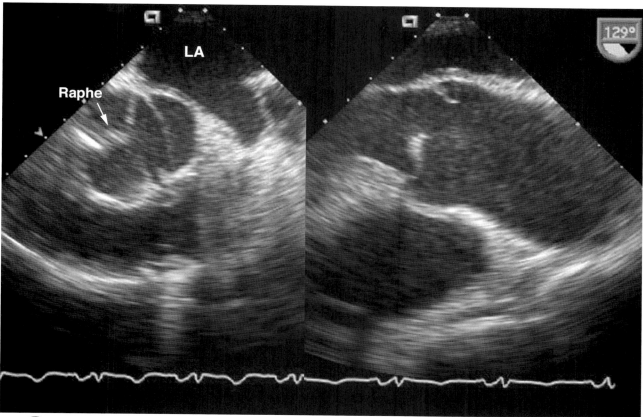

Fig 3-63. In the short-axis view of the aortic valve at 30 degrees (*left*), only two leaflets are seen with a prominent raphe in the larger rightward and anterior cusp (arrow). In the long-axis view at 129 degrees (*right*), asymmetrical closure of the leaflets with prolapse of the anterior aortic valve leaflet is seen.

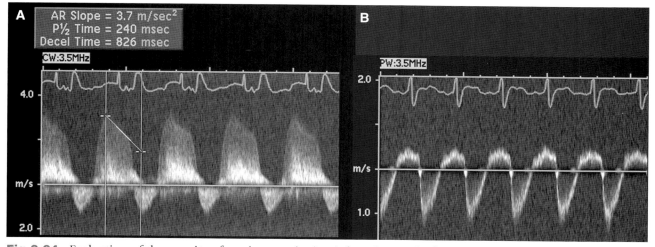

Fig 3-64. Evaluation of the severity of aortic regurgitation is based on pulsed, continuous wave (**CW**) and color Doppler evaluation. The CW Doppler signal recorded from a transgastric apical approach (**A**) shows relatively equal intensity of forward and reverse flow across the aortic valve with a deceleration slope >3 m/s^2. The descending thoracic aorta pulsed Doppler (**B**) shows holodiastolic flow reversal. Both these findings are consistent with severe, possibly acute aortic regurgitation.

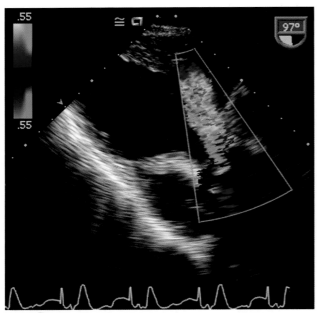

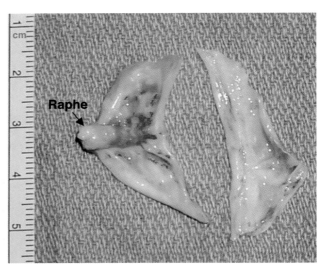

Fig 3-66. Examination of the valve removed at surgery shows the close correspondence between the details of valve anatomy appreciated on TEE and the actual pathology of the valve (see **Fig 3-63**).

Fig 3-65. Color flow imaging from an apical transgastric approach. The LV is somewhat foreshortened but color flow in the outflow tract demonstrates a wide vena contracta, also confirming severe aortic regurgitation.

Comments

A subset of patients with a bicuspid aortic valve present in young adulthood with severe aortic regurgitation. The ACC/AHA consensus guidelines recommend aortic valve replacement for severe aortic regurgitation associated with symptoms or with evidence of early ventricular dysfunction. Criteria for early ventricular dysfunction in asymptomatic adults with aortic regurgitation are an end-systolic dimension >55 mm or an ejection fraction <50%. With a bicuspid aortic valve and a normal root diameter, valve repair is rarely feasible.

With acute aortic regurgitation, left ventricular size typically is not increased. The acute volume load of the left ventricle is associated with a marked increase in end-diastolic pressure with clinical symptoms of congestive heart failure and pulmonary edema. Intra-operative echocardiography is valuable for confirming the presence and severity of aortic regurgitation, for visualization of aortic valve and root anatomy and for evaluation of ventricular systolic function before and after valve replacement.

Suggested Reading

1. Otto CM. Timing of aortic valve surgery. Heart 2000; 84:211–18.
2. Bonow RO, Carabello BA, Chatterjee K et al. ACC/AHA 2006 Practice guidelines for the management of patients with valvular heart disease: executive summary. A report of the American College of Cardiology/American Heart Association Task Force on Practice Guidelines (Writing Committee to Revise the 1998 Guidelines for the Management of Patients With Valvular Heart Disease). J Am Coll Cardiol 2006; 48:598–675.

4

Endocarditis

Native Valve Endocarditis

Case 4-1
Aortic Valve Endocarditis

This 46-year-old man with a 5-week history of fatigue and anemia suffered bilateral cerebral embolic events. He had no prior medical history other than a cardiac murmur. Blood cultures were positive for *Streptococcus viridans* and echocardiography showed aortic valve vegetations with severe aortic regurgitation. He was transferred to our medical center for surgical intervention.

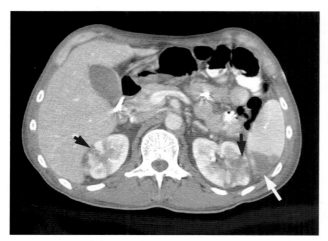

Fig 4-1. An abdominal CT scan showed multiple renal infarcts (**black arrows**) and a splenic infarct (**white arrow**) consistent with embolic events.

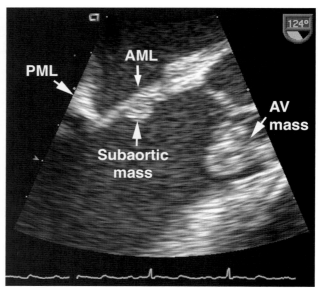

DVD **Fig 4-2.** In a long-axis view of the aortic valve (**AV**) and anterior mitral leaflet (**AML**), a vegetation is seen on the AV with another area of thickening on the AML, in the subaortic region. The posterior aortic root is thickened, suggestive of abscess. **PML** = posterior mitral leaflet.

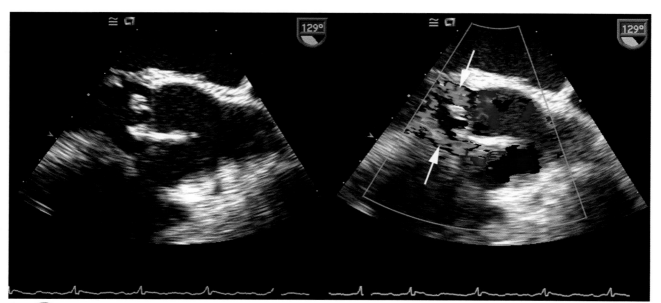

DVD **Fig 4-3.** With slight turning of the transducer in the long-axis plane, additional vegetations are seen in the center of the aortic valve. Color Doppler (*right*) demonstrates at least two regurgitant jets (**arrows**).

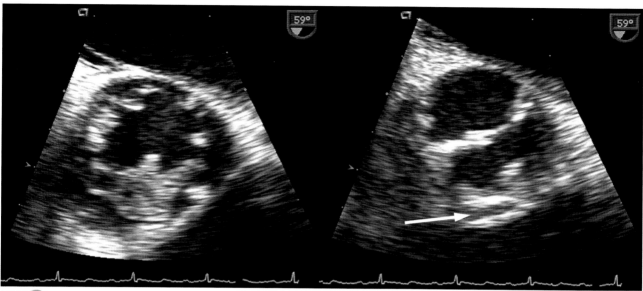

Fig 4-4. A short-axis view of the aortic valve in systole shows severe valve destruction, and large vegetations (*left*). In diastole, an echolucent area consistent with a paravalvular abscess (**arrow**) is seen. The number of leaflets cannot be determined due to the superimposed infection.

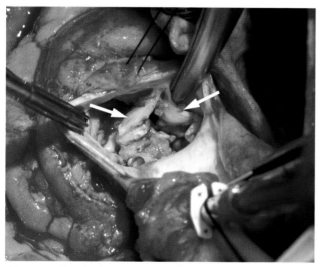

Fig 4-5. Surgical inspection of the aortic valve shows a bicuspid valve with large vegetations (**arrows**) and extensive valve destruction.

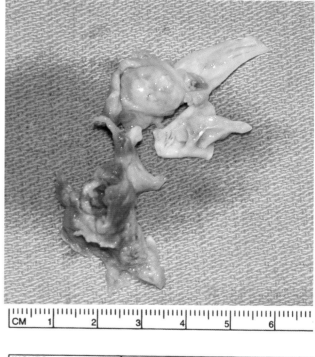

Fig 4-6. The explanted valve tissue with infection and inflammation.

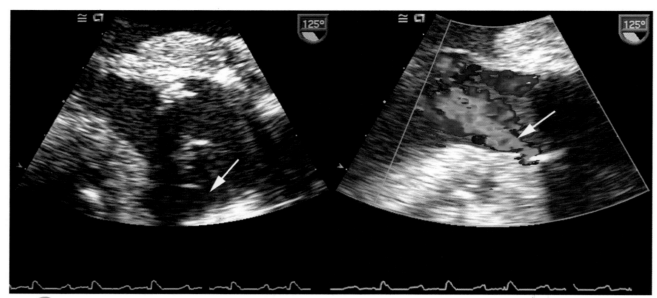

DVD **Fig 4-7.** After weaning from cardiopulmonary bypass, a long-axis view of the new tissue valve shows slight discontinuity in the annulus anteriorly (**arrow**, *left*) with color Doppler demonstrating a jet of paravalvular regurgitation (**arrow**, *right*).

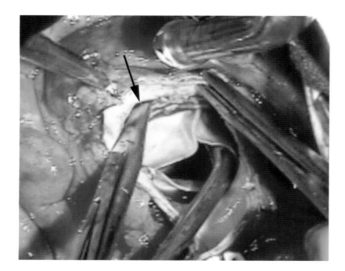

Fig 4-8. On a second bypass pump run, the site of the paravalvular leak was identified. The forceps tips are in the defect in this photograph (**arrow**).

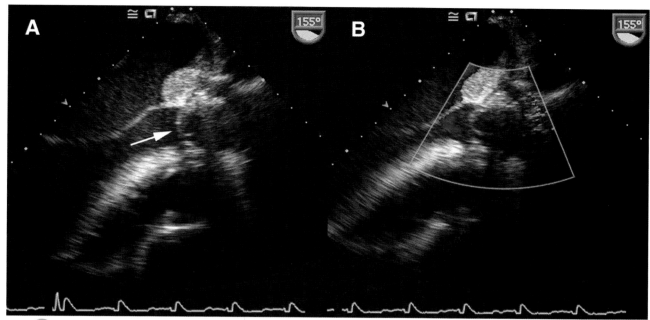

Fig 4-9. Due to the necrotic infected tissue, an aortic homograft was used to replace the valve and reconstruct the outflow tract and aortic root. A long-axis view of the homograft shows normal coaptation (**arrow**) (A), and no significant regurgitation (B). (The surgical procedure is represented on the DVD.)

His postoperative course was complicated by multiple septic embolic. After a prolonged hospital stay, he was discharged to a skilled nursing facility for further rehabilitation after his strokes.

Comments

The clinical diagnosis of endocarditis is based on a combination of clinical, bacteriologic and echocardiographic findings, known as the Duke criteria. In brief, definite endocarditis is present when there is evidence of persistent bacteremia plus echocardiographic findings consistent with endocardial infection. When only one, but not both of these criteria are present, other minor clinical criteria are used to support the diagnosis of endocarditis. A vegetation is recognized on echocardiography as an irregular mass attached to a valve leaflet but with motion independent of the normal valve motion. Vegetations are typically located on the upstream side of valves, e.g. the ventricular side of the aortic valve and the atrial side of the mitral valve. Valvular regurgitation is present in over 90% of cases, due to tissue destruction. Stenosis due to a large vegetation is rare. Transesophageal echocardiography has a very high (nearly 100%) sensitivity and specificity for detection of valvular vegetations. Other echocardiographic findings that may be mistaken for a valvular vegetation include beam width artifact, normal valve tissue (i.e. myxomatous valve disease, Lambl's excrescence), prosthetic valve thrombus, papillary fibroelastoma and non-bacterial thrombotic endocarditis.

Suggested Reading

1. Bayer AS, Bolger AF, Taubert KA et al. Diagnosis and management of infective endocarditis and its complications. *Circulation* 1998; 98:2936–48.

2. Mylonakis E, Calderwood SB. Infective endocarditis in adults. N Engl J Med 2001; 345(18):1318–30.

Case 4-2
Aortic and Mitral Valve Vegetations

This 35-year-old man presented with a 6-week history of malaise and a 2-week history of fevers, chills and right upper quadrant abdominal pain. After an abdominal ultrasound, he was started on antibiotics for ascending cholangitis. However, he continued to deteriorate clinically with sepsis and multiple blood cultures positive for *Haemophilus influenzae*. After further respiratory and hemodynamic compromise, he underwent echocardiography, which was consistent with aortic and mitral valve endocarditis with severe aortic regurgitation and moderate mitral regurgitation. He declined into cardiogenic shock and his mental status declined. Head CT showed focal right frontal lobe hypodensities consistent with embolic stroke. Because of his hemodynamic instability, he was taken to the operating room for emergency aortic valve replacement.

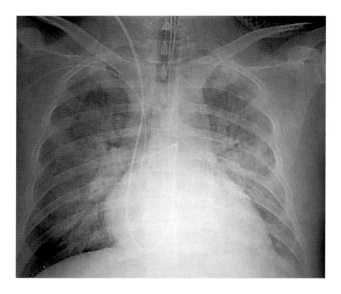

Fig 4-10. PA chest radiography shows cardiac enlargement and pulmonary edema.

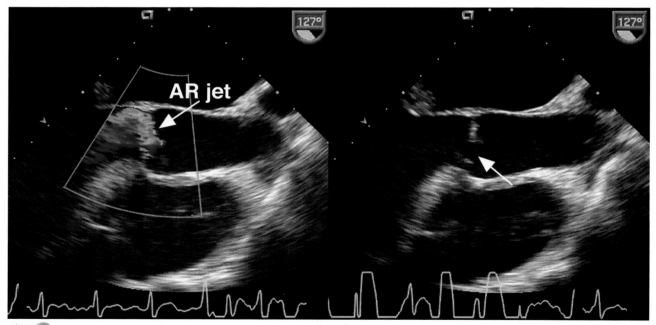

DVD **Fig 4-11.** Long-axis TEE view of the aortic valve and ascending aorta demonstrates normal aortic root size and anatomy. However, there is a discontinuity in the anterior leaflet of the aortic valve (**arrow**) with color Doppler showing a wide jet of aortic regurgitation through this region.

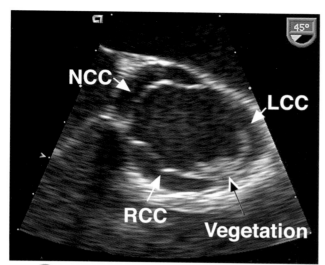

DVD ▶ Fig 4-12. The short-axis TEE view of the aortic valve demonstrates a valvular vegetation at the junction between the right (**RCC**) and left coronary cusps (**LCC**). The posteriorly located non-coronary cusp (**NCC**) appears normal in this view.

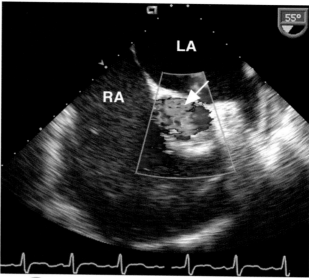

DVD ▶ Fig 4-13. Color Doppler in a short-axis view of the left ventricular outflow tract shows aortic regurgitation (mosaic green pattern, **arrow**) filling about two-thirds of the cross-sectional area of flow.

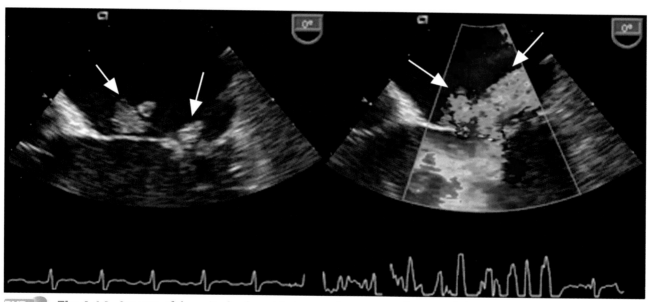

DVD ▶ Fig 4-14. Images of the mitral valve at 0 degrees demonstrate large mobile masses on both leaflets. In real time, these masses move independently from the valve leaflets and are consistent with vegetations. Color Doppler shows a wide jet of mitral regurgitation with both anteriorly and posteriorly directed jets (**arrows**).

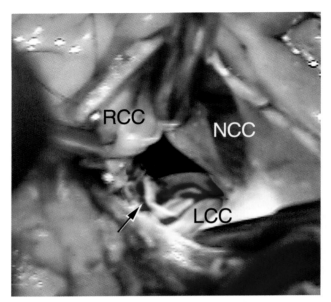

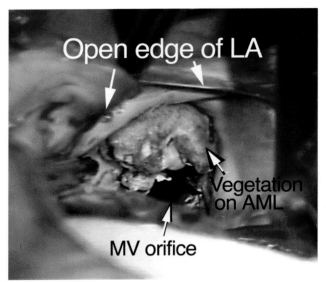

Fig 4-15. At surgical inspection, the 1 cm diameter vegetation at the junction of the left and right coronary cusps of the aortic valve is seen (**arrow**).

Fig 4-16. With the left atrium opened, the large vegetation on the anterior mitral leaflet can be appreciated. Both anterior and posterior leaflets were extensively destroyed by the infectious process. The man underwent mechanical aortic and mitral valve replacements. Although his postoperative course was complicated, 2 years after surgery he is doing well clinically on medical therapy for a left ventricular ejection fraction of 36% with moderate paravalvular aortic regurgitation.

Comments

Vegetations are described on echocardiography in terms of location, size, mobility and echodensity. The exact location on the valve may help determine if valve repair, rather than replacement, is possible. Vegetation size and mobility are markers of increased risk of complications of endocarditis. The density of a vegetation may provide clues about the chronicity of disease, with denser, calcified vegetations suggesting chronic or healed endocarditis.

In patients with underlying valve disease, bacteremia may result in direct infection at more than one site. Even when one valve is primarily infected, vegetations may occur on other valves due to direct extension of the infection. An example is an aortic annular abscess eroding into the base of the anterior mitral leaflet.

Infection of one valve may also damage an adjacent valve, leading to subsequent infection. For example, aortic regurgitation impinging on the anterior mitral leaflet results in endothelial disruption with a higher likelihood of bacterial adherence at that site. Thus, one of the primary goals of intraoperative TEE in patients undergoing valve surgery for endocarditis is to exclude infection on the other "uninvolved" valves.

Suggested Reading

1. Evangelista A, Gonzalez-Alujas MT. Echocardiography in infective endocarditis. Heart 2004; 90(6):614–17.

2. Reynolds HR, Jagen MA, Tunick PA et al. Sensitivity of transthoracic versus transesophageal echocardiography for the detection of native valve vegetations in the modern era. J Am Soc Echocardiogr 2003; 16:67–70.

Case 4-3
Mitral Valve Endocarditis with Perforated Anterior Leaflet

This 48-year-old man with a history of intravenous (IV) drug use was transferred to our medical center with *Staphylococcus aureus* mitral valve endocarditis complicated by evidence for cerebral and peripheral emboli, and a myocardial infarction due to embolic coronary artery occlusion. He was referred for mitral valve surgery.

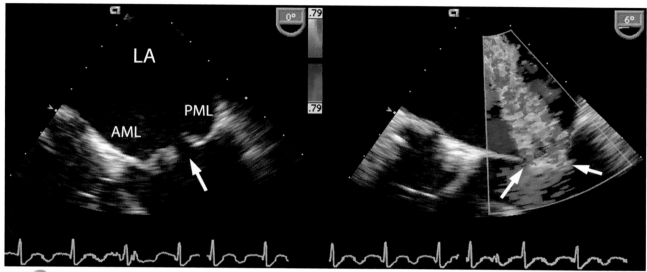

DVD **Fig 4-17.** The TEE four-chamber view of the mitral valve at 0 degrees (*left*) demonstrates an abnormal echodensity on the anterior leaflet (**AML**) that moves independently on the DVD images. In addition, there is an area of apparent discontinuity in the valve closure (**arrow**). Color Doppler (*right*) shows two jets of mitral regurgitation which coalesce into a broad jet of mitral regurgitation that is directed centrally in the enlarged left atrium. One jet appears to originate in the region of discontinuity in the valve closure, whereas the other appears to traverse the AML.

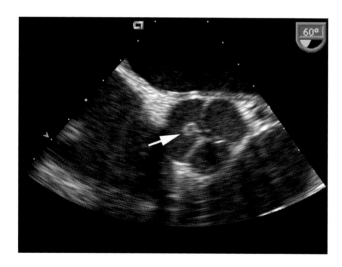

DVD **Fig 4-18.** A short-axis view of the aortic valve shows a small vegetation on the non-coronary cusp (**arrow**).

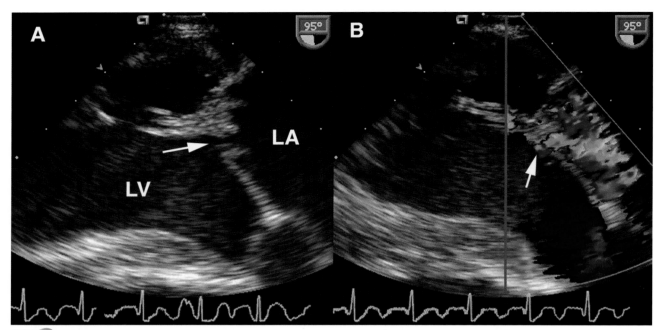

Fig 4-19. (*A*) A two-chamber view of the mitral valve, left ventricle (**LV**) and left atrium (**LA**) obtained from a transgastric view at 90 degrees shows the discontinuity in the anterior mitral leaflet in systole (**arrow**). (*B*) Color Doppler demonstrates flow through this region, indicating this is not artifactual "echo-drop-out" but an actual anatomic defect.

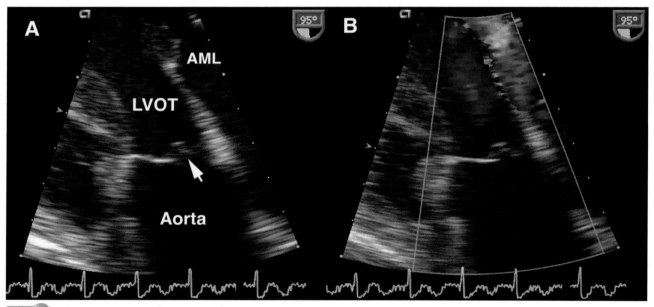

Fig 4-20. From the image plane in **Fig 4-19**, the probe is turned towards the patient's right side to obtain this view of the left ventricular outflow tract (**LVOT**) and aorta (*A*). The small vegetation on the aortic valve is again demonstrated (**arrow**), confirming that this is a real finding, not an imaging artifact, but there is no demonstrable aortic regurgitation with color Doppler (*B*).

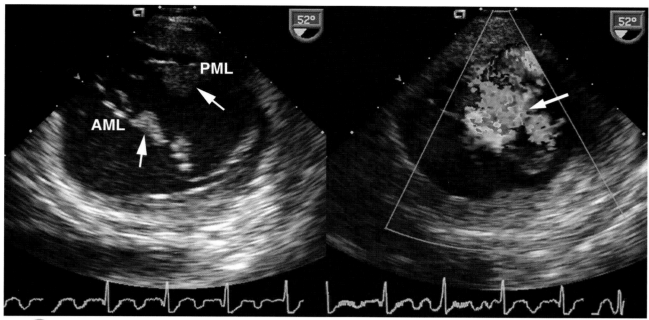

DVD **Fig 4-21.** A transgastric short-axis view of the mitral valve shows vegetations on both anterior and posterior leaflets (**arrows**) in diastole (*left*). In systole, color Doppler (*right*) demonstrates a broad jet of central mitral regurgitation (**arrow**).

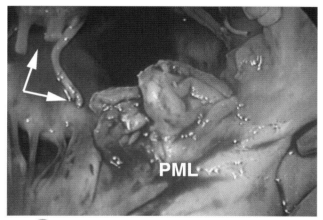

DVD **Fig 4-22.** Surgical inspection shows a large vegetation and inflammation of the posterior mitral leaflet. Fragments of chordae attached to the infected anterior mitral leaflet are seen (**arrows**).

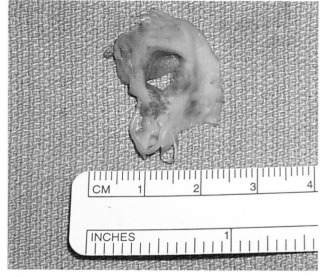

Fig 4-23. The resected anterior leaflet, with chords at the bottom of the photograph, revealed a large perforation.

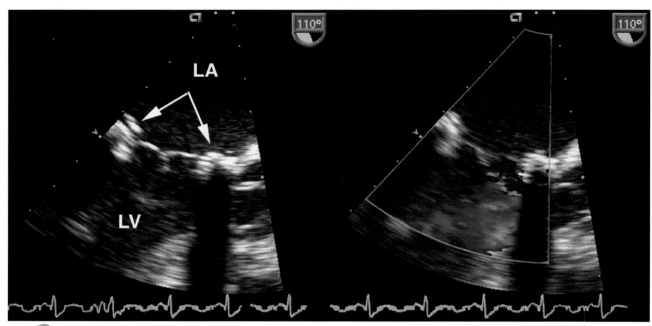

Fig 4-24. After valve replacement and weaning from cardiopulmonary bypass, the TEE image of the mitral valve shows the valve ring (**arrows**) with marked shadowing and the thin leaflets with normal motion. Color Doppler shows normal flows with no regurgitation. The man is doing well 18 months after surgery on no cardiac medications except for aspirin.

Comments

The clinical sequelae of endocarditis are due to two primary processes: tissue destruction and embolization. Tissue destruction leads to valve regurgitation and paravalvular abscess formation, whereas embolization leads to cerebrovascular events. Cerebral embolization occurs in 10–30% of patients with endocarditis, and coronary artery embolism occurs in about 10% of patients. Risk factors for embolization are infection with *Staph aureus*, fungal endocarditis and mitral valve involvement. Several studies also have suggested that larger (>1 cm in diameter) and more mobile veg-etations are at higher risk of embolization. However, earlier surgical intervention based on the appearance of the vegetation remains controversial.

Suggested Reading

1. Di Salvo G, Habib G, Pergola V et al. Echocardiography predicts embolic events in infective endocarditis. J Am Coll Cardiol 2001; 37:1069–76.
2. Vilacosta I, Graupner C, San Roman JA et al. Risk of embolization after institution of antibiotic therapy for infective endocarditis. J Am Coll Cardiol 2002; 39:1489–95.

Case 4-4
Mitral Valve Endocarditis with Perforated Posterior Leaflet

This 61-year-old man with a history of chronic renal failure on hemodialysis was transferred to our medical center with worsening congestive heart failure in the setting of *Staph aureus*, coagulase-negative, mitral valve endocarditis.

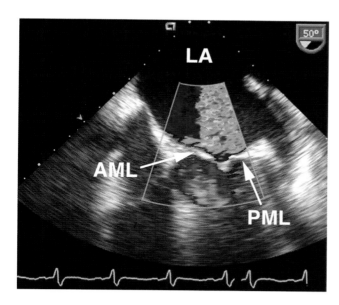

Fig 4-25. A TEE view at 50 degrees demonstrates relatively normal leaflets but a broad jet of mitral regurgitation. In this situation, careful examination in other image planes is needed to identify the mechanism and origin of the regurgitant jet.

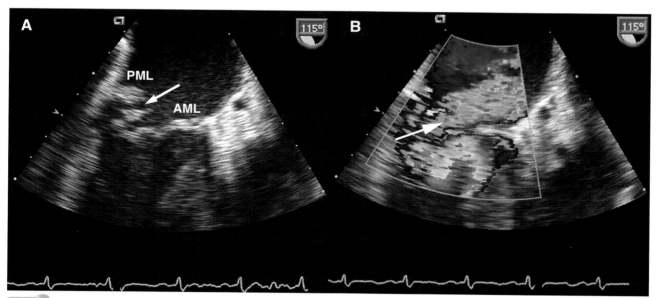

Fig 4-26. (*A*) With further rotation of the image plane to 115 degrees, the end-systolic images show a mass in the posterior annulus with discontinuity and flail of the posterior mitral leaflet (**arrow**). (*B*) Color Doppler shows a wide jet of regurgitation through this region with a vena contracta (**arrow**) of 0.8 cm.

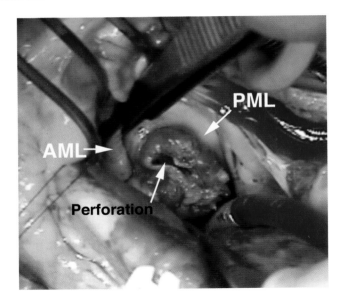

DVD **Fig 4-27.** Surgical inspection of the mitral valve from the left atrial perspective showed severe inflammation of the posterior leaflet with an area of perforation and a partial flail segment.

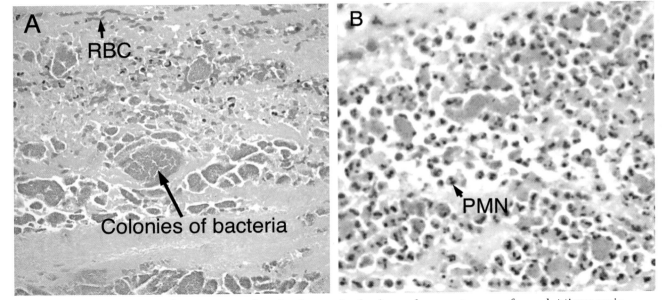

Fig 4-28. The posterior leaflet was resected and a tissue mitral valve replacement was performed. Microscopic examination showed colonies of bacteria (cocci) with destruction of the leaflet architecture (*A*) and numerous active inflammatory cells (*B*). PMN = polymorphonuclear leukocytes, RBC = red blood cells.

Comments

The treatment of endocarditis is based on antibiotic therapy and surgical intervention. Although decision making in each patient integrates multiple factors, there are three generally accepted indications for surgical intervention in patients with endocarditis: heart failure due to valve regurgitation, persistent infection (abscess or persistent positive blood cultures) and recurrent embolic events. Some centers advocate earlier surgical intervention in selected patients to prevent further tissue destruction and embolic events.

Suggested Reading

1 Knyshov GV, Rudenko AV, Vorobyova AM et al. Surgical treatment of acute infective valvular endocarditis (18 years experience). J Card Surg 2001; 16:388–91.

2. d'Udekem Y, David TE, Feindel CM et al. Long-term results of surgery for active infective endocarditis. Eur J Cardiothorac Surg 1997; 11:46–52.

Case 4-5
Another Perforated Posterior Leaflet

This 48-year-old man with a history of kidney and pancreas transplantation was transferred to our medical center with Group A streptococcal septic arthritis of the left knee complicated by acute renal failure. Echocardiography showed a large mitral valve vegetation with severe mitral regurgitation. His hospital course was complicated by an embolic stroke and embolic ischemic coronary events. He was referred for mitral valve replacement for endocarditis with severe mitral regurgitation and heart failure.

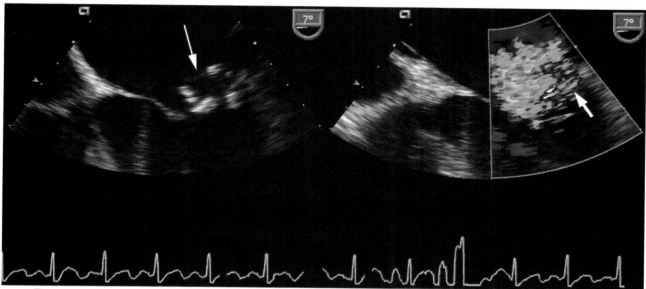

Fig 4-29. Intraoperative TEE shows a severely deformed posterior mitral leaflet (**arrow**) with real-time images showing a large vegetation and partial flail segments. These findings are demonstrated in the four-chamber plane (*left*) consistent with involvement of the central (**P2**) scallop of the posterior leaflet. Color Doppler (*right*) shows part of the regurgitant jet originating in the base of the posterior leaflet, suggesting that perforation of the leaflet is present.

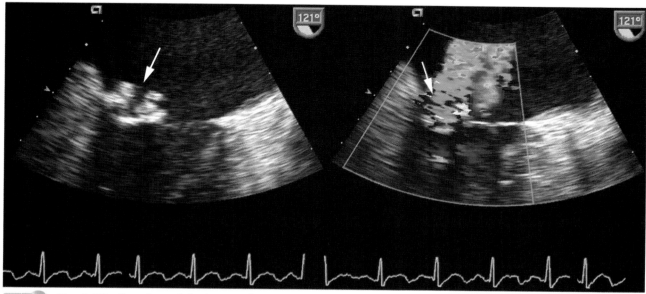

Fig 4-30. Rotation of the image plane to 121 degrees, in a two-chamber orientation, provides another view of the deformed posterior leaflet with a central gap (**arrow**) on 2D imaging that corresponds to the origin of the regurgitant jet on color Doppler (*right*).

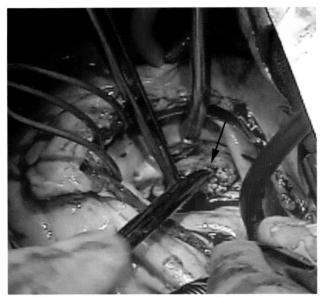

DVD **Fig 4-31.** At surgery there was a large vegetation on the central scallop of the posterior leaflet with a flail leaflet segment and perforation (**arrow**) of the posterior leaflet.

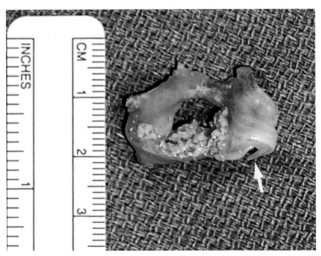

Fig 4-32. The excised posterior leaflet with the vegetation and large perforation. Some chordal structures are included in this specimen, at the right side of the photograph (**arrow**).

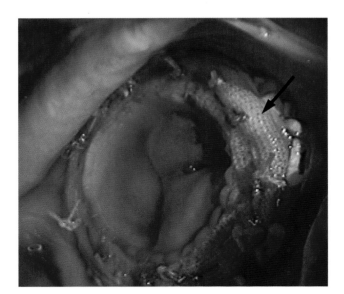

DVD **Fig 4-33.** The surgical view of the 33 mm stented tissue prosthesis used to replace the mitral valve. The anterior chordal structures were preserved but the posterior leaflet and chords were excised completely due to evidence of infection. There was no evidence of paravalvular abscess. The arrow indicates a patch that was used to reinforce an area of the mitral annulus that had been eroded by infection.

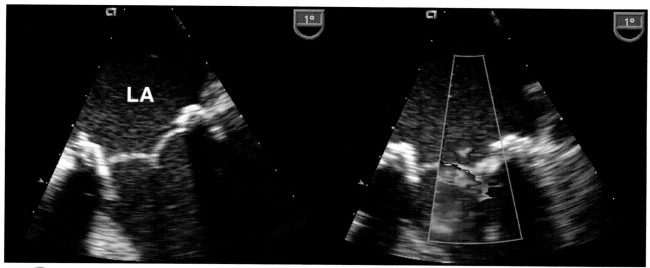

DVD **Fig 4-34.** After weaning from cardiopulmonary bypass, the tissue valve is seen in the four-chamber view with the leaflets closed in systole (*left*) and no significant regurgitation on color Doppler (*right*).

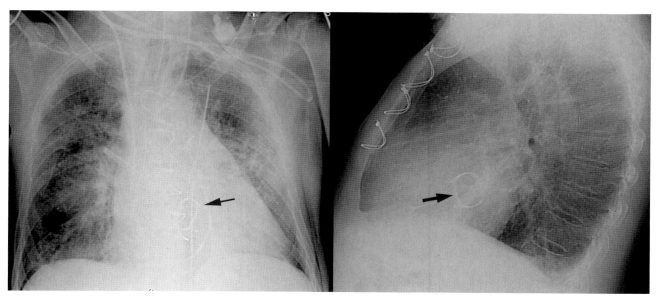

Fig 4-35. Postoperative chest radiograph with the ring of the mitral prosthesis seen in the normal mitral valve positions (**arrows**).

Comments

This patient had both severe valve regurgitation and recurrent embolic events as indications for surgical intervention. Unfortunately, the extent of tissue destruction was so severe that valve repair was not possible. Many surgeons prefer to implant a tissue (instead of mechanical) valve in patients with active endocarditis due to concerns about reinfection of the valve prosthesis and chronic anticoagulation.

Suggested Reading

1. Siniawski H, Lehmkuhl H, Weng Y et al. Stentless aortic valves as an alternative to homografts for valve replacement in active infective endocarditis complicated by ring abscess. Ann Thorac Surg 2003; 75(3):803–8.

2. Delay D, Pellerin M, Carrier M et al. Immediate and long-term results of valve replacement for native and prosthetic valve endocarditis. Ann Thorac Surg 2000; 70(4):1219–23.

Case 4-6
Pulmonic Valve Vegetation

This 39-year-old man with a history of IV drug use was transferred to our medical center with *Staph aureus* endocarditis involving the tricuspid and pulmonic valves.

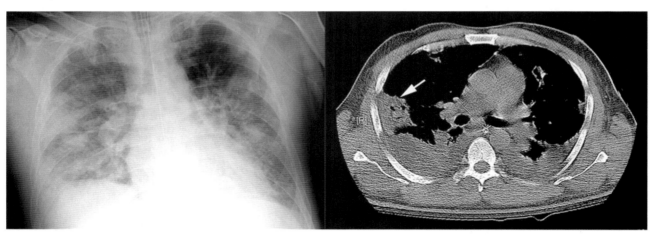

Fig 4-36. Chest X-ray (*left*) shows bilateral patchy lung consolidation. CT scan (*right*) reveals bilateral scattered densities with gas collections (**arrow**), most compatible with septic emboli.

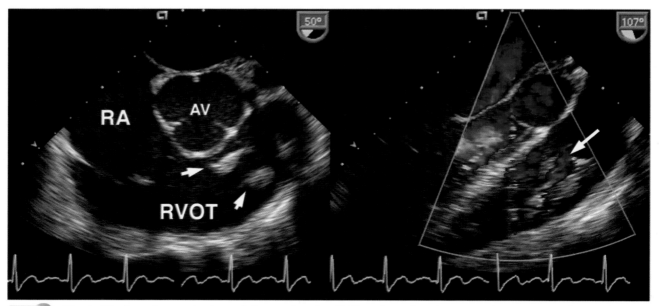

DVD ▶ **Fig 4-37.** In a short-axis view of the aortic valve (*left*), pulmonic valve vegetations are seen (**arrows**) in the RVOT. In a view at 107 degrees rotation (*right*), the pulmonic valve vegetations are seen, with color Doppler evidence of pulmonic regurgitation (**arrow**).

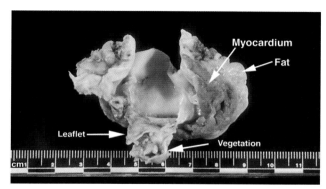

Fig 4-38. The excised pulmonic valve is accompanied by myocardium and epicardial fat. There is a large vegetation attached to one of the pulmonic leaflets, which has ruptured.

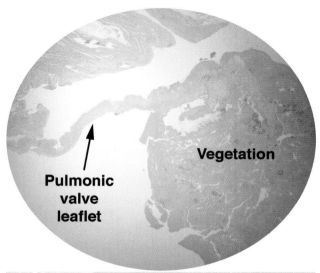

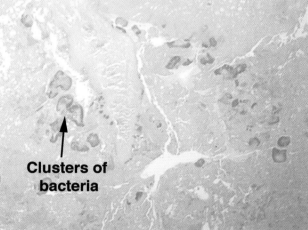

Fig 4-39. Pathologic examination shows attachment of the vegetation to the pulmonic leaflet (*top*). Clusters of bacteria are seen in the leaflet tissue (*bottom*).

This patient underwent tricuspid valve replacement with a pericardial prosthesis and pulmonic valve replacement with a pulmonic root homograft prosthesis. At surgery, both the tricuspid and pulmonic valves had large vegetations with severe valve destruction.

Comments

Endocarditis due to IV drug use affects the tricuspid valve in 75% of cases, with pulmonic valve involvement being much less common. Over 50% of cases of right-sided endocarditis are due to *Staph aureus*. With uncomplicated right-sided endocarditis, a shorter course of IV antibiotics is needed, compared with left-sided endocarditis. However, about 25% of patients also have involvement of left-sided heart valves. Complications of tricuspid valve endocarditis include septic pulmonary emboli and valve destruction leading to tricuspid regurgitation. The initial clinical prognosis is good with an in-hospital mortality of only 3–9%. However, long-term outcomes are poor, related to other medical and social issues, with a 10-year survival of only 10%. Tricupsid regurgitation may be well tolerated in the short term, but most patients eventually develop right heart failure and low output symptoms with uncorrected severe tricuspid regurgitation.

Suggested Reading

1. Hecht SR, Berger M. Right-sided endocarditis in intravenous drug users. Prognostic features in 102 episodes. *Ann Intern Med* 1992; 117:560–6.

Complications of Native Valve Endocarditis

Case 4-7
Aortic Annular Abscess

This 30-year-old man with no prior cardiac history transferred to our hospital with streptococcal aortic valve endocarditis and a possible paravalvular abscess.

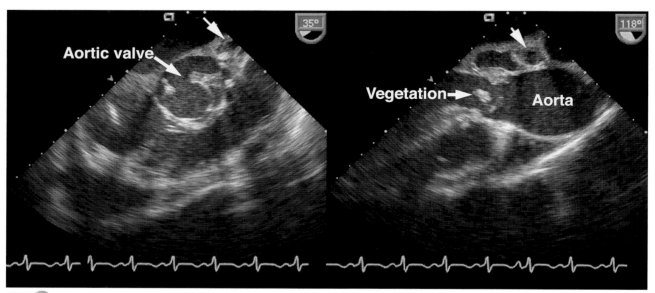

DVD **Fig 4-40.** A short-axis (*left*) and long-axis (*right*) view of the aortic valve demonstrate thickened valve leaflets and a complex echo-free space (arrows) consistent with an abscess.

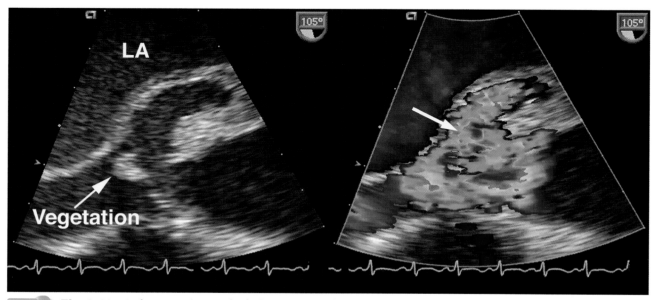

DVD **Fig 4-41.** A close-up view with slight rotation of the image plane demonstrates the connection between the echo-free space posterior to the aorta with the aortic root, just distal to the aortic valve. Color Doppler (*right*) shows flows in and out of this cavity.

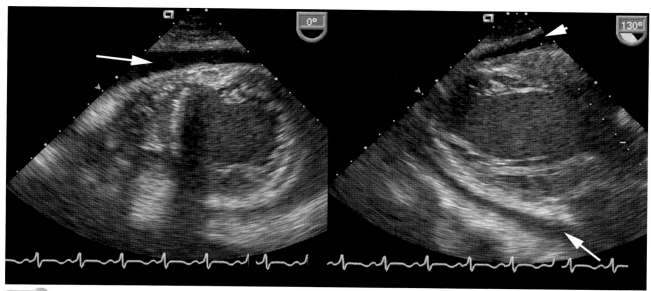

DVD **Fig 4-42.** The transgastric short-axis (*left*) and two-chamber (*right*) views show a small to moderate pericardial effusion (**arrows**). In real time, bi-ventricular systolic function is reduced.

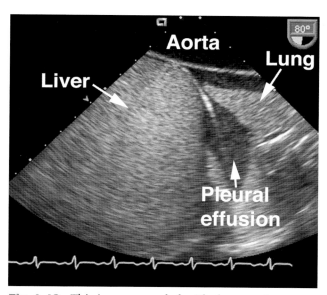

Fig 4-43. This image recorded with the transducer at the gastroesophageal junction with the transducer turned posteriorly towards the descending aorta shows compressed lung, with a surrounding pleural effusion, and the liver.

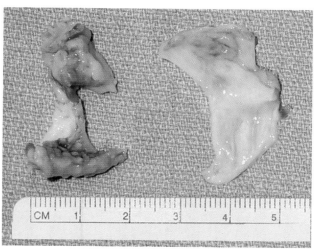

Fig 4-44. At surgery, there were large valve vegetations with a paravalvular abscess. A strip of pericardium was used to reconstruct the annulus and a 24 mm cryopreserved aortic allograft was implanted. The coronary buttons were anastomosed to the side of the graft. The resected bicuspid aortic valve shows diffuse thickening of the leaflet on the right. The leaflet on the left shows severe valve destruction due to endocarditis.

Comments

Paravalvular abscess formation complicates 20–25% of aortic valve and about 15% of mitral valve endocarditis cases. On echocardiography, an intracardiac abscess may appear either echodense or echolucent, depending on whether the abscess cavity communicates with the bloodstream. For example, when aortic valve infection spreads to the sinuses of Valsalva, the sinus dilates and may be irregular in contour. Abscess may also appear as increased thickening in the paravalvular region, which can be difficult to distinguish from normal tissue. The sensitivity of transesophageal echocardiography for detection of abscess is about 90%, compared with <50% for transthoracic imaging.

Clinically, patients with paravalvular abscess have evidence of persistent infection, including fever and persistently positive blood cultures. An aortic paravalvular abscess at the base of the septum may result in prolongation of the PR interval on ECG, or higher degrees of heart block, due to infection or edema of the conduction system. Mitral paravalvular abscess may rupture into the pericardium, resulting in purulent pericarditis.

Suggested Reading

1. Choussat R, Thomas D, Isnard R et al. Perivalvular abscesses associated with endocarditis; clinical features and prognostic factors of overall survival in a series of 233 cases. Perivalvular Abscesses French Multicentre Study. Eur Heart J 1999; 20:232–41.

2. San Roman JA, Vilacosta I, Sarria C et al. Clinical course, microbiologic profile, and diagnosis of periannular complications in prosthetic valve endocarditis. Am J Cardiol 1999; 83:1075–9.

Case 4-8
Aneurysm of the Aortic Mitral Intervalvular Fibrosa

This 29-year-old man had an aortic coarctation and patent ductus arteriosus repair at 9 months of age. He then had repair of a ventricular septal defect at age 2 years. At age 6 years, he had aortic valve endocarditis and underwent aortic valve replacement with a 17 mm mechanical tilting disk valve. He now presents with new-onset atrial fibrillation and episodes of a wide complex tachycardia. Echocardiography showed an aneurysm of the mitral aortic intervalvular fibrosa (MAIVF), severe mitral regurgitation and a small ventricular septal defect. He was referred for surgical intervention.

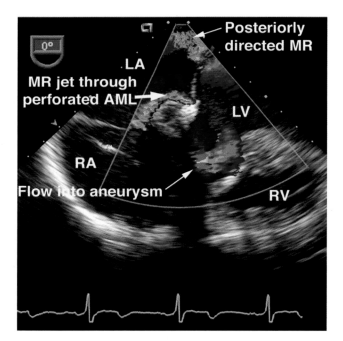

DVD **Fig 4-45.** In this oblique four-chamber view, there are two jets of mitral regurgitation, one at the base of the anterior leaflet and one posteriorly directed jet. In addition, color flow is seen in systole adjacent to the basal septum. In other views, this flow signal was consistent with an aneurysm of the MAIVF.

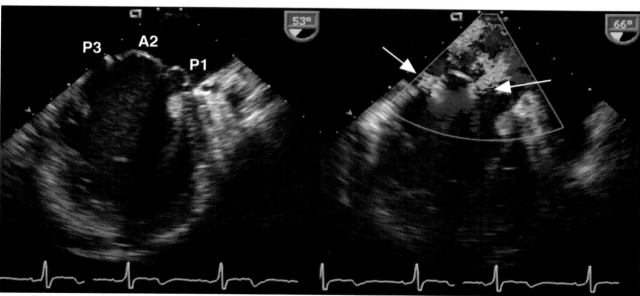

Fig 4-46. In a mitral commissural view (*left*), the medial (**P3**) and lateral (**P1**) scallops of the posterior mitral leaflet and central portion of the anterior leaflet (**A2**) are seen. Color flow (*right*) demonstrates mitral regurgitation through the leaflet coaptation plane at both the medial and lateral commissures (**arrows**).

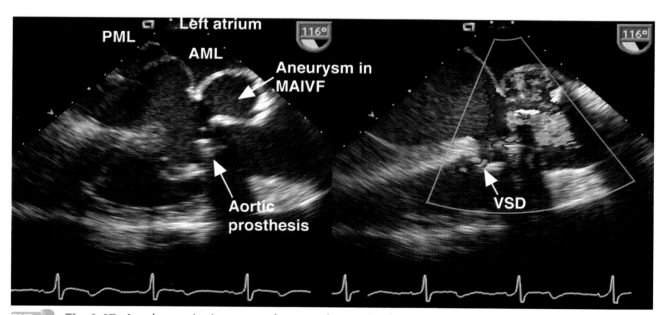

Fig 4-47. In a long-axis view at 116 degrees, a large echo-free space is seen posterior to the aortic root contiguous with the base of the anterior mitral leaflet, consistent with an aneurysm of the MAIVF. The aortic prosthesis causes shadowing. Color Doppler (*right*) demonstrates flow in and out of the aneurysm from the left ventricular outflow tract. A small ventricular septal defect (**VSD**) is also present.

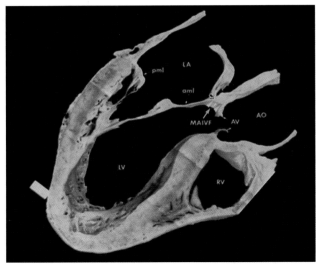

Fig 4-48. This normal anatomic specimen is oriented in the long-axis plane as seen in **Fig 4-47**. Note that the fibrous skeleton of the heart is characterized by continuity between the posterior wall of the aortic root and the bases of the anterior mitral leaflet. With infection of this region, an aneurysm can form that extends posterior to the aortic root. (Reproduced with permission from Karalis DG et al. Transesophageal echocardiographic recognition of subaortic complications in aortic valve endocarditis. Circulation 1992; 86:353–62. ©1992 American Heart Association.)

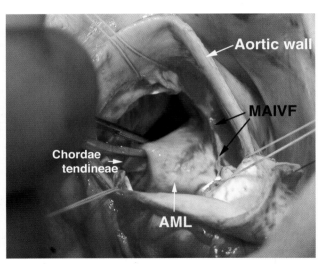

Fig 4-50. For comparison, in a patient with isolated aortic valve disease in whom the valve has been removed, a normal MAIVF is seen as the juncture between the aortic annulus and the anterior leaflet of the mitral valve.

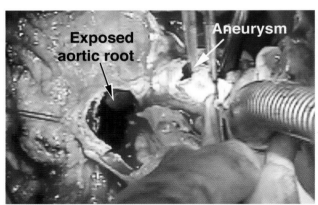

DVD **Fig 4-49.** At surgery, with the aortic root opened and the prosthetic valve removed, the aneurysm can be seen laterally and posteriorly. The aneurysm was resected and the infected anterior mitral leaflet excised. A mechanical mitral valve replacement was performed followed by patch closure of the aneurysm and enlargement of the LV outflow tract with placement of a 21 mm mechanical aortic valve prosthesis. The patient also had an epicardial implantable defibrillator placed at the time of surgery.

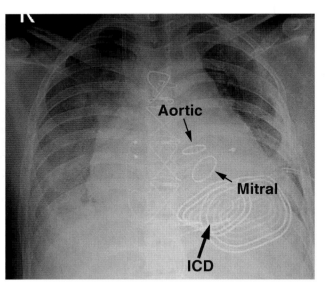

Fig 4-51. Postoperative chest X-ray shows the positions of the aortic and mitral prostheses, and the previously placed pericardial ICD pads.

Comments

The fibrous "skeleton" of the heart consists of the rings of fibrous tissue that surround the tricuspid and mitral annulus and the region where these rings meet. The junction of the annular rings, and the base of the interatrial septum, form the central fibrous body. The segment of the mitral annulus that joins the base of the aorta is the MAIVF. When infection from the aortic or mitral valve extends into this area of common tissue that joins the two valves, the tissue becomes weakened with formation of a space that opens into the LV at the base of the anterior mitral leaflet and extends posteriorly to the aortic root, protruding into the left atrium. This space is called an aneurysm or, more correctly, a pseudoaneurysm, with the walls formed by infected fibrous tissue. This aneurysm is a variant of paravalvular abscess and usually requires surgical repair for eradication of the infected tissue.

Suggested Reading

1. Afridi I, Apostolidou MA, Saad RM, Zoghbi WA. Pseudoaneurysms of the mitral-aortic intervalvular fibrosa: dynamic characterization using transesophageal echocardiographic and Doppler techniques. J Am Coll Cardiol 1995; 25(1):137–45.

2. Bansal RC, Graham BM, Jutzy KR et al. Left ventricular outflow tract to left atrial communication secondary to rupture of mitral-aortic intervalvular fibrosa in infective endocarditis: diagnosis by transesophageal echocardiography and color flow imaging. J Am Coll Cardiol 1990; 15(2):499–504.

3. Karalis DG, Bansal RC, Hauck AJ et al. Transesophageal echocardiographic recognition of subaortic complications in aortic valve endocarditis. Circulation 1992; 86:353–62.

Pacer Infections

Case 4-9
Pacer Lead Infection

This 56-year-old man with an atrioventricular pacer placed 4 years ago for sick sinus syndrome presented with septic arthritis. Blood cultures were positive for *Staph aureus* and transthoracic echocardiography showed vegetations on the tricuspid valve and pacer leads. He was referred for surgical explantation of the pacer and pacer leads.

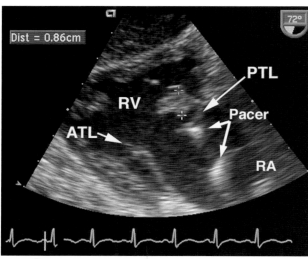

DVD **Fig 4-52.** In a transgastric position with the image plane rotated to 72 degrees and the probe turned towards the patient's right side, a right ventricular inflow view is obtained. A large mobile mass is seen in the region where the pacer lead (bright echo) crosses the posterior tricuspid leaflet (**PTL**). The anterior tricuspid leaflet (**ATL**) appears relatively normal.

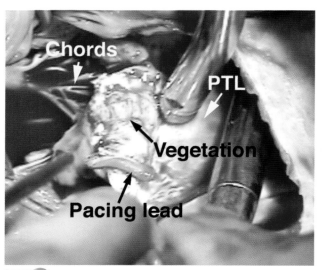

DVD **Fig 4-53.** With the right atrium opened, a large vegetation is seen attached to the tricuspid leaflet and pacer lead. There was severe leaflet destruction and perforation with a paravalvular abscess.

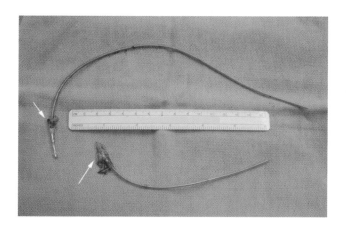

Fig 4-54. The tricuspid valve was replaced with a stented tissue prosthesis and the pacer and pacer leads were removed and replaced. The explanted atrial and ventricular pacer leads with attached areas of infection (**arrows**) are shown. The patient's hospital course was complicated by renal failure requiring dialysis.

Comments

Infection of permanent pacer leads is rare. The clinical presentation is similar to native right-sided endocarditis, with fever, bacteremia, systemic signs and pulmonary emboli. Vegetations attached to the pacer wires are identified in only about 7% of patients on transthoracic imaging, but can be seen on TEE in over 90% of patients. Treatment usually includes removal of the entire infected pacer system.

Suggested Reading

1. Klug D, Lacroix D, Savoye C et al. Systemic infection related to endocarditis on pacemaker leads: clinical presentation and management. Circulation 1997; 95:2098–107.

2. Duval X, Selton-Suty C, Alla F et al. Association pour l'Etude et la Prevention de l'Endocardite Infectieuse. Endocarditis in patients with a permanent pacemaker: a 1-year epidemiological survey on infective endocarditis due to valvular and/or pacemaker infection. Clin Infect Dis 2004; 39(1):68–74.

Prosthetic Valve Endocarditis

Case 4-10
Tissue Tricuspid Valve Endocarditis

This 47-year-old woman, with a history of tricuspid valve replacement for severe regurgitation due to Ebstein's anomaly and placement of a permanent pacer for complete heart block 10 years ago, presented with fever and chills. Blood cultures were positive for *Staph aureus*. She had progressive clinical deterioration in her status, with respiratory failure, renal failure and pancreatitis. Echocardiography showed vegetations on the tricuspid valve and pacer leads. She was transferred to our medical center for surgical intervention.

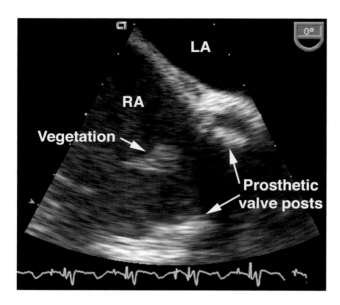

DVD **Fig 4-55.** In a close-up image from a high TEE four-chamber view, a mobile mass consistent with a vegetation is seen on the atrial side of a tissue tricuspid valve prosthesis.

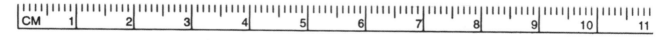
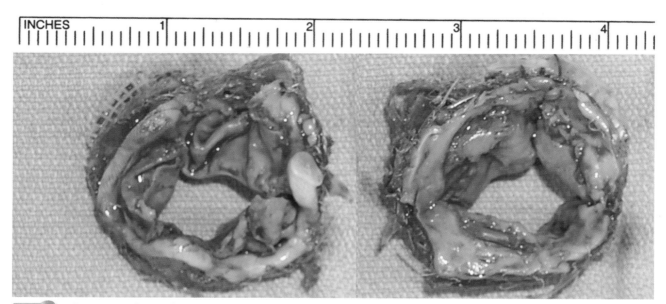

DVD **Fig 4-56.** The explanted valve has been photographed from both the ventricular (*left*) and atrial (*right*) sides of the valve. Valve leaflet destruction by endocarditis is seen.

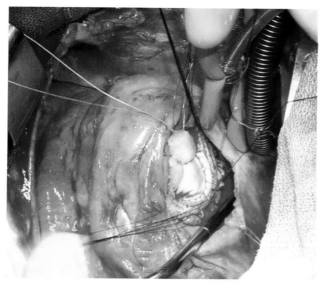

Fig 4-57. A new normal-appearing tricuspid valve prosthesis was sutured in the tricuspid annulus. The pacer and pacer leads were also explanted and replaced.

Comments

The diagnosis of prosthetic valve endocarditis is based on the same criteria as native valve endocarditis, with the caveat that visualization of valve vegetations is more difficult. With tissue prosthetic valves, infection may result in typical valvular vegetations, as in this case, although often transesophageal imaging is needed for identification. However, with mechanical valves, echocardiography may fail to detect infection because (1) infection is often limited to the sewing ring and annulus, and thus not evident on imaging, and (2) shadowing and reverberations from the metal sewing ring and valve occluders limit visualization of the valve or any adherent vegetations. Paravalvular abscess formation is common with prosthetic valve endocarditis, occurring in 60–70% of infected aortic prosthetic valves and in 20–25% of infected mitral prosthetic valves.

Suggested Reading

1. Piper C, Korfer R, Horstkotte D. Prosthetic valve endocarditis. Heart 2001; 85(5):590–3.
2. Mourvillier B, Trouillet JL, Timsit JF et al. Infective endocarditis in the intensive care unit: clinical spectrum and prognostic factors in 228 consecutive patients. Intensive Care Med 2004; 30(11):2046–52.

Case 4-11
Mechanical Mitral Valve Endocarditis

This 67-year-old woman had undergone mitral valve replacement 5 years ago. Over the past 5 years, she had a complicated clinical course with persistent heart failure, chronic atrial fibrillation and severe pulmonary hypertension. About 2 weeks ago she presented with a 2-week history of fatigue, vague neurologic symptoms and the sudden onset of severe substernal chest pressure associated with ECG changes of acute anterior myocardial infarction. Emergent coronary angiography revealed a proximal left anterior descending artery occlusion. She subsequently became febrile and TEE showed a large mitral valve vegetation. She was then transferred to our medical center for surgical intervention.

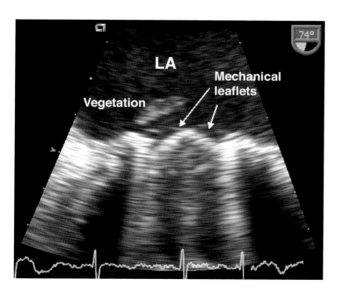

DVD **Fig 4-58.** In a magnified image of the mitral valve in the four-chamber view, the closed bileaflet mechanical valve with shadowing and reverberations obscuring the left ventricle is seen. In addition, a large, mobile mass of echoes, with motion independent from the valve leaflet motion, is seen on the left atrial side of the valve, consistent with a vegetation.

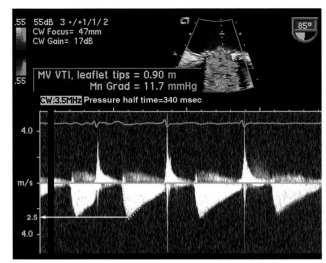

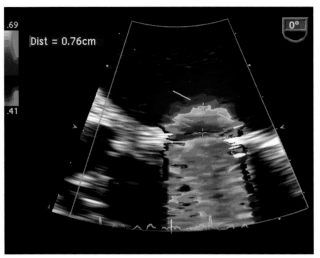

Fig 4-59. Pulsed Doppler interrogation of the antegrade transmitral flow shows a peak velocity of 2.5 m/s, a mean gradient of 12 mmHg and a pressure half-time of 340 ms. Using an empiric constant of 220, estimated mitral valve area is 0.65 cm².

Fig 4-60. Color flow imaging shows the acceleration of flow proximal to the mitral orifice. The instantaneous transmitral volume flow rate is calculated as the aliasing velocity (41 cm/s) × the surface area of the aliasing hemisphere ($2 \times \pi \times (0.76 \text{ cm})^2 = 3.6 \text{ cm}^2$) = 149 ml/s. Dividing by the peak antegrade mitral velocity (2.5 m/s from **Fig 4-59**), the estimated mitral orifice area is 0.60 cm².

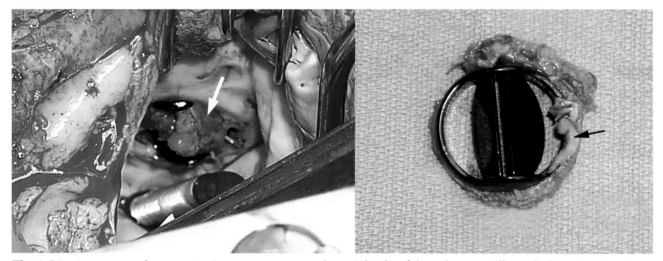

Fig 4-61. At surgery, a large vegetation was present on the atrial side of the valve, partially occluding the mitral orifice (**arrow**) (*left*). The resected valve shows that the mechanical valve itself is normal (*right*). The site of attachment of the vegetation to the annulus is indicated by the arrow. Blood cultures and the resected vegetation grew coagulase-negative staphylococcus. The patient expired 10 days postoperatively with multiorgan system failure.

Comments

Endocarditis typically leads to valve regurgitation due to leaflet destruction. However, a large vegetation, as in this case, or infection involving the hinge points of a mechanical valve, can result in functional valve stenosis. Evaluation of the hemodynamic severity of valve obstruction follows the same principles as for any stenotic valve.

In addition to cerebral ischemic events or systemic emboli, fragments of valvular vegetations may embolize to the coronary arteries, resulting in acute myocardial infarction, as in this case. When the coronary angiogram suggests an embolic occlusion in a patient with a valve prosthesis, evaluation for infection or thrombus formation on the valve is needed.

Suggested Reading

1. Eltzschig HK, Lekowski RW Jr, Shernan SK et al. Intraoperative transesophageal echocardiography to assess septic coronary embolism. Anesthesiology 2002; 97(6):1627–9.

2. Voss F, Bludau HB, Haller C. Mitral valve endocarditis: an uncommon cause of myocardial infarction. Z Kardiol 2003; 92(8):686–8.

Case 4-12
Homograft Aortic Valve Endocarditis

This 35-year-old man had an aortic homograft valve replacement for endocarditis 2 years ago. He now presented with fevers and sweats, with six sets of blood cultures positive for *Strep viridans*. Echocardiography showed severe aortic regurgitation, and he was referred for repeat aortic valve replacement.

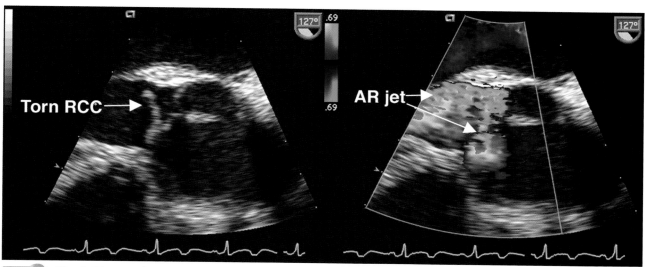

DVD **Fig 4-62.** In a long-axis view, a flail leaflet (**arrow**) of the tissue prosthesis is seen. Color Doppler (*right*) shows an eccentric jet of regurgitation with a vena contracta width of 5 mm.

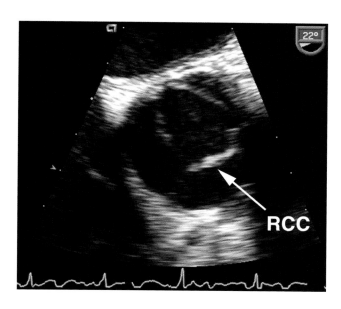

Fig 4-63. The short-axis view of the aortic prosthesis in systole shows normal opening of all three leaflets. The right coronary cusp (**RCC**) appears thickened.

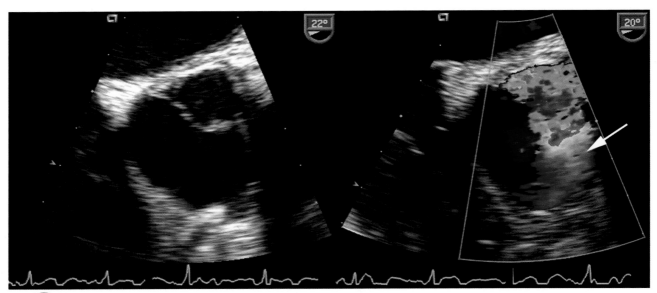

Fig 4-64. In diastole, the short-axis view shows the abnormal leaflet closure. Color flow (*right*) shows regurgitation through the region of the flail leaflet (**arrow**); the jet is then deflected posteriorly.

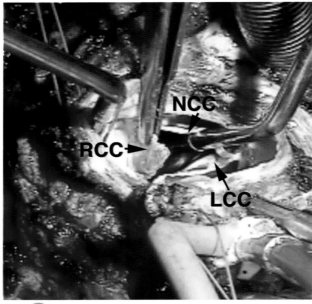

Fig 4-65. At surgery, the flail right coronary cusp can be seen.

Comments

Infection of a tissue aortic valve prosthesis may result in acute severe aortic regurgitation due to rupture or destruction of the valve leaflet tissue. A flail aortic valve leaflet is recognized as a linear echo that prolapses into the LVOT in diastole, associated with severe regurgitation. A flail leaflet can occur with valve degeneration, even in the absence of infection, so the diagnosis of endocarditis depends on the combination of typical echocardiographic findings and evidence of bacteremia. When endocarditis is present, a vegetation can mimic a flail leaflet; the differentiating features are that the flail leaflet is more echodense and linear in appearance compared with a less echodense, more irregularly shaped vegetation. Both prolapse into the LVOT in diastole and both show independent motion.

Suggested Reading

1. Yankah AC, Klose H, Petzina R et al. Surgical management of acute aortic root endocarditis with viable homograft: 13-year experience. Eur J Cardiothorac Surg 2002; 21(2):260–7.

2. Ronderos RE, Portis M, Stoermann W, Sarmiento C. Are all echocardiographic findings equally predictive for diagnosis in prosthetic endocarditis? J Am Soc Echocardiogr 2004; 17(6):664–9.

Case 4-13
Mechanical Aortic Valve Endocarditis

This 44-year-old man presented with ascending cholangitis, and was subsequently diagnosed with *Haemophilus influenzae* endocarditis. His clinical course was complicated by a right frontal cerebrovascular accident (CVA), renal failure, atrial fibrillation and cardiogenic shock. He underwent aortic and mitral valve replacement in conjunction with a prolonged course of IV antibiotic therapy. However, 5 months after surgery, he had recurrent arrhythmias and worsening heart failure symptoms. Echocardiography showed severe prosthetic aortic regurgitation, and he was referred for surgical intervention.

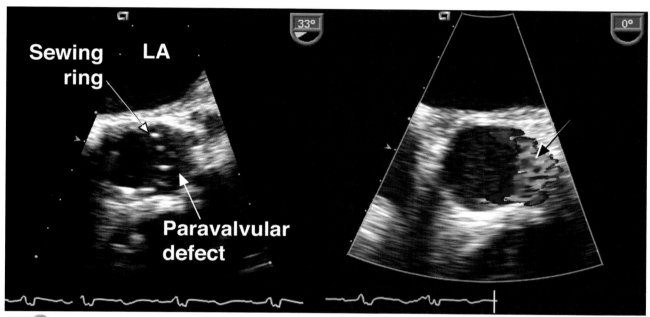

Fig 4-66. In a short-axis view (*left*) of the mechanical aortic prosthesis at 33 degrees rotation, a crescent-shaped echolucent area is seen along the lateral aspects of the valve, consistent with a paravalvaular abscess or valve dehiscence. Color Doppler (*right*) demonstrates diastolic flow filling this region (**arrow**).

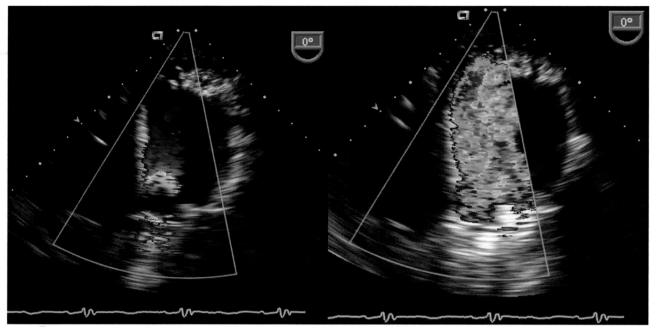

DVD **Fig 4-67.** From the transgastric apical position with the image plane at 0 degrees, the probe is flexed to obtain an anteriorly angulated four-chamber view. There is normal acceleration of flow proximal to the aortic prosthesis in systole (*left*) with the diastolic image (*right*) showing turbulent flow filling the outflow tract, consistent with severe aortic regurgitation.

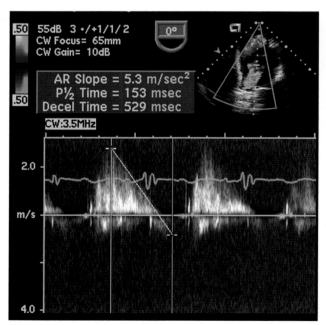

Fig 4-68. A continuous wave Doppler signal of the aortic regurgitation was recorded in the same image plane as in **Fig 4-67**. Although the intercept angle is not parallel (so velocity is underestimated) and signal strength is poor, the steep diastolic deceleration slope suggests acute regurgitation.

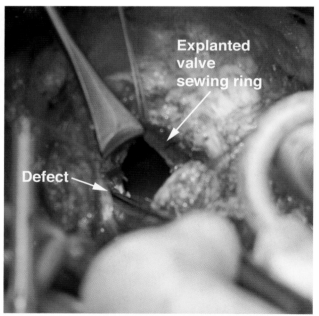

Fig 4-69. In this intraoperative photograph, the mechanical valve has been removed except for a residual rim of the sewing ring. The probe is in the paravalvular defect.

Comments

A small amount of paravalvular regurgitation is seen in up to 10% of mechanical valve replacements, even in the absence of endocarditis. However, new or worsening paravalvular regurgitation suggests infection of the sewing ring.

The severity of prosthetic valve regurgitation in patients with prosthetic valve endocarditis is evaluated using the same approaches as for evaluation of native valves. However, often only a semiquantitative measure of severity is needed because the decision about timing of surgical intervention is typically based on clinical events and the presence of valve dysfunction, rather than a specific measure of regurgitant severity.

For aortic regurgitation, the most useful quick methods to evaluate regurgitant severity are (1) the intensity and diastolic slope of the CW Doppler curve and (2) the presence of holodiastolic flow reversal in the proximal abdominal aorta. Color Doppler is more helpful for defining the site and mechanism of regurgitation than for quantitation of hemodynamics in this situation.

Suggested Reading

1. Davila-Roman VG, Waggoner AD, Kennard ED et al; Artificial Valve Endocarditis Reduction Trial echocardiography study. Prevalence and severity of paravalvular regurgitation in the Artificial Valve Endocarditis Reduction Trial (AVERT) echocardiography study. J Am Coll Cardiol 2004; 44(7):1467–72.

Case 4-14
Infected Bentall Aortic Valve and Root

This 12-year-old boy with congenital aortic stenosis was treated with a valvuloplasty at age 5 months, mechanical aortic valve replacement with a Konno procedure at age 2 years, and aortic homograft valve replacement at age 8 years. Two months ago he underwent aortic valve (23 mm St Jude mechanical) and root replacement with reimplantation of the coronary arteries (Bentall procedure). His postoperative course was complicated by respiratory failure, complete heart block, mediastinitis and coagulase-negative staphylococcal endocarditis with severe mitral regurgitation. He was treated initially with high-dose IV antibiotics and chest drainage. After placement of an intra-aortic balloon pump, he was taken back to the operating room for emergent mitral valve replacement.

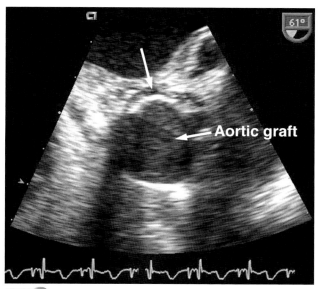

DVD **Fig 4-70.** In a short-axis view of the aortic graft, an echo-free space posterior to the aortic graft (**arrow**) is suggestive of an infective process.

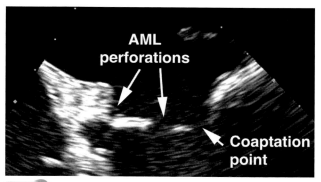

DVD **Fig 4-71.** In a TEE four-chamber view, the anterior mitral leaflet appears discontinuous. Given that the mitral leaflet is relatively perpendicular to the ultrasound beam in this view, these discontinuities are suggestive of two valve perforations.

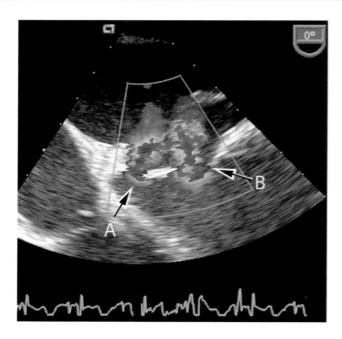

DVD **Fig 4-72.** Color Doppler shows regurgitant flow through the perforation at the base of the anterior mitral leaflet (**A, arrow**). There is also a jet through the coaptation point (**B, arrow**), which most likely merges with a jet through the midleaflet perforation seen in **Fig 4-71.**

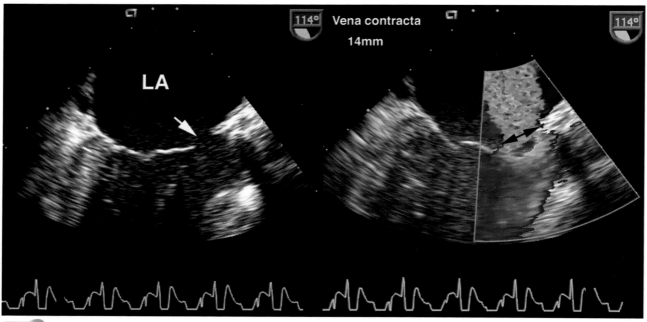

DVD **Fig 4-73.** The long-axis view of the aortic prosthesis and mitral valve showing a perforation at the base of the anterior mitral valve leaflet (**arrows**) with color flow showing severe mitral regurgitation with a vena contracta width of 14 mm and a prominent PISA.

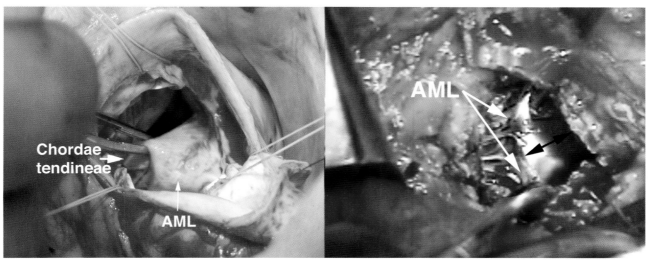

Fig 4-74. At surgery, the aortic graft was infected with an aortic paravalvular abscess. The abscess had extended into the base of the anterior mitral valve leaflet with perforation and severe mitral regurgitation. In this intraoperative photograph, the infected aortic conduit and aortic valve have been explanted with excision of the coronary buttons. Compared with the normal anterior mitral leaflet (**AML**) shown in a different patient (*left*), there is a perforation (**arrow**) at the base of the anterior leaflet, with rupture of some of the chords attached to the anterior leaflet. The posterior leaflet and chords were normal.

Comments

Early prosthetic valve endocarditis is defined as valve infection occurring within 60 days of implantation. The most common organisms causing early prosthetic valve endocarditis are staphylococcus, fungi or gram-negative bacilli. As in this case, eradication of infection usually requires removal of the infected prosthesis, as well as prolonged IV antibiotic therapy. With early surgical intervention for prosthetic valve endocarditis, operative mortality is about 10% and long-term survival is about 80% at 5 years.

Suggested Reading

1. Lytle BW, Priest BP, Taylor PC et al. Surgical treatment of prosthetic valve endocarditis. *J Thorac Cardiovasc Surg* 1996; 111:198–207.

2. Yu VL, Fang GD, Keys TF et al. Prosthetic valve endocarditis: superiority of surgical valve replacement versus medical therapy only. *Ann Thorac Surg* 1994; 58:1073–7.

Case 4-15
Aortic to Left Atrial Fistula

This 68-year-old man with a mechanical aortic valve replacement 5 years ago presented in septic shock.

Evaluation showed an infected prosthetic valve, and he was referred for surgery.

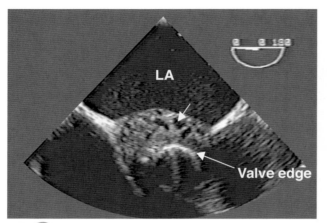

Fig 4-75. In a high TEE view at 0 degrees, an inhomogeneous mass of echoes is surrounding the valve prosthesis (**arrow**). In real time, the prosthesis is seen to be freely mobile, or "rocking."

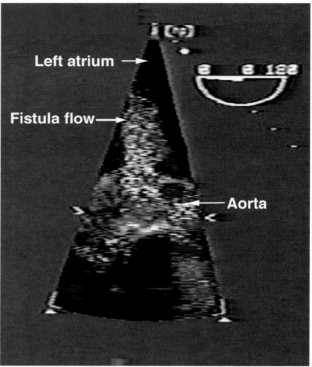

Fig 4-77. Color Doppler demonstrates continuous flow from the aorta into the left atrium through this fistula.

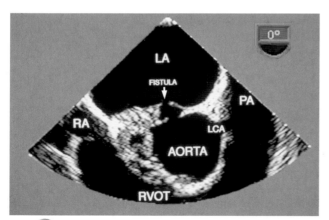

Fig 4-76. With the probe moved slightly cephalad, an echo-free space within this mass, with probable communication with the left atrium, is seen.

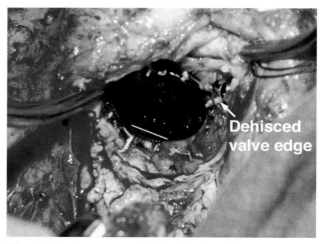

Fig 4-78. At surgery, a dehisced valve edge was seen.

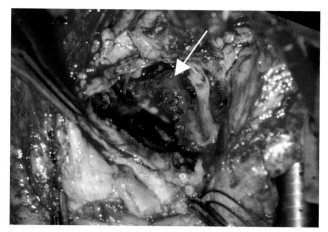

Fig 4-79. After explantation of the mechanical valve, a large paravalvular abscess was seen (**arrow**).

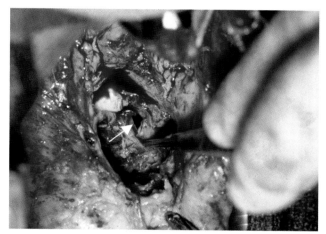

Fig 4-80. In the midst of the perivalvular inflammation, a perforation is seen (**arrow**) that communicates posteriorly with the left atrium.

Comments

Aortic annular abscesses can rupture into any of the four cardiac chambers due to the central location of the aortic valve in the heart. The potential patterns of rupture can be best appreciated by considering the short-axis view of the aortic valve. Most often, rupture occurs from the aorta into the left ventricle, resulting in aortic regurgitation. However, abscess in the region of the left or non-coronary cusp can rupture posteriorly into the left atrium, as in this case. Abscess in the region of the non-coronary cusp can rupture into the right atrium, and abscess in the region of the right coronary cusp can rupture into the right ventricular outflow tract. An aortic annular abscess may also rupture into the mediastinum, resulting in a pseudo-aneurysm if the rupture is contained by the mediastinal tissue and/or local adhesions.

Suggested Reading

1. Lastowiecka E, Biederman A, Szajewski T, Rydlewska-Sadowska W. The rupture of periaortic infective aneurysm into the left atrium and the left ventricular outflow tract: preoperative diagnosis by transthoracic echocardiography. Echocardiography 2002; 19(3):173–6.

2. Esen AM, Kucukoglu MS, Okcun B et al. Transoesophageal echocardiographic diagnosis of aortico-left atrial fistula in aortic valve endocarditis. Eur J Echocardiogr 2003; 4(3):221–2.

5

Prosthetic Valves

Bioprosthetic Valves: Normal

Case 5-1
Bioprosthetic Aortic Valve

Example of the insertion of a normal stented bioprosthetic valve in the aortic position.

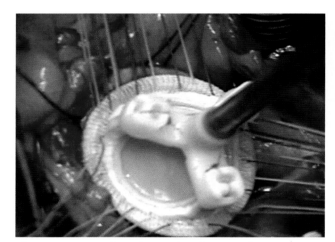

Fig 5-1. Sutures have been placed at equidistant intervals in the sewing ring and aortic annulus. The valve is lowered into position before the sutures are tied. (Perimount bovine pericardial valve, Edwards Lifesciences, Irvine, California.)

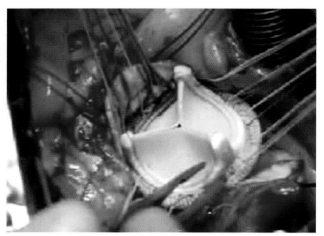

Fig 5-2. With the valve-holding device removed, the three struts at the commissures of the valve are well seen. Note the height of the struts parallels the normal anatomy of the native aortic valve, with the valve commissures more cephalad than the valve sewing ring, resulting in the typical curvature of the valve leaflets. The normal overlap between the leaflets in the closed position is greatest adjacent to the commissures and least in the center of the valve.

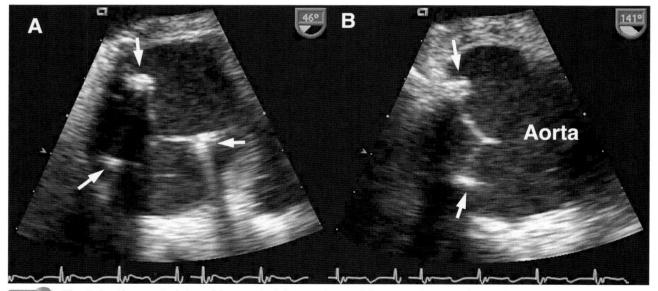

DVD **Fig 5-3.** Short-axis (A) and long-axis (B) TEE views of the aortic bioprosthesis show the three struts in short axis and two struts in long axis (**arrows**) with the thin leaflets in the closed position in diastole.

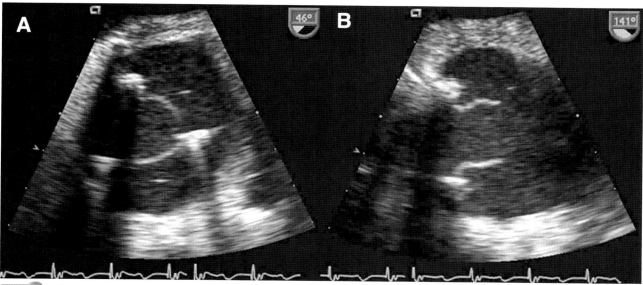

Fig 5-4. In systole, the short-axis (*A*) and long-axis (*B*) TEE views show the open leaflets during ventricular ejection.

Comments

The two major categories of prosthetic valves are tissue valves and mechanical valves. Bioprosthetic (or tissue) valve leaflets are fashioned from bovine pericardium or a porcine aortic valve. The leaflets are supported by a rigid ring around the annulus with metal or polymer stents that support the commissures of the valve leaflets. Implantation of these "stented" bioprostheses involves sewing an appropriately sized valve into the annulus, with the valve height and symmetry ensured by the annular ring and struts. In contrast, stentless tissue valves are supported only by a cylinder of flexible fabric or tissue. Implantation of stentless valves involves placement and suturing both at the annulus, and at the top of the commissures at the appropriate height.

Tissue valves open with a central circular orifice with a valve opening and closing motion similar to a native trileaflet aortic valve. However, the antegrade velocities (and pressure gradient) are higher than expected for a native valve because the sewing ring reduces the effective orifice area. At smaller valve sizes, the degree of functional stenosis can be significant, with a smaller effective orifice area than a similar-size mechanical valve. Thus, the optimal valve choice in each patient depends on the size of valve that can be implanted, in addition to considerations of valve durability and long-term anticoagulation. If the implanted valve is too small for the patient size, patient–prosthesis mismatch (defined as an indexed effective valve area $<0.85 \text{ cm}^2/\text{m}^2$) is associated with increased short-term mortality and suboptimal long-term outcomes.

Suggested Reading

1. Yoganathan AP, Travis BR. Fluid dynamics of prosthetic valves. In: Otto CM, ed. Clinical Practice of Echocardiography. Philadelphia: WB Saunders, 2002.

2. Pibarot P, Dumesnil JG. Hemodynamic and clinical impact of prosthesis–patient mismatch in the aortic valve position and its prevention. J Am Coll Cardiol 2000; 36(4):1131–41.

3. Blais C, Dumesnil JG, Baillot R et al. Impact of valve prosthesis–patient mismatch on short-term mortality after aortic valve replacement. Circulation 2003; 108(8):983–8.

4. Van den Brink RB. Evaluation of prosthetic heart valves by transesophageal echocardiography: problems, pitfalls and timing pf echocardiography. Semin Cardiothoracic Vasc Anesth 2006; 10(1):89–100.

Case 5-2
Bioprosthetic Mitral Valve

Example of the implantation of a normal bio-prosthetic mitral valve.

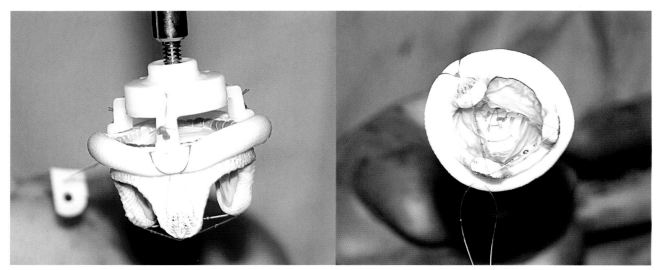

Fig 5-5. A stented mitral bioprosthesis (Medtronic Mosaic Mitral Prosthesis, Minneapolis, Minnesota), attached to the holder, is seen from a lateral view (*left*) and from the ventricular aspect of the valve (*right*) with the leaflets in the open position. The blue sutures maintain the shape of the prosthesis and provide orientation but are removed at the time of implantation.

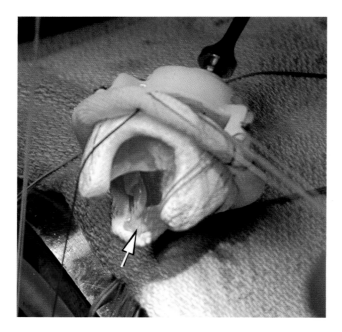

Fig 5-6. An oblique photograph of the valve demonstrates the 3D anatomy of the prosthesis. The commissures (**arrow**) are located at the superior aspect of each stent to maintain the 3D curve of each leaflet.

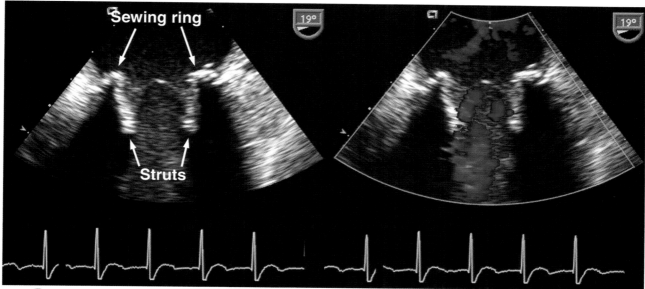

DVD **Fig 5-7.** With the valve implanted, the four-chamber TEE view shows the sewing ring, struts and valve leaflets in systole. There are prominent acoustic shadows from the sewing ring on the 2D image (*left*). Color Doppler (*right*) shows no mitral regurgitation.

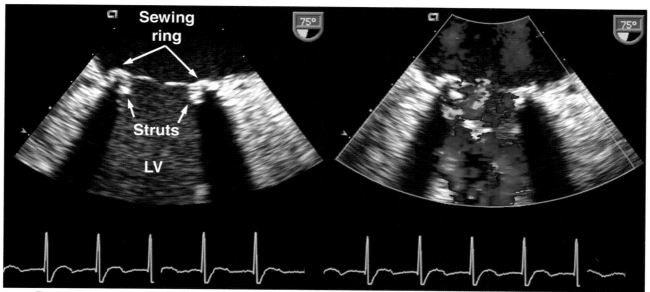

DVD **Fig 5-8.** The TEE view in a two-chamber orientation at 75 degrees rotation appears similar to the 0 degree view due to the radial symmetry of this valve.

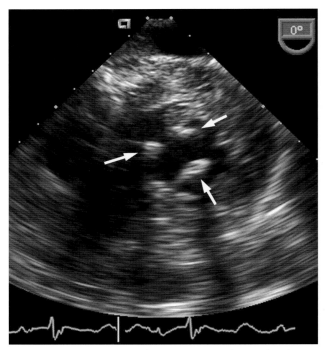

Fig 5-9. A transgastric short-axis view shows the three struts (**arrows**) of the mitral bioprosthesis.

Comments

In the mitral position, mechanical valves are often used, as many of these patients are on chronic anticoagulation for atrial fibrillation. When bioprosthetic valves are used, stented valves are needed, rather than stentless valves, given the anatomy of the mitral annulus and left ventricle. The appearance of the valve in the mitral position is similar to a native aortic valve, with the stents protruding into the LVOT. Occasionally, the stents may produce some degree of outflow tract obstruction, particularly if the ventricle is small and hypertrophied. The flow through the mitral prosthesis is similar to a normal mitral valve, with an early diastolic peak (E-velocity), normal deceleration time and an atrial velocity peak (A-velocity) if the patient is in sinus rhythm. Velocities are only slightly higher than for a native valve, due to the large effective valve area and low left atrial to left ventricular pressure gradient in diastole.

Suggested Reading

1. Zabalgoitia M. Echocardiographic recognition and quantitation of prosthetic valve dysfunction. In: Otto CM, ed. Clinical Practice of Echocardiography. Philadelphia: WB Saunders, 2002.

Case 5-3
Bioprosthetic Tricuspid Valve

Example of normal bioprosthetic valves in the tricuspid and pulmonic valve positions.

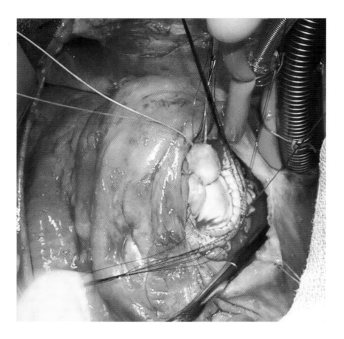

Fig 5-10. Surgical view of a tricuspid valve bioprosthesis from the right atrial side.

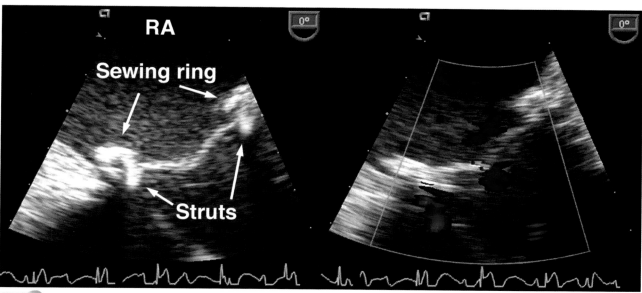

DVD **Fig 5-11.** In a four-chamber orientation at 0 degrees rotation, the tricuspid bioprosthetic sewing ring and struts are seen. The valve leaflets close at a slight angle in systole (*left*) with no detectable regurgitation on color Doppler (*right*).

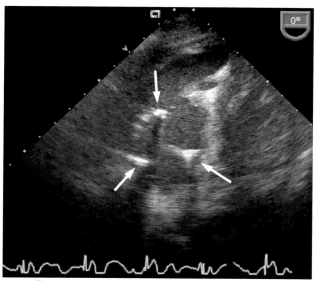

DVD **Fig 5-12.** A transgastric short-axis view of the tricuspid bioprosthesis shows the three struts (**arrows**) and the closed leaflets in systole.

Comments

Replacement of right-sided valves is less common than left-sided valves in adults. Mechanical valves in the tricuspid position have a high rate of valve thrombosis, whereas tissue valves have rapid valve deterioration. Thus, tricuspid valve repair is preferred whenever possible. Bioprosthetic tricuspid valves have an appearance and flow dynamics similar to a mitral bioprosthesis. A small degree of central regurgitation is normal with bioprosthetic valves in any position, although not seen in this case.

Suggested Reading

1. Connolly HM, Miller FA Jr, Taylor CL et al. Doppler hemodynamic profiles of 82 clinically and echocardiographically normal tricuspid valve prostheses. Circulation 1993; 88(6):2722–7.

Bioprosthetic Valves: Dysfunction

Case 5-4
Bioprosthetic Aortic Valve Degeneration

This 41-year-old man, with a 23 Carpentier–Edwards standard porcine prosthesis implanted 11 years ago for congenital aortic stenosis, presents now with severe aortic regurgitation and was referred for repeat aortic valve replacement.

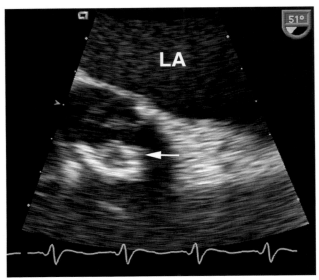

DVD **Fig 5-13.** In a short-axis view of the aortic bioprosthesis, a small area of increased echodensity is seen. In real time, this area is seen to have independent motion (**arrow**).

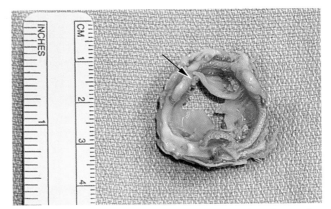

Fig 5-15. Photograph of the explanted valve shows the detachment of the leaflet from the sewing ring at one of the valve struts (**arrow**), resulting in a flail leaflet.

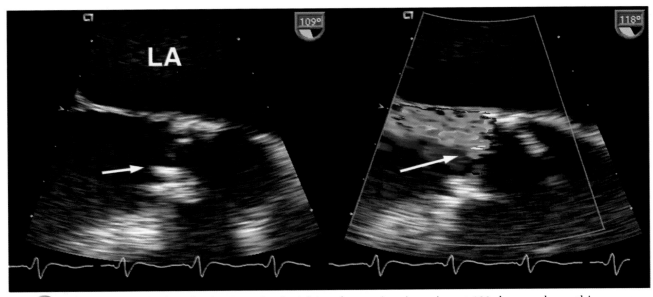

DVD **Fig 5-14.** 2D (*left*) and color Doppler (*right*) in a long-axis orientation at 109 degrees shows this area on the valve leaflet prolapsing into the LVOT (**arrows**) in diastole with associated moderate-to-severe regurgitation.

Comments

The major disadvantage of tissue valves is structural deterioration. The prevalence of primary valve failure 15 years after valve implantation is about 20% for aortic bioprostheses and nearly 40% for mitral bioprostheses. Mechanisms of valve failure include (1) tissue deterioration, resulting in loss of leaflet integrity (as in this case) with consequent regurgitation, and (2) tissue calcification, resulting in valve stenosis or regurgitation.

In a patient with a bioprosthetic valve, the differential diagnosis of a mobile mass in or near the valve should always include a flail leaflet, as well as valve vegetation or thrombosis. Often, transesophageal imaging is needed to fully define the mechanism of valve dysfunction.

Suggested Reading

1. Hammermeister K, Sethi GK, Henderson WG et al. Outcomes 15 years after valve replacement with a mechanical versus a bioprosthetic valve: final report of the Veterans Affairs randomized trial. J Am Coll Cardiol 2000; 36(4):1152–8.

Case 5-5
Bioprosthetic Mitral Valve Degeneration

This 40-year-old woman first underwent mitral valve replacement at age 23 years for rheumatic mitral valve disease, with a repeat mitral valve replacement at age 30 years with a stented bioprosthetic valve. At age 36 years, she developed heart failure symptoms after the birth of her son, followed by the new onset of atrial fibrillation. Her medical course has been complicated by diabetes, hypothyroidism, anemia and sleep apnea. Echocardiography showed a flail prosthetic valve leaflet with severe mitral regurgitation. She was referred for repeat valve replacement.

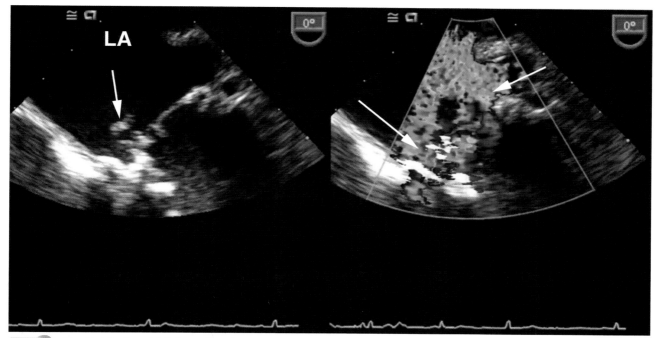

DVD **Fig 5-16.** In a TEE four-chamber view at 0 degrees, a mass attached to the mitral valve leaflet prolapses into the left atrium in systole (*left*) with color Doppler (*right*) showing at least two regurgitant jets, one paravalvular medially and one through the central area of the valve leaflets (**arrows**).

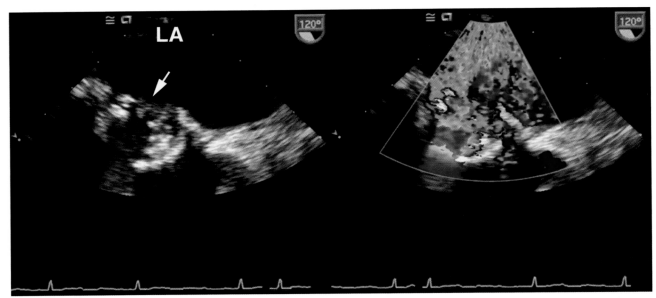

DVD **Fig 5-17.** In a long-axis view at 120 degrees, the marked irregularity of the leaflets of the stented valve (**arrow**) and the severe regurgitation are again seen.

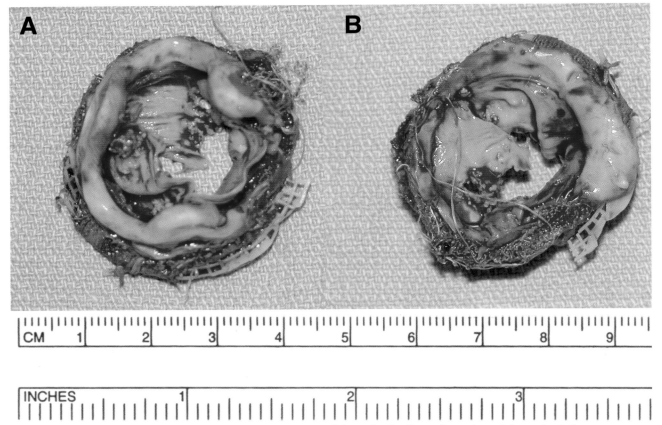

Fig 5-18. The explanted valve shows severe destruction of the valve leaflets when viewed from the left ventricular (*A*) or left atrial (*B*) side of the valve.

Comments

This woman had structural failure of a mitral bioprosthesis only 10 years after valve replacement, with symptoms consistent with prosthetic valve dysfunction as early as 6 years after valve implantation. The longevity of a bioprosthetic valve is inversely related to patient age at the time of surgery. For example, the 10-year rate of freedom from structural deterioration in patients over age 70 years old is about 90% compared with only 10% in patients aged 16–39 years and 35% in patients aged 40–49 years.

It remains controversial whether pregnancy accelerates the rate of bioprosthetic valve deterioration, but careful monitoring of bioprosthetic valve function during pregnancy is warranted given the rapid rate of structural deterioration in women in this age range.

Suggested Reading

1. Yun KL, Miller DC, Moore KA et al. Durability of the Hancock MO bioprosthesis compared with standard aortic valve bioprostheses. Ann Thorac Surg 1995; 60(2 Suppl):S221–8.

Case 5-6
Bioprosthetic Mitral Valve Regurgitation

This 79-year-old woman had a history of bioprosthetic mitral valve replacement 8 years ago. She was transferred to our medical center with severe symptomatic valvular aortic stenosis and a recent history of dark urine. She was thought to have hemolytic anemia with a hemoglobin of 9.7 g/dl, a hematocrit of 27% and a reticulocyte count of 5.5%. Her urine was positive for occult blood but was negative for red blood cells. She had a markedly elevated lactate dehydrogenase level and a bilirubin level of 1.9 mg/dl. Echocardiography showed severe aortic stenosis and moderate mitral regurgitation. She was referred for aortic valve replacement and possible re-do mitral valve replacement.

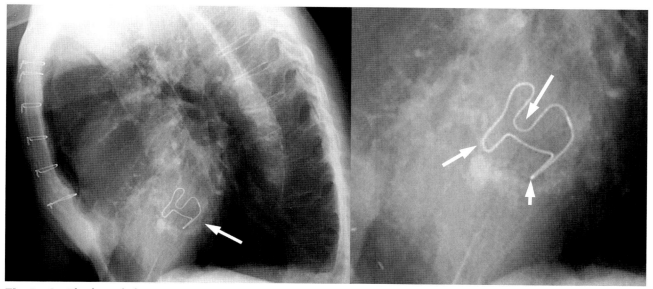

Fig 5-19. The lateral chest radiograph (*left*) shows the position of the stented mitral valve replacement. An enlarged view of the valve (*right*) shows the wire reinforcement of each of the three valve stents (**arrows**).

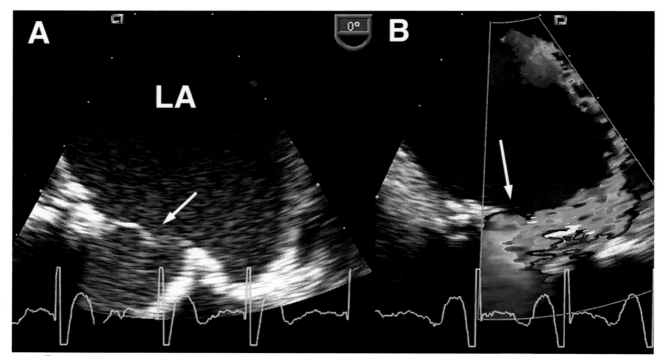

DVD **Fig 5-20.** (*A*) The initial four-chamber view of the mitral prosthesis in a magnified view shows thin leaflets with a normal closure contour (**arrow**). (*B*) However, with color Doppler, a wide jet of regurgitation is seen through the valve (**arrow**).

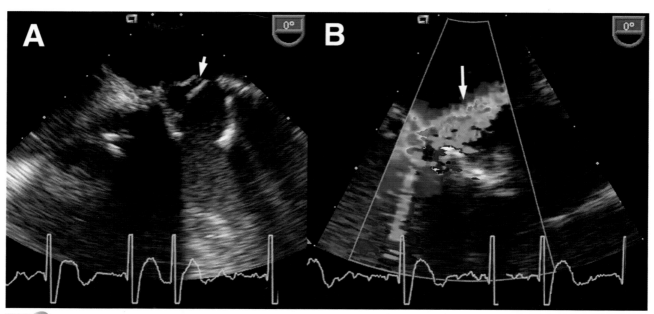

DVD **Fig 5-21.** (*A*) In the four-chamber view with slight anterior angulation, linear mobile structures associated with the valve stent are seen (**arrow**), with the regurgitant jet (*B*) going through this segment of the valve (**arrow**).

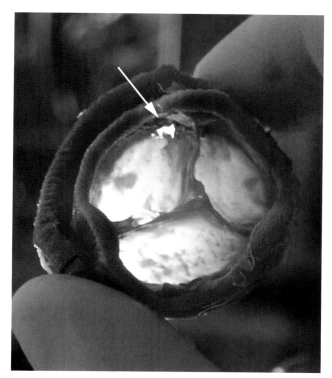

Fig 5-22. The explanted valve shows thin translucent leaflets with only a mild amount of lipid deposition (irregular yellow patches) but with a tear in the leaflet at the junction with the sewing ring at the 12 o'clock position (**arrow**).

Comments

This patient presented with signs and symptoms of hemolytic anemia, most likely due to the regurgitant jet through the bioprosthetic valve. Hemolytic anemia typically occurs with a mitral paravalvular regurgitant jet. The volume of regurgitation is often small, but the high-velocity flow adjacent to the rough-edged sewing ring results in red cell disruption and fragmentation due to rapid acceleration and high shear stress. This case is unusual in that the regurgitation occurred through the valve prosthesis rather than through a paravalvular defect. However, the mechanism of hemolysis is typical, with the blood cells in the high-velocity jet hitting the exposed sewing ring.

Suggested Reading

1. Vesey JM, Otto CM. Complications of prosthetic heart valves. Curr Cardiol Rep 2004; 6(2):106–11.
2. Yeo TC, Freeman WK, Schaff HV, Orszulak TA. Mechanisms of hemolysis after mitral valve repair: assessment by serial echocardiography. J Am Coll Cardiol 1998; 32(3):717–23.

Case 5-7
Mitral Bioprosthetic Paravalvular Regurgitation

This 70-year-old female had a history of two mitral valve replacements in the past due to paravalvular regurgitation and hemolytic anemia after the initial surgery. She again presents with severe anemia due to hemolysis, requiring frequent blood transfusions. Outpatient evaluation showed a recurrent paravalvular regurgitant jet and she was referred for valve surgery.

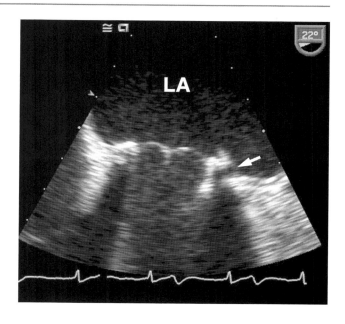

DVD **Fig 5-23.** This four-chamber view (at 22 degrees) of the tissue mitral prosthesis shows the thin leaflets closed in diastole. At the base of the lateral strut, there is an area of apparent discontinuity between the annulus and the sewing ring (**arrow**) that might be due to shadowing or to an actual area of valve dehiscence.

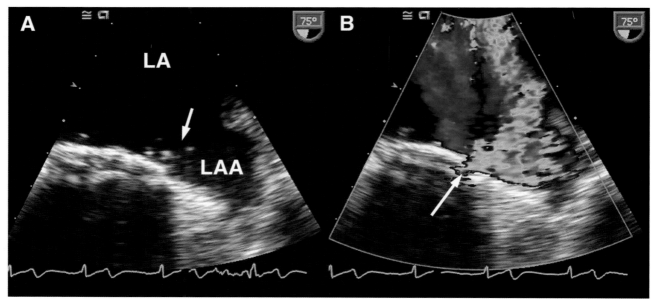

Fig 5-24. In a two-chamber orientation at 75 degrees rotation (*A*), there are some fine mobile echoes on the left atrial side of the prosthesis at this site, consistent with disrupted sutures (**arrow**). Color flow (*B*) demonstrates a paravalvular regurgitant jet that originates at the site of discontinuity seen on 2D imaging (**arrow**).

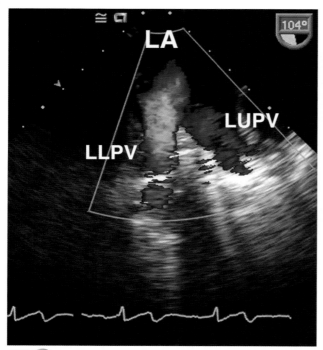

Fig 5-25. In this diastolic frame, both left upper (**LUPV**) and left lower pulmonary veins (**LLPV**) are identified with the image plane rotated to 104 degrees and the probe turned towards the patient's left side.

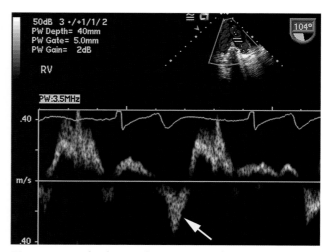

Fig 5-26. Pulsed Doppler recording from the LUPV demonstrates the late systolic flow reversal due to significant eccentric mitral regurgitation.

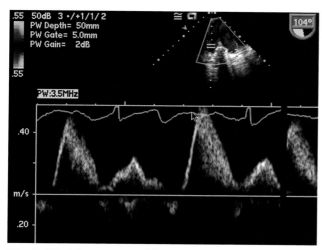

Fig 5-27. The pattern of flow is normal in the LLPV due to the eccentric mitral regurgitant jet that is directed superiorly in the left atrium.

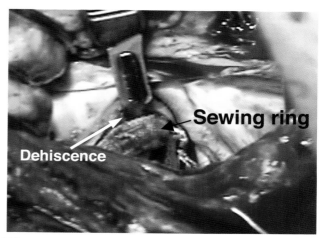

Fig 5-28. At surgery, the tissue mitral valve was partially dehisced with prominent mitral annular calcification. An intraoperative view from the left atrial side of the valve shows the area of dehiscence between the sewing ring and annulus.

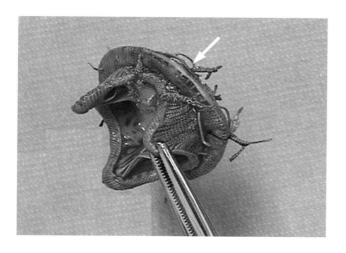

Fig 5-29. On the explanted valve an area of disruption of the fabric covering the sewing ring is seen with interrupted sutures (**arrow**).

Comments

The primary causes of paravalvular regurgitation are (1) fibrosis and calcification of the annulus, resulting in disruption of sutures due to the mechanical stress between the valve sewing ring and annulus, and (2) paravalvular infection. This patient has a typical history for annular fibrosis and calcification that results in repeat mitral valve replacements due to recurrent paravalvular regurgitation.

The diagnosis of paravalvular regurgitation is based on demonstration of a color Doppler jet outside the sewing ring. These jets typically are eccentric, as in this case, hugging the wall of the left atrium. With these eccentric jets, systolic flow reversal is present only in the pulmonary veins within the jet's direction. It can be difficult to distinguish valvular from paravalvular regurgitation; identification of the vena contracta on the ventricular side of the sewing ring aids in this distinction. The clinical significance of the paravalvular leak may be due to the severity of regurgitation (i.e. regurgitant volume and effective regurgitation orifice area) or the severity of intravascular hemolysis, as in this case.

Suggested Reading

1. Davila-Roman VG, Waggoner AD, Kennard ED et al; Artificial Valve Endocarditis Reduction Trial echocardiography study. Prevalence and severity of paravalvular regurgitation in the Artificial Valve Endocarditis Reduction Trial (AVERT) echocardiography study. J Am Coll Cardiol 2004; 44(7):1467–72.

2. Rallidis LS, Moyssakis IE, Ikonomidis I, Nihoyannopoulos P. Natural history of early aortic paraprosthetic regurgitation: a five-year follow-up. Am Heart J 1999; 138(2 Pt 1):351–7.

Case 5-8
Bioprosthetic Aortic Valve Dehiscence

In this 47-year-old man with a history of IV drug use, aortic valve replacement with a stented tissue valve had been performed 4 years previously for *Staphylococcus aureus* endocarditis with severe aortic regurgitation. He now presents with *Streptococcus viridans* bacteremia and evidence for prosthetic valve endocarditis with a paravalvular abscess, after 2 weeks of IV antibiotic therapy.

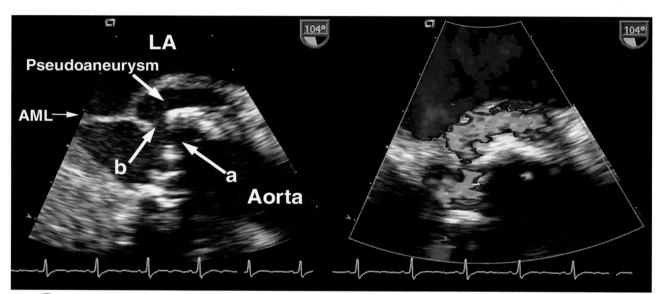

DVD **Fig 5-30.** A long-axis view at 104 degrees (*left*) shows deformity of the aortic valve with discontinuity in the leaflet (*a*) and a space originating between the base of the anterior mitral leaflet (**AML**) and the aorta (*b*) with an echo-free space between the posterior aortic root and the left atrium (**LA**) consistent with a pseudoaneurysm. Color flow (*right*) shows the communication between the left ventricle and this space, often called an aneurysm of the mitral aortic intervalvular fibrosa (**MAIVF**).

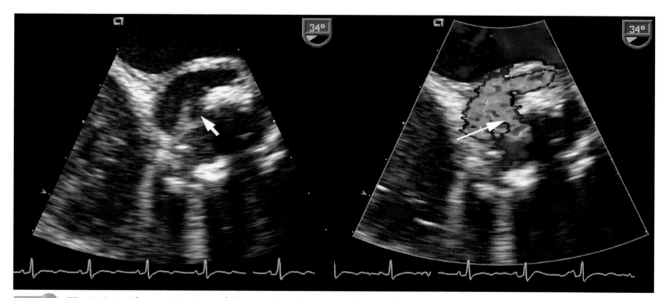

DVD **Fig 5-31.** Short-axis view of the aortic valve at 34 degrees shows an area of discontinuity (*left*, **arrow**) with color Doppler evidence of flow into the pseudoaneurysmal space (*right*, **arrow**).

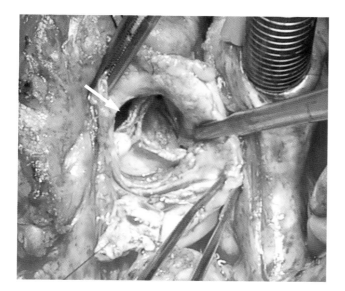

Fig 5-32. At surgery the areas of valve dehiscence between the stented tissue valve and annulus were seen (**arrow**). The valve was removed and replaced with an aortic homograft. Bilateral coronary bypass grafts were used because the coronary ostium could not be reimplanted due to friable tissue. He could not be weaned from bypass and expired.

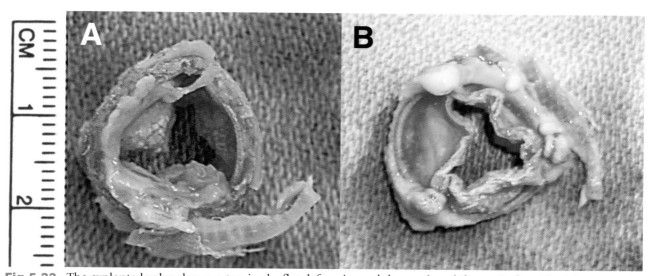

Fig 5-33. The explanted valve shows extensive leaflet deformity and destruction: (*A*) ventricular side; (*B*) aortic side.

Comments

Prosthetic heart valves have a higher prevalence of endocarditis than native valves due to the abnormal flow dynamics and the presence of foreign material in the bloodstream. The risk of prosthetic valve endocarditis is approximately 0.5% per year. Early prosthetic valve infection, occurring within 2 months of valve implantation, is most often due to *Staph epidermidis*. Late prosthetic valve endocarditis, as in this patient, has a bacteriologic spectrum similar to that seen for native valve endocarditis, with *Strep viridans* and *Staph aureus* being most common. Infection of bioprosthetic valves can affect the leaflets, with typical valvular vegetations, or can affect the sewing ring. Infection of the sewing ring often leads to abscess formation, which is most accurately diagnosed by TEE. An abscess may be echodense or echolucent; diagnosis is especially difficult with prosthetic valves, not only due to shadowing and reverberations by the valve ring/struts but also due to postoperative changes in the paravalvular region.

In this case, the abscess involved the aortic annulus at its junction with the base of the anterior mitral valve leaflet. Dehiscence of the sewing ring sutures resulted in an infected cavity between the posterior aortic root and anterior mitral leaflet that communicated with the LVOT. This aneurysm of the MAIVF is an uncommon but serious complication of prosthetic valve endocarditis.

Suggested Reading

1. Afridi I, Apostolidou MA, Saad RM, Zoghbi WA. Pseudoaneurysms of the mitral–aortic intervalvular fibrosa: dynamic characterization using transesophageal echocardiographic and Doppler techniques. J Am Coll Cardiol 1995; 25(1):137–45.

2. Zoghbi WA. Echocardiographic recognition of unusual complications after surgery on the great vessels and cardiac valves. In: Otto CM, ed. Clinical Practice of Echocardiography. Philadelphia: WB Saunders, 2002: 551–70.

Case 5-9
Tissue Mitral Valve Endocarditis

This 52-year-old male had undergone mitral valve replacement 15 years ago for endocarditis, with repeat mitral valve replacement 2 months ago for tissue degeneration of the prosthesis. His postoperative course was complicated by sternal wound infection, adult respiratory distress syndrome (ARDS), *Staph aureus* sepsis and acute renal failure. At that time, both transthoracic and transesophageal echocardiography showed normal valve function with no evidence of infection. He was treated with IV antibiotics and sternal wound debridement but had progressive clinical deterioration. He is now transferred to our medical center in acute cardiogenic shock with severe mitral regurgitation, presumed due to prosthetic valve endocarditis.

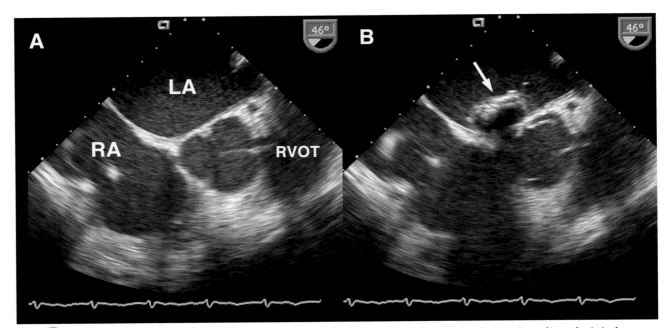

Fig 5-34. A short-axis view at the level of the aortic valve (at 46 degrees rotation) in diastole (*A*) shows the closed aortic valve and normal left atrium (**LA**). A catheter is present in the right atrium (**RA**). In systole (*B*), a large echodense mass prolapses into the LA (**arrow**), presumably from the mitral valve prosthesis.

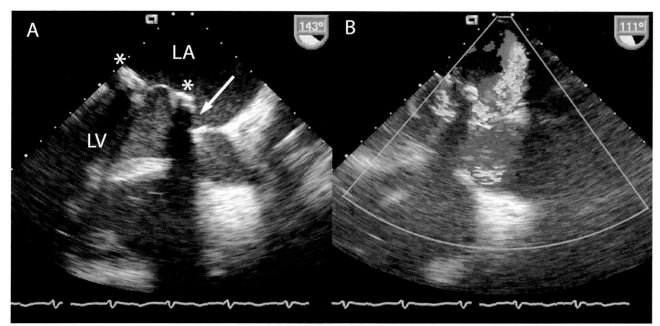

Fig 5-35. The long-axis view (at 143 degrees rotation) confirms that the prolapsing mass (**asterisks**) is attached to the mitral leaflet. The arrow indicates where the valve has become dehisced from the annulus (*left*). Color flow (*right*) demonstrates significant mitral regurgitation. At surgery, the mitral valve prosthesis was encircled by vegetations and was dehisced from the annulus, being held in place only by two remaining pledgets in the posterior–lateral aspect of the annulus. Pathologic examination demonstrated vegetations with Gram-positive coccal bacterial forms. Cultures of the valve tissue showed no growth. Although cultures of mediastinal tissue grew *Candida albicans*, there were no fungal forms seen in the valve tissue.

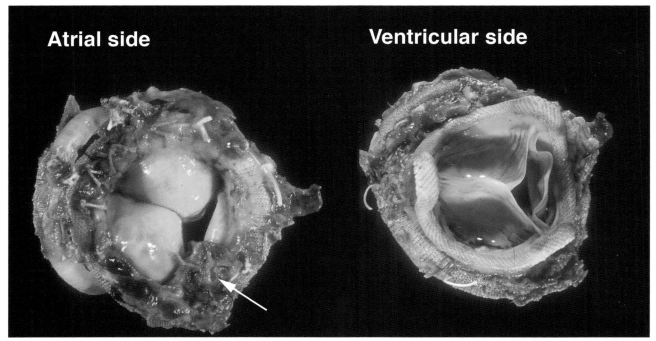

Fig 5-36. Pathologic examination of the valve revealed inflammatory tissue circumferentially around the metallic rim of the valve, as well as a lesion projecting over one of the cusps (**arrow**). Pathologic examination was consistent with bacterial vegetation. All three cusps were intact.

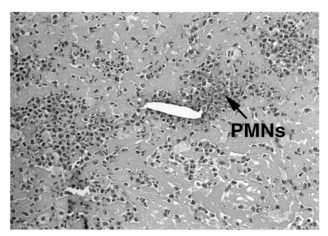

Fig 5-37. Microscopic examination of the tissue around the annulus revealed active inflammation with sheets of polymorphonuclear leukocytes (**PMNs**).

Comment

This patient has early prosthetic valve endocarditis with a large vegetation on the valve leaflet and infection of the sewing ring, resulting in valve dehiscence. Most cases of prosthetic valve endocarditis require removal of the prosthesis, in addition to prolonged antibiotic therapy. In this patient with fungal infection of the mediastinum and a large vegetation on the prosthetic valve, fungal endocarditis was suspected. However, the pathologic examination was most consistent with *Staph aureus* endocarditis, emphasizing that large vegetations may be seen with bacterial, as well as fungal, endocarditis. *Staph aureus* is a very virulent organism and there is a high prevalence of paravalvular abscess and poor outcomes in patients with *Staph aureus* endocarditis.

Suggested Reading

1. Sett SS, Hudon MP, Jamieson WR, Chow AW. Prosthetic valve endocarditis. Experience with porcine bioprostheses. J Thorac Cardiovasc Surg 1993; 105:428.

2. John MVD, Hibberd PL, Karchmer AW et al. Staphylococcus aureus prosthetic valve endocarditis: optimal management and risk factors for death. Clin Infect Dis 1998; 26:1302.

Mechanical Prosthetic Valves: Normal

Case 5-10
Bileaflet Mitral Valve

Example of a normal bileaflet mitral valve prosthesis.

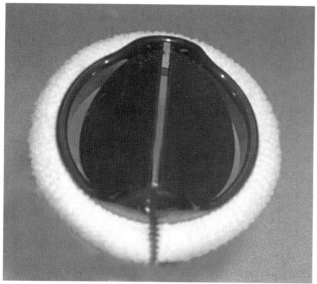

Fig 5-38. Photograph of a bileaflet mitral valve from the left atrial side of the valve with the leaflets slightly open. The two semicircular occluders (or leaflets) are free at the edges, with attachment only at small "hinges" near the center of the valve. The sewing ring is covered with cloth to allow attachment of sutures.

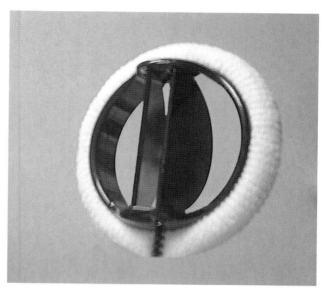

Fig 5-39. A photograph of the valve in the open position from the left atrial side shows the narrow slit-like central orifice and the larger lateral semicircular orifices on both sides of the valve.

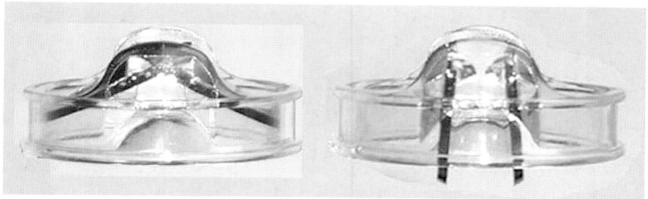

Fig 5-40. This clear plastic model of a bileaflet valve in the closed position (*left*) and open position (*right*) shows the normal positions of the valve leaflets relative to the sewing ring.

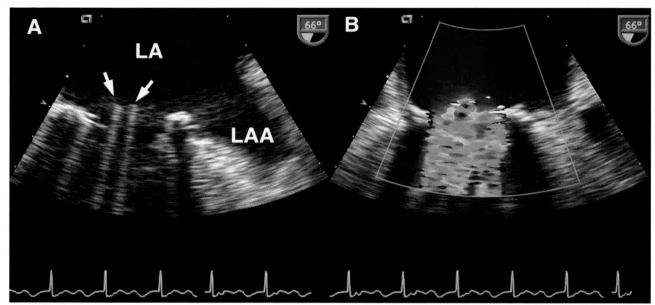

Fig 5-41. In an echocardiographic two-chamber view at 66 degrees rotation, the diastolic image (A) of the valve shows the parallel alignment of the open leaflets (**arrows**). Color Doppler (B) shows flow through the narrow central orifice and larger lateral orifices.

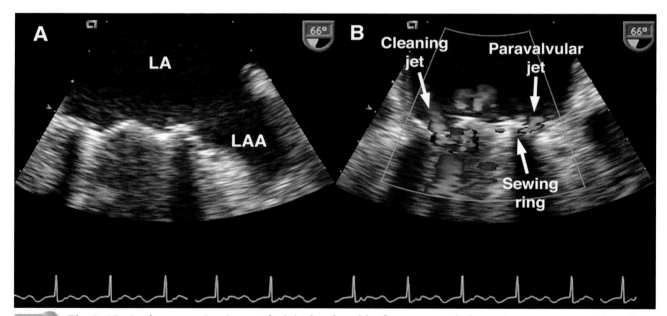

Fig 5-42. In the same view in systole (A), the closed leaflets are at a slight angle to each other. Note the shadows cast by the sewing ring and reverberations due to the disk occluders that obscure the left ventricle in this view. Color Doppler (B) shows the typical small eccentric jets due to closure of the leaflets. A small paravalvular jet is also seen—this closed spontaneously, shortly after separating from cardiopulmonary bypass.

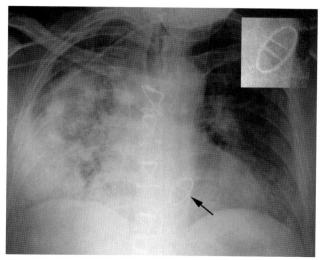

Fig 5-43. Posteroanterior (**PA**) chest X-ray shows the open bileaflet mechanical valve in the mitral position (**arrow**, see also the inset).

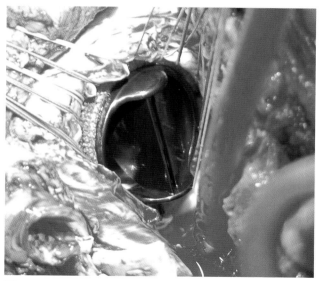

Fig 5-44. The bileaflet valve after insertion, viewed via the open left atrium.

Comment

The most common types (and examples) of mechanical valves are (1) bileaflet valves (St Jude Medical, CarboMedics), (2) single tilting disk valves (Bjork–Shiley, Medtronic Hall) and (3) ball-cage valves (Starr–Edwards). The normal fluid dynamics of bileaflet mechanical valve prosthesis are characterized by a small amount of regurgitation due to the closure of the valve occluders. With a bileaflet valve, there are typically two converging jets from the pivot points, a small central jet, and a variable number of peripheral jets, with little signal aliasing. In addition, these normal regurgitant jets are small in size, originating from within the sewing ring.

In contrast, pathologic regurgitation occurs in unexpected locations, often paravalvular, and is usually associated with larger, more eccentric jets. Prosthetic valve regurgitation is evaluated using the same approaches as for native valves, including measurement of the vena contracta width, evaluation of the intensity and shape of the continuous wave Doppler curve, and calculation of regurgitant volume and orifice area. However, evaluation of prosthetic valves, particularly in the mitral position, requires transesophageal imaging because shadowing and reverberations from the prosthesis preclude evaluation from the transthoracic approach. Detection of the proximal isovelocity surface area (PISA) on the ventricular side of the valve is helpful for identification of the origin of the regurgitant jet, but measurements are often difficult due to PISA asymmetry and poor image quality.

Suggested Reading

1. Baumgartner H, Khan S, DeRobertis M et al: Color Doppler regurgitant characteristics of normal mechanical mitral valve prostheses in vitro. Circulation 1992; 85:323–32.

2. Flachskampf FA, O'Shea JP, Griffin BP et al. Patterns of normal transvalvular regurgitation in mechanical valve prostheses. J Am Coll Cardiol 1991;18:1493–8.

Case 5-11
Bileaflet Aortic Valve

Example of a normal bileaflet mechanical aortic valve replacement.

As compared to the bileaflet valve in the mitral position, the valve in the aortic position is flipped on its vertical axis.

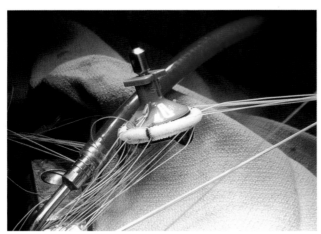

Fig 5-45. The mechanical valve is positioned in the holder, with only the sewing ring of the valve visible. Sutures have been placed equidistant around the sewing ring for attaching the prosthesis to the aortic annulus.

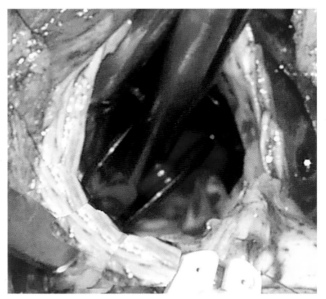

Fig 5-46. The bileaflet valve in the aortic position with the forceps opening the two leaflets. Note the narrow slit-like central orifice and the two larger semicircular orifices.

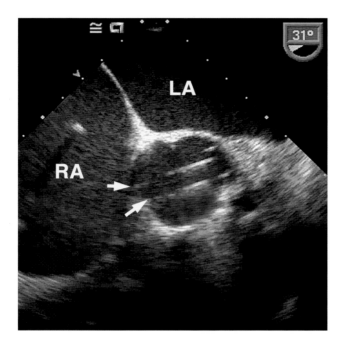

Fig 5-47. In a view similar to the surgical view, this echocardiographic short-axis view of the aortic valve at 31 degrees rotation shows the two leaflets open in systole (**arrows**) with the central slit-like orifice and two larger semicircular orifices anteriorly and posteriorly.

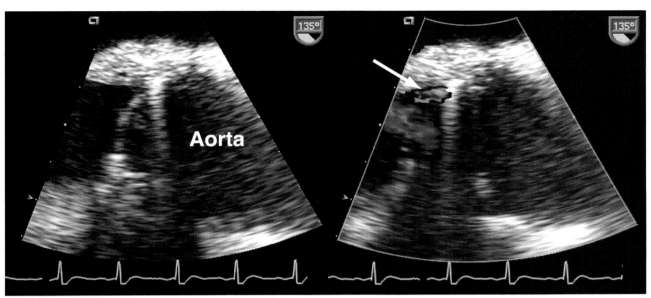

Fig 5-48. Long-axis view at 135 degrees. In real time, the normal leaflet motion is seen with some shadowing and reverberations by the proximal aspect of the valve. Color Doppler (*right*) shows a small amount of regurgitation (**arrow**), as expected for this valve type.

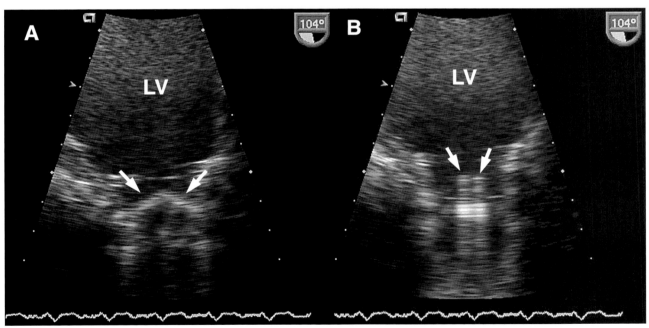

Fig 5-49. A transgastric apical view of left ventricle (**LV**) and ascending aorta in a long-axis view shows the bileaflet valve in the aortic position in diastole (*A*) and systole (*B*). Note that in the normal closed position, the leaflets (**arrows**, *left*) are at a slight angle to each other whereas the open leaflets (**arrows**, *right*) assume a parallel orientation.

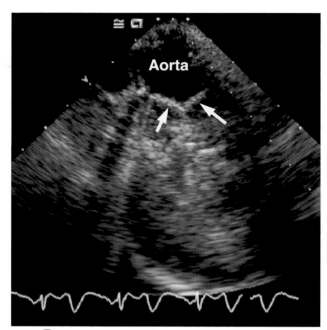

Fig 5-50. With a sterile transducer placed epicardially during surgery on the ascending aorta, this view of the aortic prosthesis was obtained. The closed leaflets (**arrows**) are at a slight angle, as seen in the apical view.

Comments

The bileaflet valve consists of two pyrolytic carbon disks attached to a rigid ring by two small hinges. This design results in a small central slit-like orifice and two larger lateral semicircular orifices when the valve is open. As for tissue valves, the hemodynamics of a normally functioning mechanical valve are inherently stenotic, compared with a normal native valve, with tables available listing the expected transvalvular velocities, pressure gradients and expected orifice areas for each valve type and size. Even higher velocities may be recorded with normally functioning valves due to the fluid dynamics of the central slit-like orifice. Effective orifice areas can be calculated using the continuity equation, as for native valves. Because the velocity and pressure gradient across a prosthesis valve depend on transvalvular flow rate, as well as valve type and size, a baseline examination when valve function is clinically normal is useful for distinguishing valve stenosis from normal hemodynamics, on serial examinations.

Suggested Reading

1. Reisner SA, Meltzer RS. Normal values of prosthetic valve Doppler echocardiographic parameters: a review. J Am Soc Echocardiogr 1988; 1:201–10.

2. Baumgartner H, Khan S, DeRobertis M et al. Effect of prosthetic aortic valve design on the Doppler-catheter gradient correlation: an in vitro study of normal St. Jude, Medtronic-Hall, Starr-Edwards and Hancock valves. J Am Coll Cardiol 1992; 19:324–32.

3. Blais C, Dumesnil JG, Baillot R et al. Impact of valve prosthesis–patient mismatch on short-term mortality after aortic valve replacement. Circulation 2003; 108(8):983–8.

Case 5-12
Bileaflet Tricuspid and Pulmonic Valves

Example of a bileaflet mechanical valve in the tricuspid position.

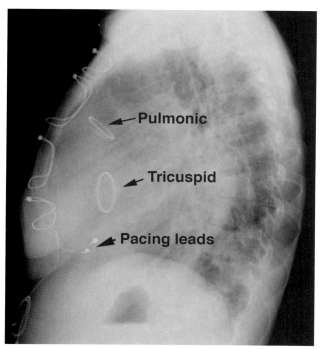

Fig 5-51. The lateral chest radiograph in this patient demonstrates the sewing ring of both a prosthetic pulmonic and prosthetic tricuspid valve. Epicardial pacing leads and sternal closure wires are also seen.

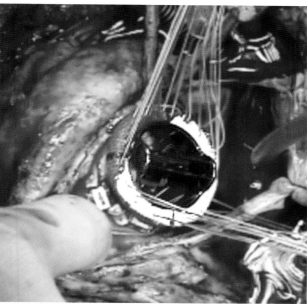

DVD **Fig 5-52.** An intraoperative view from the right atrium of the mechanical valve being sutured into the tricuspid annulus. Note that the sutures are passed through small rectangular pledgets (near the tip of the surgeon's finger) to secure the valve to the annulus. These pledgets can sometimes be seen on echocardiography.

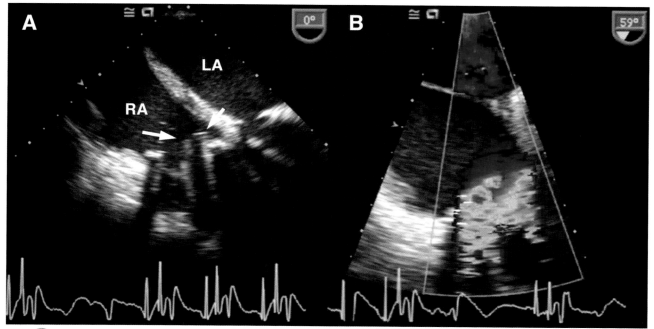

DVD **Fig 5-53.** (A) In a four-chamber view at 0 degrees the mechanical valve is present in the tricuspid position in diastole with the leaflets open (**arrows**). (B) Color Doppler in a short-axis view at 59 degrees rotation shows normal antegrade flow across the valve.

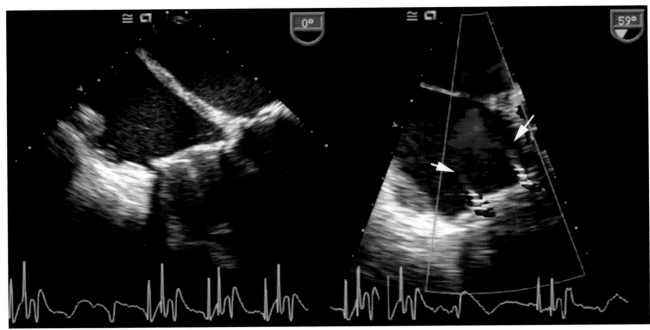

DVD **Fig 5-54.** In the same two views as in **Fig 5-53**, the closed valve leaflet and normal prosthetic regurgitation (**arrows**) are seen.

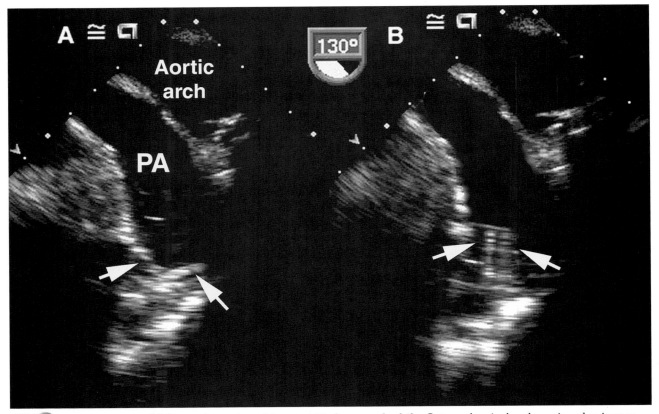

DVD **Fig 5-55.** In a high esophageal position at 130 degrees, the bileaflet mechanical pulmonic valve is seen closed in diastole (*A*, **arrows**) and open in systole (*B*, **arrows**).

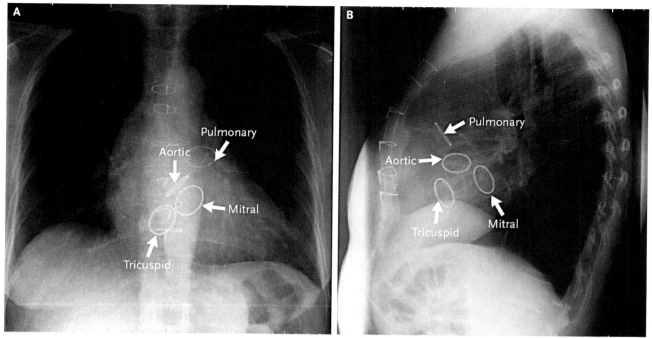

Fig 5-56. The normal positions of prosthetic valves in the cardiac silhouette are demonstrated in this posterolateral and lateral chest X-ray. (Reproduced with permission from van den Brink B. Four artificial heart valves. N Engl J Med 2005; 353:712. ©Massachusetts Medical Society.)

Comments

Although the most straightforward way to determine the type and location of valve prostheses in a patient is to review the medical record or the valve card patients are given to carry with them, in some cases valve position and type must be inferred from physical examination or chest radiography. As shown in this example, a standard posteroanterior and lateral chest radiograph allows identification of valve position, based on the normal position of the valves within the cardiac silhouette (**Fig 5-56**).

A valve prosthesis in the tricuspid position has an appearance and flow dynamics similar to the prosthetic mitral valve, although velocities and pressure gradients may be even lower because a larger prosthesis can be placed in the tricuspid annulus. In addition to the mean pressure gradient, evaluation of mechanical atrioventricular valves includes measurement of the pressure half-time. The empiric constant of 220, derived from studies of native mitral stenosis, can also be used for central orifice bioprosthetic valves and for mechanical valves to estimate valve area.

Suggested Reading

1. Vongpatanasin W, Hillis LD, Lange RA. Prosthetic heart valves. N Engl J Med 1996; 335:407–16.

2. Otto CM. Prosthetic valves. In Otto CM, ed. Textbook of Clinical Echocardiography, 3rd edn. Philadelphia: Elsevier Saunders, 2004: 355–83.

Case 5-13
Tilting Disk Mitral Valve

Example of a normal tilting disk mechanical valve in the mitral position.

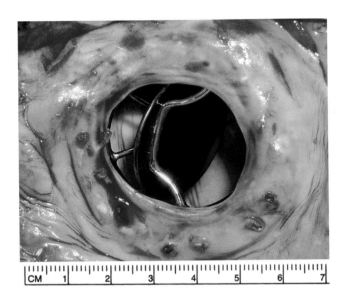

Fig 5-57. Photograph from the left atrial side of a single tilting disk mechanical valve in the mitral position. Note the angled metal struts on both sides of the valve that retain the concave-shaped disk. In this view, the valve is in the open position with the disk at a slight angle relative to the sewing ring, resulting in a small orifice (*on the left*) and a larger orifice (*on the right*).

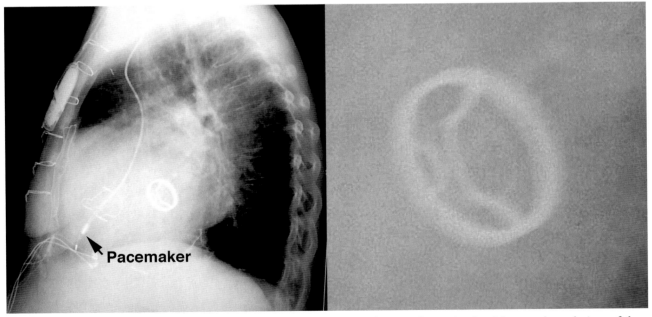

Fig 5-58. A lateral chest radiograph shows the normal position of a mitral prosthesis with an enlarged view of the valve on the right. This patient also has sternal wires and a transvenous pacer lead in the right ventricular apex.

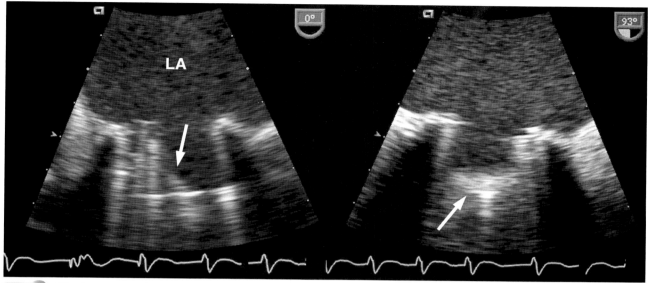

DVD **Fig 5-59.** In a four-chamber (*left*) and two-chamber (*right*) TEE view of the mitral prosthesis, the normal angle of opening of the single disk (**arrows**) in diastole is seen. There are reverberations from the disk and shadowing from the sewing ring that obscure the left ventricle.

Case 5-14
Tilting Disk Aortic Valve

Example of a normal tilting disk mechanical valve in the aortic position.

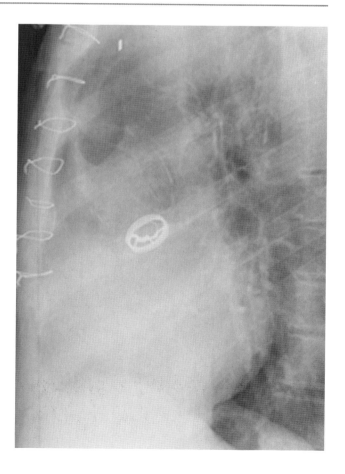

Fig 5-60. The lateral chest radiography shows the normal position of the aortic prosthesis.

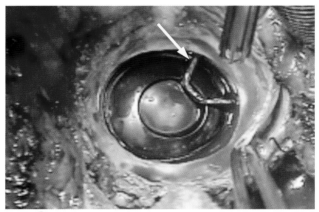

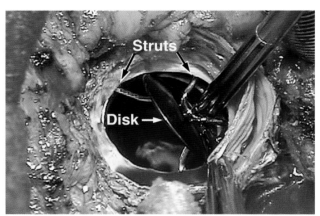

DVD **Fig 5-61.** A surgical view of the closed valve from the aorta shows the ridge on this particular type of valve and one of the metal struts (**arrow**). There are several different designs for the struts and occluders for single disk valves.

DVD **Fig 5-62.** A suction device has been used to open the valve, revealing the other strut and showing the normal range of motion of the disk.

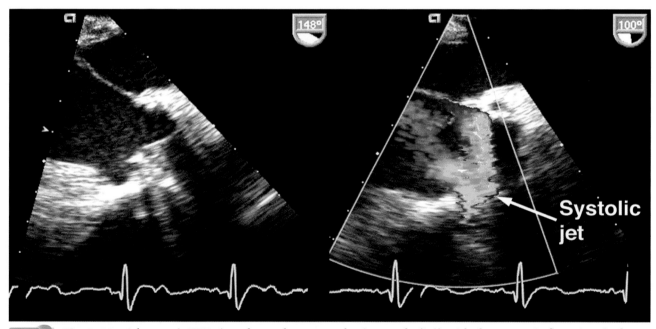

DVD **Fig 5-63.** A long-axis TEE view shows the open valve in systole (*left*) with the eccentric flow signal of antegrade flow seen with color Doppler (*right*).

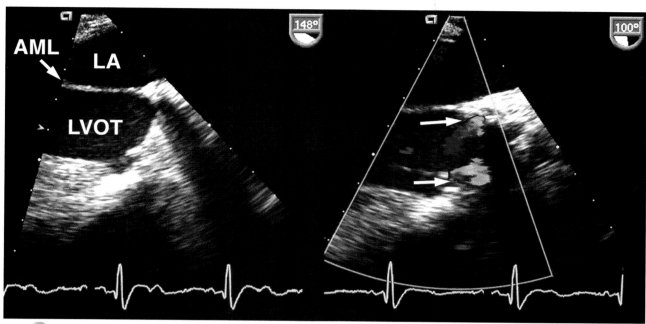

Fig 5-64. The long-axis view in diastole shows the closed valve (*left*) with color Doppler demonstrating two small jets of regurgitation (**arrows**) (*right*) at valve closure.

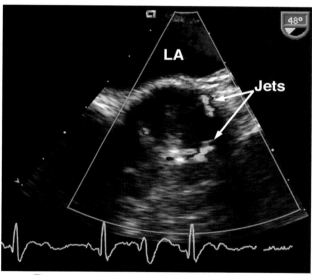

Fig 5-65. These small jets of aortic regurgitation are also seen in a short-axis view of the LVOT, immediately adjacent to the valve plane.

Comments (for Cases 5-13 and 5-14)

Tilting disk valves either have a ridge on the disk (as in these cases) or a central hole with central strut that maintains disk position as the valve opens and closes. The antegrade flow patterns vary with the exact type of valve, but basically consist of two asymmetric antegrade flow streams over and under the tilting disk in the open position. As the disk closes, there is a normal small amount of valve regurgitation between the disk and the sewing ring. Tilting disk valves that have a central strut and hole normally show a large central jet and one or two small peripheral jets.

Suggested Reading

1. Flachskampf FA, O'Shea JP, Griffin BP et al. Patterns of normal transvalvular regurgitation in mechanical valve prostheses. J Am Coll Cardiol 1991; 18:1493–8.

Case 5-15
Ball-Cage Valve with Replacement with a Valved Conduit

This 59-year-old man underwent aortic valve replacement 30 years ago with a 26 mm Starr–Edwards ball-cage prosthesis. He now presents with an ascending aortic aneurysm measuring 65 mm in maximum diameter.

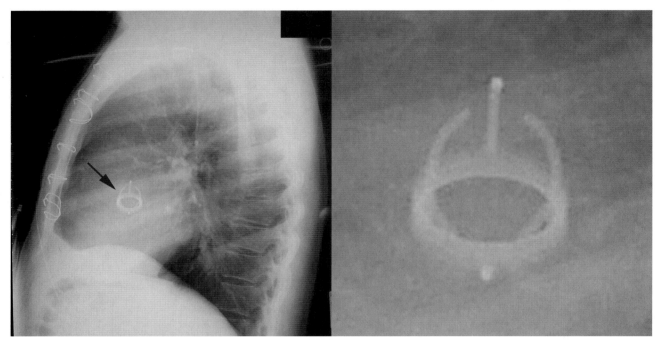

Fig 5-66. The lateral chest radiograph shows the valve in the aortic position (close up on the right) and retrosternal fullness, consistent with a dilated aorta. This ball-cage valve is unusual in that the three struts are open at the top. Most models have three bare metal struts that meet at the top of the "cage" and do not have any struts below the sewing ring.

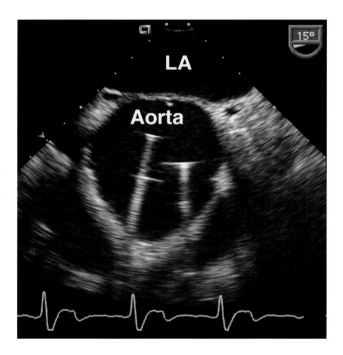

DVD **Fig 5-67.** A short-axis echocardiographic view of the ascending aorta shows marked dilation with the three struts from the valve cage. The echoes appear as dense lines due to beam width artifact from strong reflectors, with reverberations emanating from each strut. The reverberations from two of the struts overlap.

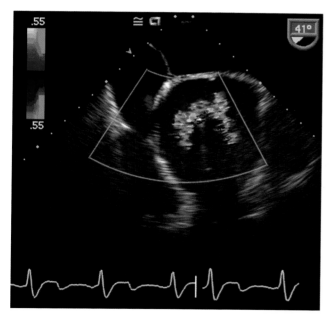

Fig 5-68. Color Doppler in the short-axis view shows flow around the ball occluder. The signal appears crescent shaped due to shadowing of the more distal part of the color Doppler signal by the occluder.

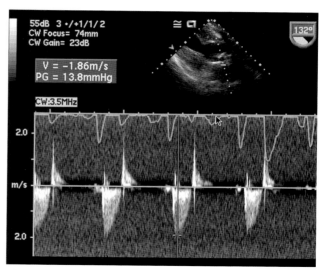

Fig 5-70. This view then allows Doppler recording of the transgastric aortic jet velocity at 1.9 m/s, although this is probably an underestimate as the angle between the direction of blood flow and the ultrasound beam is probably not parallel.

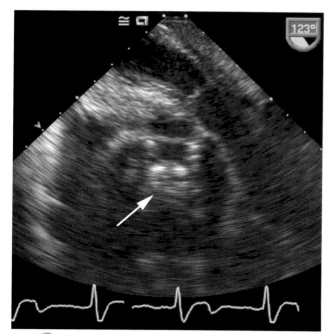

Fig 5-69. From a transgastric short-axis view, the image plane has been rotated to 123 degrees and the probe turned medially to show the valve prosthesis. In real time, movement of the ball occluder (**arrow**) is noted.

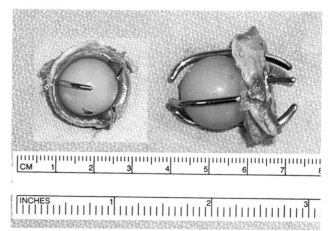

Fig 5-71. The valve was removed and a valved conduit used to replace the ascending aorta and valve. The resected valve shows the bare metal struts and plastic ball occluder. This particular model also has struts that extend below the sewing ring.

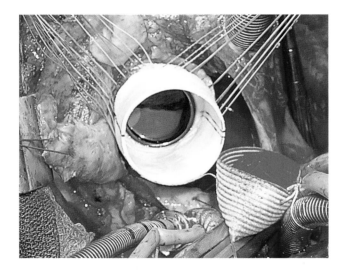

Fig 5-72. The composite mechanical bileaflet valve and fabric root replacement in situ at the time of surgery.

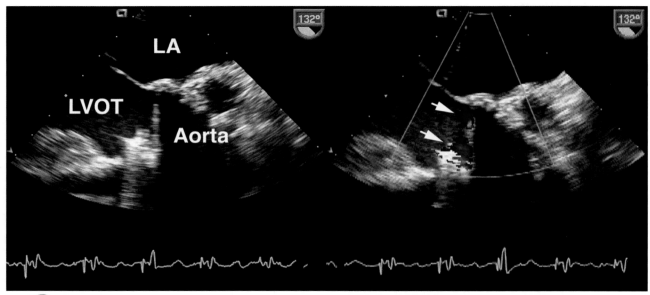

DVD **Fig 5-73.** An echocardiographic long-axis view of the new valve. The two color Doppler jets (*right*, **arrows**) are normal. This procedure, often called a Bentall procedure, also included reimplantation of the right and left coronary ostium with small buttons of tissue into the Dacron aortic graft. Pathology of the aorta was consistent with severe cystic medial necrosis.

Comments

It is likely that the original reason for valve replacement when this patient was 29 years old was severe aortic regurgitation due to a bicuspid aortic valve. In a subset of patients with a bicuspid aortic valve, the aortic root is also abnormal, with a high prevalence of aortic dilation and an increased risk of aortic dissection. The strongest risk factor for aortic root dilation after aortic valve replacement is a bicuspid aortic valve.

The ball-cage valve in this patient was very durable, functioning normally 30 years after implantation, with the valve removed at this surgery because of the need to do a composite root and valve replacement. Ball-cage valves are used less often than bileaflet or tilting disk valves, but may be seen in an occasional patient. The design of the ball-cage valve has changed over time, so that the echocardiographer should be aware of possible variations in valve appearance. Verification of the valve design by the manufacturer can be helpful when these patients are seen.

Suggested Reading

1. Godje OL, Fischlein T, Adelhard K et al. Thirty-year results of Starr–Edwards prostheses in the aortic and mitral position. Ann Thorac Surg 1997; 63(3):613–19.

2. Orszulak TA, Schaff HV, Puga FJ et al. Event status of the Starr–Edwards aortic valve to 20 years: a benchmark for comparison. Ann Thorac Surg 1997; 63(3):620–6.

3. Fedak PW, Verma S, David TE et al. Clinical and pathophysiological implications of a bicuspid aortic valve. Circulation 2002; 106(8):900–4.

Mechanical Prosthetic Valves: Dysfunction

Case 5-16
Paravalvular Aortic Regurgitation

This 55-year-old man had undergone aortic valve replacement 6 months earlier with a bileaflet mechanical valve. He now presented with a new diastolic murmur and an echocardiogram showing severe aortic regurgitation. He was referred for surgical treatment.

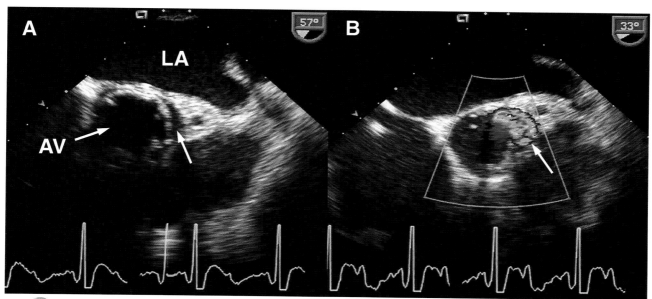

DVD **Fig 5-74.** The short-axis TEE view (*A*) at 57 degrees shows a crescent-shaped echolucent area (**arrow**) around the left coronary cusp aspect of the sewing ring. Color Doppler (*B*) shows diastolic flow in this region consistent with aortic regurgitation (**arrow**). This represents the vena contracta in short axis at the level of the valve.

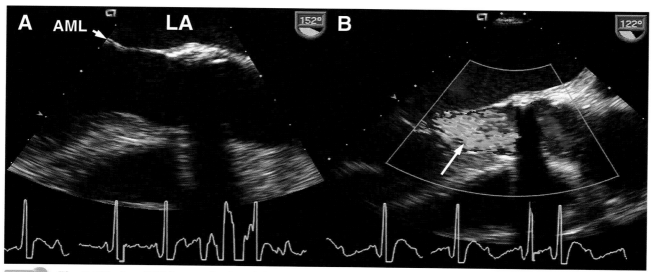

DVD **Fig 5-75.** In a TEE long-axis view (*A*) at 152 degrees there is shadowing from the mechanical valve, but color Doppler (*B*) shows a broad jet (**arrow**) of aortic regurgitation that fills the LVOT.

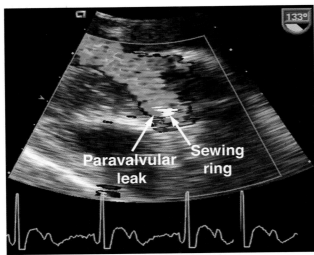

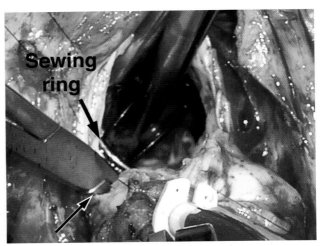

DVD **Fig 5-76.** A transgastric long-axis view was obtained starting in a transgastric short-axis view at 0 degrees and then rotating the image plane to 133 degrees and turning the transducer medially. Color Doppler shows a broad aortic regurgitant jet. This view is helpful with prosthetic aortic valves, as the valve does not shadow the outflow tract from this angle.

Fig 5-77. At surgery, the valve appeared intact. However, on very close inspection there was an area of dehiscence (**arrow**, instrument in dehisced area) extending from just below the left main coronary artery laterally to the junction of the left and right native commissure. Given the fact that there was no evidence of infection, this was thought to be a mechanical failure and amenable to repair.

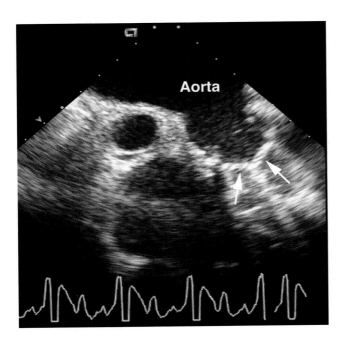

DVD **Fig 5-78.** Epiaortic scanning after correction of paravalvular leak in diastole shows the normal slightly obtuse closure angle of leaflets (not 180 degrees) (**arrows**).

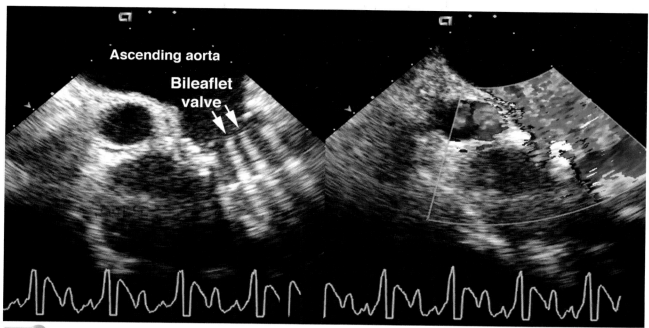

Fig 5-79. Epiaortic scanning after correction in systole shows full excursion of the mechanical leaflets (*left*) and normal antegrade flow (*right*).

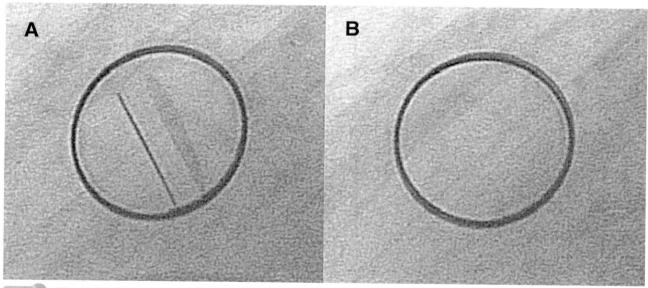

Fig 5-80. Postoperative fluoroscopy shows the leaflets fully opened in systole (*A*) and not visible during diastole (*B*) due to the relative angle of the valve leaflets and the X-ray source.

Comments

Mechanical valves have a very low rate of primary structural deterioration, with the interface between the valve sewing ring and the native annular tissue being the most vulnerable location for dysfunction. In this patient, the sutures attaching the valve to the aortic annulus were disrupted. Early after surgery, suture disruption may occur due to friction if there is any movement of the valve ring or if the annulus is fibrotic or calcified, which is the most likely explanation in this case. Later after surgery, mechanical disruption of the sutures is less likely due to tissue growth onto the sewing ring. The most common cause of late paravalvular regurgitation is infection, with paravalvular abscess formation.

Regurgitation of a mechanical aortic valve is often best evaluated from a transthoracic approach because the valve is well seen from this position and the outflow tract is not shadowed by the valve. With transesophageal imaging for prosthetic aortic valves, care is needed to demonstrate aortic regurgitation. As in this case, transgastric views may be helpful for color Doppler demonstration of regurgitation. Continuous wave Doppler examination can also be diagnostic.

The epiaortic imaging and fluoroscopy of the valve demonstrate the normal opening and closing of this bileaflet valve.

Suggested Reading

1. Karalis DG, Chandrasekaran K, Ross JJ Jr et al. Single-plane transesophageal echocardiography for assessing function of mechanical or bioprosthetic valves in the aortic valve position. Am J Cardiol 1992; 69:1310–15.

2. Puvimanasinghe JP, Steyerberg EW, Takkenberg JJ et al. Prognosis after aortic valve replacement with a bioprosthesis: predictions based on meta-analysis and microsimulation. Circulation 2001; 103(11):1535–41.

Case 5-17
Paravalvular Mitral Regurgitation

This 55-year-old man had a complex cardiac history with three previous mitral valve surgical procedures. He was admitted for hemolytic anemia with symptoms of lightheadedness and one episode of syncope.

Transthoracic echocardiography showed paravalvular mitral regurgitation and he was referred for surgical consideration.

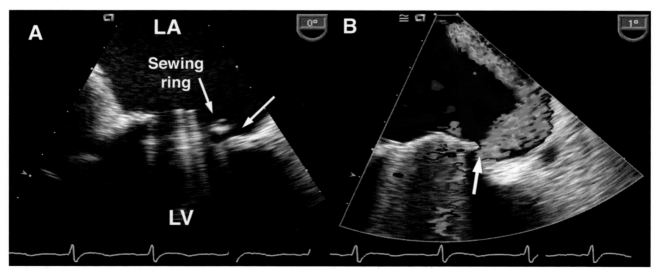

Fig 5-81. A four-chamber TEE view at 0 degrees shows the bileaflet mitral valve open in diastole (*A*) with an area of apparent discontinuity (**arrow**) at the lateral sewing ring. Color Doppler during systole (*B*, **arrow**) shows a large jet of paravalvular mitral regurgitation originating at this site that is eccentric in direction and extends along the lateral wall of the left atrium. The vena contracta width of 5 mm (**arrow**) is consistent with at least moderate regurgitation.

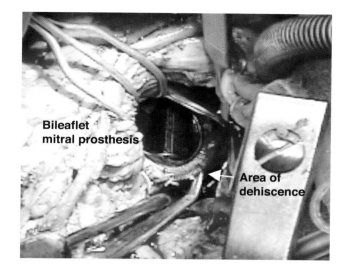

Fig 5-82. At surgery, a view from the left atrial side of the valve showed the area of paravalvular dehiscence.

Comments

This patient had recurrent paravalvular regurgitation due to a calcified and fibrotic annulus, resulting in disruption of the sutures, without evidence of infection. Regurgitation of mechanical prosthetic valves in the mitral position is best evaluated by transesophageal imaging. In this case, it is obvious that regurgitation is pathologic because it originates outside the sewing ring, the vena contracta is wide and the jet is eccentric and turbulent. Compare the pathologic regurgitant jet in this example with the normal regurgitant jet seen in Case 5-10.

Hemolytic anemia is most common with paravalvular regurgitation of the mechanical valve in the mitral position, as in this case. The severity of regurgitation is often only mild to moderate, as in this case, with symptoms due to anemia, not regurgitation. Some cases of hemolytic anemia can be treated conservatively with folate and iron replacement and occasional transfusion, but more severe anemia, refractory to medical therapy, requires surgical intervention.

Suggested Reading

1. Garcia MJ, Vandervoort P, Stewart WJ et al. Mechanisms of hemolysis with mitral prosthetic regurgitation. Study using transesophageal echocardiography and fluid dynamic simulation. J Am Coll Cardiol 1996; 27(2):399–406.

2. Skoularigis J, Essop MR, Skudicky D et al. Frequency and severity of intravascular hemolysis after left-sided cardiac valve replacement with Medtronic Hall and St. Jude Medical prostheses, and influence of prosthetic type, position, size and number. Am J Cardiol 1993; 71(7):587–91.

3. Maraj R, Jacobs LE, Ioli A, Kotler MN. Evaluation of hemolysis in patients with prosthetic heart valves. Clin Cardiol 1998; 21(6):387–92.

Case 5-18
Impaired Occluder Motion, Mitral Position

This 59-year-old man had aortic and mitral valve replacements 19 years ago for endocarditis. He now presents with decreased exercise tolerance and increasing shortness of breath over the past 1–2 years. Physical examination was unremarkable, but echo- cardiography demonstrated functional mitral stenosis with a mean gradient of 16 mmHg and a pressure half-time valve area of 1.4 cm². Pulmonary pressures were mildly elevated at 40 mmHg.

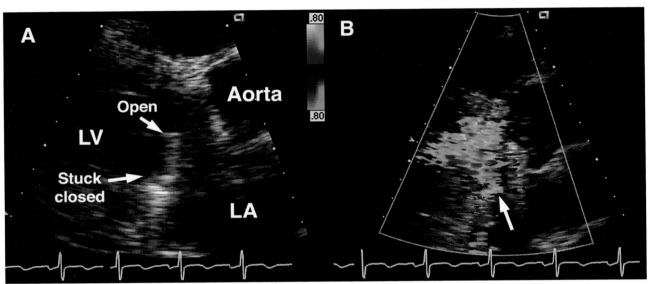

DVD ▶ Fig 5-83. Transthoracic images are shown because esophageal pathology precluded intraoperative TEE. In a parasternal long-axis TTE view (*A*) of the mitral valve prosthesis only one of the two leaflets opens in diastole. Color Doppler (*B*, **arrow**) shows antegrade flow only through the lateral half of the orifice.

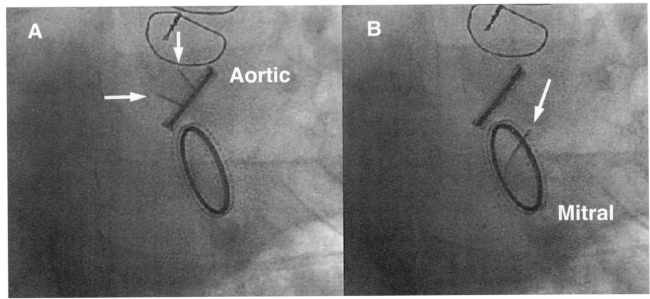

DVD ▶ Fig 5-84. Fluoroscopy of the aortic and mitral valves shows normal opening of the two aortic leaflets (**arrows**) in systole (*A*). However, in diastole (*B*) only one of the two mitral leaflets (**arrow**) opens.

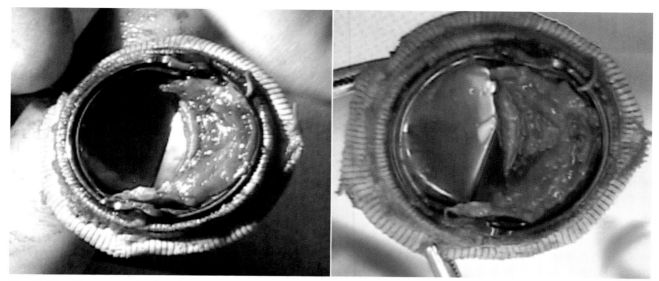

Fig 5-85. The resected valve shows severe pannus ingrowth filling half the area of the prosthetic valve. This is evident on both the ventricular (*left*) and atrial (*right*) sides.

Comments

The most common mechanisms of mechanical valve dysfunction are infection and thrombosis. Valve thrombosis may be acute, for example thrombus in the hinges of a bileaflet valve limiting disk excursion, or chronic, with a slowly enlarging thrombus leading to impairment of disk motion. In addition, tissue ingrowth (or pannus) around the annulus on the upstream side of the valve, as seen in this case, can prevent normal disk opening and/or closing. The risk factors for pannus ingrowth have not been studied. In some cases, pannus ingrowth seems to be associated with suboptimal long-term anticoagulation, suggesting a pattern of repetitive thrombosis and tissue ingrowth.

However, other cases do not appear to be related to adequacy of anticoagulation. Pathologic examination of the tissue is non-specific, showing fibrous tissue.

Suggested Reading

1. Fligner DL, Reichenbach DD, Otto CM. Pathology and etiology of valvular heart disease. In Otto CM, ed. Valvular Heart Disease. Philadelphia: Elsevier Saunders, 2004: 18–50.
2. Barbetseas J, Nagueh SF, Pitsavos C et al. Differentiating thrombus from pannus formation in obstructed mechanical prosthetic valves: an evaluation of clinical, transthoracic and transesophageal echocardiographic parameters. J Am Coll Cardiol 1998; 32(5):1410–17.

Case 5-19
Impaired Occluder Motion, Tricuspid Position

This 28-year-old woman with complex congenital heart disease is status post-tricuspid valve replacement and classic Glenn shunt for Ebstein's anomaly as a child. She has a history of several right lung arterial-venous vascular malformations with cyanosis, complete heart block with a transvenous atrial lead and an epicardial ventricular lead, and significant LV systolic dysfunction. She has been treated for congestive heart failure with an improvement in her ejection fraction from 15% to 45%. However, she continues to have persistent symptoms and signs of right-sided heart failure and is wheelchair bound due to exertional limitations. Transthoracic echocardiography shows a mean gradient of about 12 mmHg across the mechanical tricuspid valve and severe tricuspid regurgitation. She is referred to surgery for formation of a bidirectional Glenn shunt, insertion of new atrial and ventricular pacer leads and consideration of repeat tricuspid valve replacement.

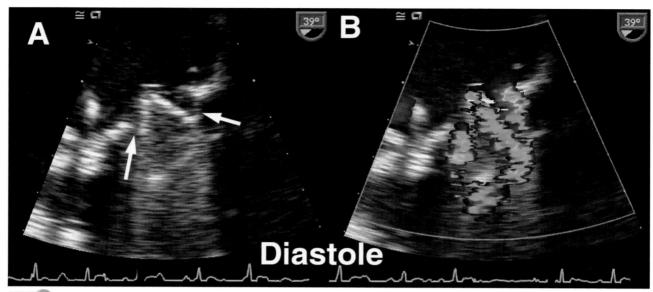

DVD ▶ **Fig 5-86.** A view of the tricuspid prosthesis at 39 degrees rotation shows a reduction in the maximum opening of the leaflets in diastole (*A*, **arrows**). Instead of a parallel alignment, the leaflets only partly open at an acute angle. Color Doppler (*B*) of antegrade flow shows three narrow jets, instead of the normal pattern of antegrade flow across a bileaflet valve.

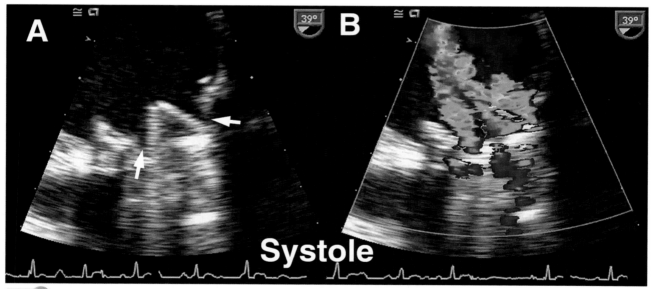

DVD ▶ **Fig 5-87.** In the same orientation, the valve leaflets fail to close in systole (*A*, **arrows**) with color Doppler (*B*) showing severe tricuspid regurgitation.

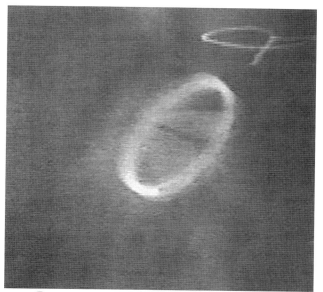

DVD **Fig 5-88.** Fluoroscopy of the valve shows the position of the leaflets; in real time, the leaflets fail to move during the cardiac cycle.

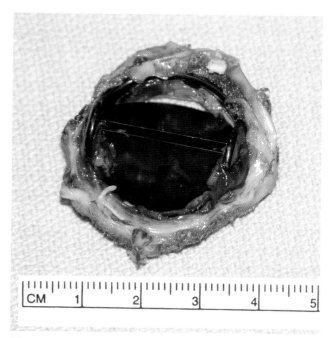

Fig 5-89. The resected valve demonstrates pannus, particularly in the region of the leaflet "hinges", with resultant restriction of leaflet motion. The valve was replaced with a 27 mm pericardial tissue prosthesis. The woman had a dramatic clinical improvement after surgery, with a substantial improvement in exercise tolerance.

Comments

In this patient with complex cyanotic congenital heart disease, it was difficult to differentiate whether symptoms were due to tricuspid valve dysfunction or inadequate pulmonary blood flow. At surgery, she had both repeat tricuspid valve surgery and restoration of the connection between the right and left pulmonary arteries so that flow from the Glenn shunt now supplies both lungs. The resected tricuspid valve was clearly dysfunctional, so it is likely that her clinical improvement was due, at least in part, to improvement in the function of the tricuspid valve. Because of the risk of tissue degeneration of valves in the tricuspid position, she will need periodic echocardiographic evaluation of tricuspid valve function.

Suggested Reading

1. Durrleman N, Pellerin M, Bouchard D et al. Prosthetic valve thrombosis: twenty-year experience at the Montreal Heart Institute. J Thorac Cardiovasc Surg 2004; 127(5):1388–92.

2. Maleszka A, Kleikamp G, Koerfer R. Tricuspid valve replacement: clinical long-term results for acquired isolated tricuspid valve regurgitation. J Heart Valve Dis 2004; 13(6):957–61.

3. Tong AT, Roudaut R, Ozkan M et al. Prosthetic Valve Thrombolysis—Role of Transesophageal Echocardiography (PRO-TEE) Registry Investigators. Transesophageal echocardiography improves risk assessment of thrombolysis of prosthetic valve thrombosis: results of the international PRO-TEE registry. J Am Coll Cardiol 2004; 43(1):77–84.

Case 5-20
Impaired Mechanical Leaflet Motion, Mitral Position

This 25-year-old man had undergone aortic coarctation repair at age 2 years. Over the past 23 years he has done well with no limitations, on no medical therapy, with periodic evaluations for a bicuspid aortic valve and mild mitral valve prolapse. He now presents with a 1-month history of increasing shortness of breath and dyspnea on exertion. Physical examination showed a grade 4 apical holosystolic murmur, and echocardiography demonstrated a partial flail anterior mitral leaflet with severe regurgitation. There also was moderate left atrial enlargement and severe pulmonary hypertension with pulmonary systolic pressures greater than 90 mmHg.

Valve repair was unsuccessful, so a mechanical mitral valve replacement was performed with preservation of the mitral leaflets and chords. However, after weaning from cardiopulmonary bypass, pulmonary systolic pressure was still in the 70–80 mm range, despite the use of pulmonary vasodilators.

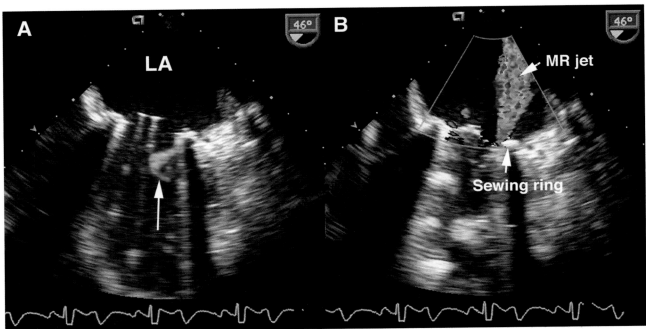

Fig 5-90. A two-chamber TEE view at 46 degrees of the mitral prosthesis shows a mass of echoes (**arrow**) at the lateral aspect of the valve in diastole with the mechanical leaflets open (*A*). A systolic frame with color Doppler (*B*) shows a moderately sized jet of regurgitation at that site. The surgeon was concerned that the native valve tissue might be interfering with normal closure of the mechanical valve.

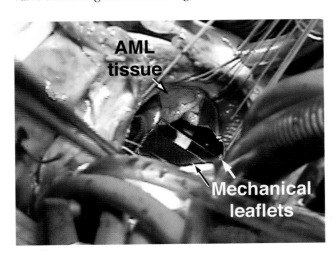

Fig 5-91. After reinstituting cardiopulmonary bypass and opening the left atrium, the redundant tissue of the native anterior mitral leaflet (**AML**) is seen to prevent motion of one of the mechanical leaflets (**arrow**). A small piece of tissue was excised from this medial segment of the anterior leaflet with preservation of all of the chords to the posterior leaflet and the lateral anterior segment. Repeat TEE after weaning from cardiopulmonary bypass showed no significant regurgitation and pulmonary pressures were reduced. He has done well long term postoperatively, with continued periodic evaluation of his bicuspid aortic valve.

Comments

Preservation of the continuity between the mitral annulus and papillary muscles helps maintain normal left ventricular systolic function after mitral valve surgery. When a valve repair is not possible, it is still preferable to preserve the native valve leaflets at the time of valve replacement. The posterior leaflet is easily retained, with a low likelihood of interference with mitral valve function. The anterior leaflet is often divided, with the two segments positioned so that they do not interfere with mechanical valve function. In this case, the redundant native anterior leaflet prevented normal valve closure, resulting in mitral regurgitation. Another described complication after valve replacement is LVOT obstruction due to the native anterior mitral leaflet. This complication is recognized on echocardiography by the presence of an increased velocity in the subaortic region. Clinically, patients with subaortic obstruction may be hypotensive and have difficulty weaning from cardiopulmonary bypass.

Suggested Reading

1. Rietman GW, van der Maaten JM, Douglas YL, Boonstra PW. Echocardiographic diagnosis of left ventricular outflow tract obstruction after mitral valve replacement with subvalvular preservation. Eur J Cardiothorac Surg 2002; 22(5):825–7.

2. Gallet B, Berrebi A, Grinda JM et al.. Severe intermittent intraprosthetic regurgitation after mitral valve replacement with subvalvular preservation. J Am Soc Echocardiogr 2001; 14(4):314–16.

6

Right-Sided Valve Disease

Case 6-1
Normal Tricuspid and Pulmonic Valves

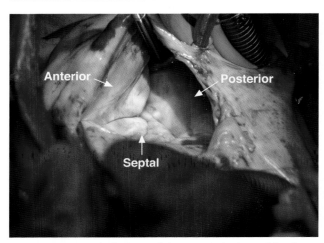

Fig 6-1. A surgical view of the normal tricuspid valve, viewed from the right atrium (and the head of the operating table), demonstrates the three normal leaflets—anterior, septal and posterior—with the normal leaflets appearing thin, smooth and with complete coaptation in diastole.

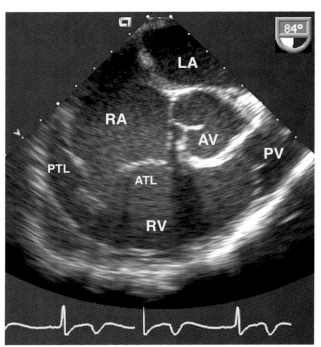

DVD **Fig 6-3.** From the four-chamber view, the image plane is rotated to about 90 degrees to obtain this orthogonal, or "right-sided inflow–outflow view" of the tricuspid valve with anterior and posterior leaflets demonstrated (**ATL**, **PTL**). In addition, the pulmonic valve (**PV**) is visualized in a long-axis plane relative to the valve.

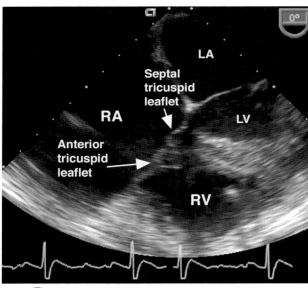

DVD **Fig 6-2.** The standard high TEE view of the tricuspid valve is obtained at 0 degrees, starting in the four-chamber view, and turning the transducer slightly towards the patient's right side. Visualization of the tricuspid valve is often enhanced by slightly advancing the probe in the esophagus from the standard four-chamber view. In this view, the septal and anterior tricuspid valve leaflets are seen.

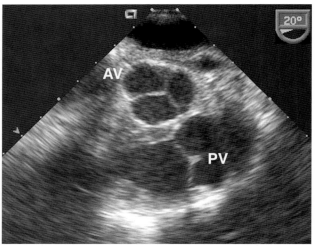

DVD **Fig 6-4.** In a short-axis view of the aortic valve, the pulmonic valve can sometimes be seen by slight withdrawal of the probe in the esophagus. Note the normal perpendicular relationship between the aortic valve (seen in short axis) and the pulmonic valve (seen in long axis).

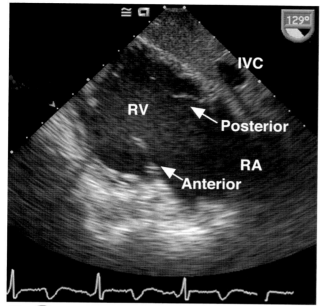

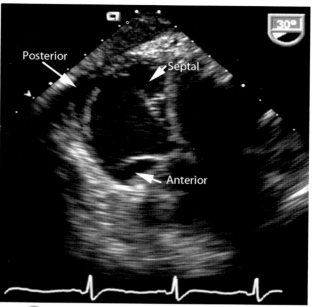

Fig 6-5. From the transgastric view, a right ventricular inflow view is obtained by starting in the short-axis view of the left ventricle, rotating the image plane to about 120 degrees, and turning the transducer slightly to the patient's right. The posterior and anterior tricuspid valve leaflets are seen.

Fig 6-7. A short-axis view of the tricuspid valve, showing all three leaflets, can sometimes be obtained from the transgastric view at a rotation of about 30 degrees.

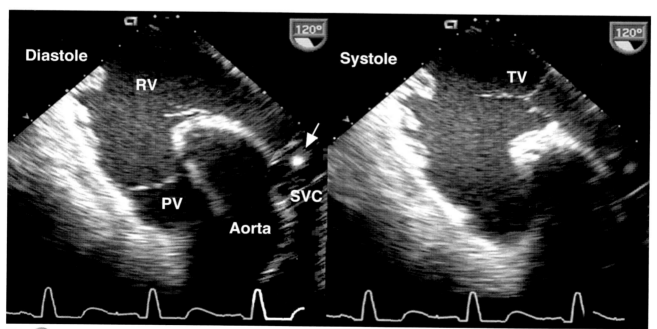

Fig 6-6. By moving the transducer to a position just on the gastric side of the gastroesophageal junction, a view of both tricuspid and pulmonic valves (shown in diastole on the left and in systole on the right) can be obtained. Note that this image plane is the same as shown in **Fig 6-3**, rotated 90 degrees counterclockwise, due to the different position of the transducer in the transgastric compared to the high esophageal position. The arrow points to a central venous catheter in the superior vena cava (**SVC**).

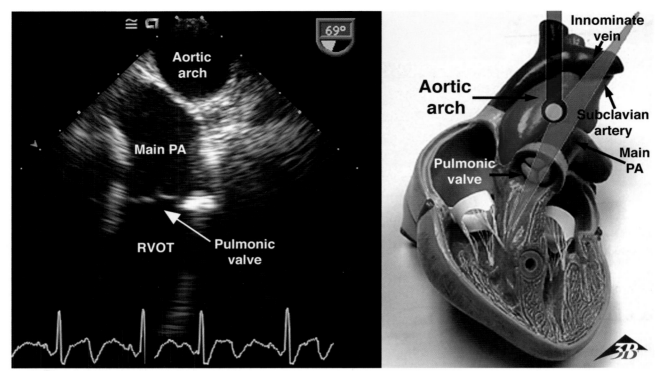

DVD   **Fig 6-8.** This view of the pulmonic valve and right ventricular outflow tract (**RVOT**) was acquired from a very high esophageal position. After imaging the descending aorta in the mid esophageal longitudinal plane (approximately 70–110 degrees), the probe is gradually withdrawn. As the level of the arch is reached, the probe is rotated counterclockwise to image the pulmonic valve and RVOT (based on Economy Heart Model 3B Scientific.) This view is useful in determining if a PA catheter has traversed the pulmonic valve.

Comments

The tricuspid valve is routinely evaluated on TEE in at least two views. Most often the four-chamber view and a short-axis ("inflow–outflow") view are used, with 2D imaging of leaflet thickness and mobility and annulus size with color Doppler evaluation of regurgitation. When regurgitation is present, severity is evaluated based on the vena contracta width. In addition, velocity is recorded using continuous wave Doppler, although velocity may be underestimated as it is not always possible to obtain a parallel intercept angle between the ultrasound beam and direction of the tricuspid regurgitant jet on a TEE examination. Additional views of the tricuspid valve are typically obtained only if initial images are abnormal or if there is clinical concern for tricuspid valve involvement.

Case 6-2
Rheumatic Valve Disease

This 49-year-old man with a prior mitral commissurotomy for rheumatic mitral valve disease presented with right-sided heart failure, atrial fibrillation, recurrent mitral stenosis and severe tricuspid regurgitation.

He was referred for mitral valve replacement, tricuspid annuloplasty and radiofrequency ablation of atrial fibrillation.

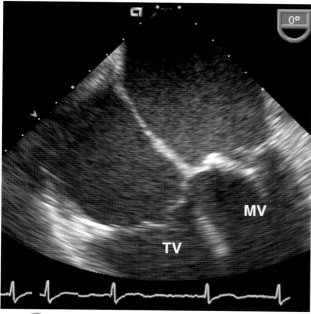

DVD **Fig 6-9.** In a four-chamber view, rheumatic mitral valve disease is seen but the tricuspid leaflets appear thin with normal mobility.

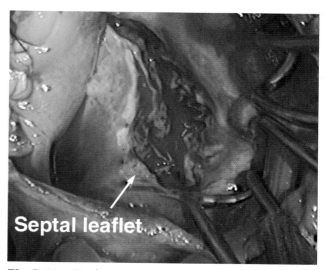

Fig 6-11. On direct inspection, the tricuspid leaflets were normal in thickness, with no evidence of commissural fusion. However, the annulus was severely dilated to 38 mm.

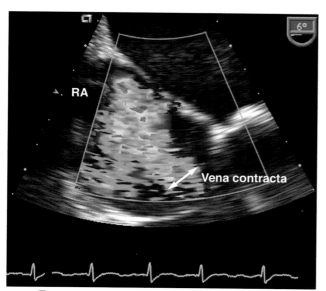

DVD **Fig 6-10.** Severe tricuspid regurgitation is demonstrated by color Doppler imaging with a wide vena contracta width of 10 mm and a large jet area relative to right atrial size.

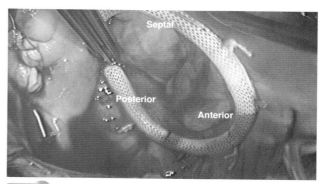

DVD **Fig 6-12.** After replacing the mitral valve, a 32 mm tricuspid valve ring was placed.

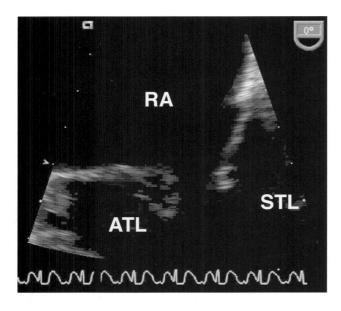

DVD ▶ **Fig 6-13.** In another patient with rheumatic mitral stenosis, the tricuspid valve imaged at 0 degrees shows thickness and tethering compatible with rheumatic tricuspid valve disease. On this systolic image, the leaflets fail to coapt. ATL = anterior tricuspid leaflet; STL = septal tricuspid leaflet.

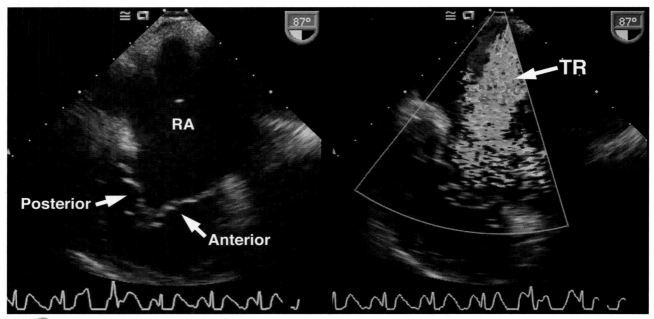

DVD ▶ **Fig 6-14.** At 87 degrees, the tricuspid leaflets are retracted with failure to coapt centrally and a jet of severe tricuspid regurgitation (**TR**) is seen.

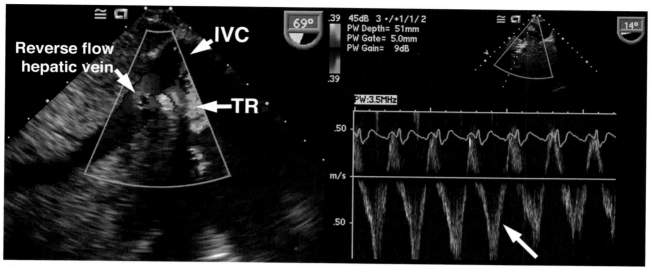

Fig 6-15. *Left:* Severe tricuspid regurgitation extends into the IVC with systolic flow reversal and extension into the hepatic vein. *Right:* pulsed wave Doppler in the hepatic vein confirms holosystolic reversal (**arrow**), indicative of severe TR.

Comments

The tricuspid valve is affected by the rheumatic process in about 5–10% of patients with rheumatic mitral valve disease. Rheumatic involvement of the tricuspid valve results in leaflet thickening, commissural fusion and fusion and shortening of the chords, although findings are often subtle compared with the mitral valve. Rheumatic involvement of the tricuspid valve can cause stenosis, due to commissural fusion, or regurgitation, due to chordal shortening and fusion, but severe stenosis is uncommon.

However, most patients with rheumatic mitral stenosis have significant tricuspid regurgitation, even when the tricuspid leaflets are unaffected by rheumatic disease. Functional tricuspid regurgitation is present in about 80% of patients with rheumatic mitral stenosis and about 40% of those with severe rheumatic mitral regurgitation.

In these patients, chronic pulmonary hypertension secondary to mitral stenosis results in right ventricular and tricuspid annular dilation. With severe annular dilation, the normal tricuspid leaflets cannot completely close in diastole, leading to tricuspid regurgitation. It is postulated that the additional right ventricular volume overload from tricuspid regurgitation leads to further right ventricular enlargement and progressive tricuspid regurgitation. In addition, there may be subtle rheumatic involvement of the tricuspid leaflets that may be better evaluated by 3D echocardiography. Most clinicians recommend tricuspid annuloplasty at the time of mitral valve repair or replacement when significant tricuspid regurgitation is present.

Suggested Reading

1. Chockalingam A, Gnanavelu G, Elangovan S et al. Clinical spectrum of chronic rheumatic heart disease in India. J Heart Valve Dis 2003; 12:577–81.

2. Henein MY, O'Sullivan CA, Li W et al. Evidence for rheumatic valve disease in patients with severe tricuspid regurgitation long after mitral valve surgery: the role of 3D echo reconstruction. J Heart Valve Dis. 2003; 12:566–72.

Case 6-3
Ebstein's Anomaly

This 40-year-old female with Ebstein's anomaly of the tricuspid valve was referred for surgical intervention because of increasing shortness of breath in association with increasing tricuspid regurgitation.

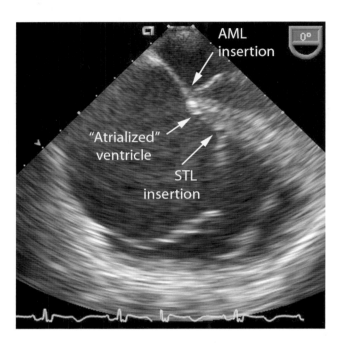

Fig 6-16. The four-chamber view shows the apical displacement of the septal leaflet of the tricuspid valve (**STL**) when compared with the insertion point of the anterior mitral valve leaflet (**AML**). The normal distance between the mitral and tricuspid insertion points is less than 1 cm. A greater distance, as in this case, suggests Ebstein's anomaly. Right atrial and ventricular enlargement can also be appreciated in this view. The segment of the right ventricular myocardium on the atrial side of the displaced tricuspid valve is considered "atrialized" because it exhibits ventricular electrical activity but is exposed to atrial pressures.

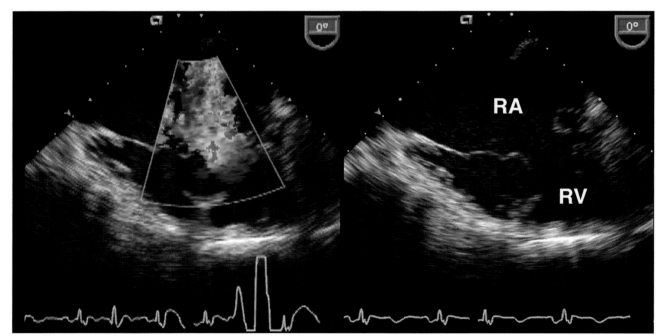

DVD **Fig 6-17.** With the probe advanced in the esophagus and turned towards the right, color flow Doppler shows severe tricuspid regurgitation with a broad vena contracta, measuring 18 mm.

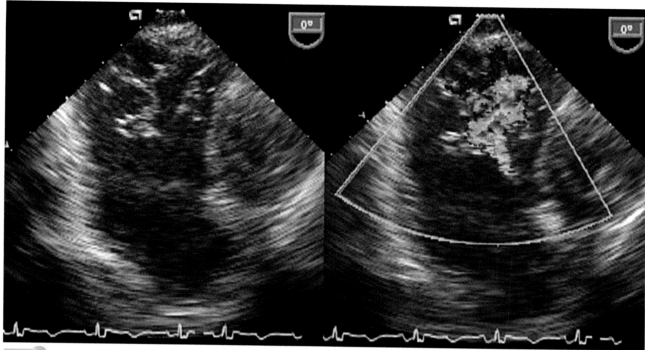

DVD **Fig 6-18.** A transgastric short-axis view of the tricuspid valve shows the severe right-sided chamber enlargement in comparison to the normal size of the left ventricle. Color flow demonstrates severe central tricuspid regurgitation.

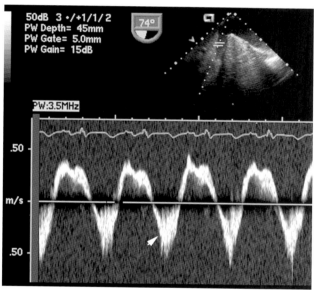

Fig 6-19. The hepatic vein is imaged from the transgastric position. Pulsed Doppler shows normal flow into the right atrium in diastole (above the baseline), with reserved flow in systole (arrowhead). This finding is consistent with severe tricuspid regurgitation. However, correlation with other measures of regurgitant severity is needed because systolic flow reversal can be seen in the absence of severe tricuspid regurgitation in patients with severely elevated venous pressures or with atrial fibrillation.

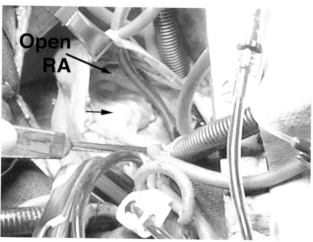

Fig 6-20. Intraoperative inspection of the valve demonstrates the apically displaced, elongated tricuspid valve leaflets (**arrow**). Valve repair was not successful in this patient, so she underwent tricuspid valve replacement.

Comments

Some patients with Ebstein's anomaly who reach adulthood without a previous surgical procedure remain asymptomatic, without clinical evidence of right heart failure, despite moderate to severe tricuspid regurgitation. In some cases, regurgitant severity increases or chronic right-sided volume overload leads to right heart failure symptoms, prompting surgical intervention.

Ebstein's anomaly may be associated with atrial septal defects in about one-third of patients, and a patent foramen ovale is common in those without an atrial septal defect. Elevated right atrial pressures due to tricuspid regurgitation may lead to right-to-left shunting at the atrial level with systemic arterial oxygen desaturation and cyanosis. Ebstein's anomaly is also associated with ventricular pre-excitation (e.g. Wolff–Parkinson–White syndrome).

Patients with Ebstein's anomaly are unlikely to have pulmonary hypertension. However, the apparent tricuspid regurgitant jet signal is often difficult to interpret due to the effect of motion of the large, displaced tricuspid valve and there may be erroneous overestimation of pulmonary pressures by Doppler. When pulmonary hypertension is suspected in patients with Ebstein's anomaly, right heart catheterization should be performed for direct measurement of pulmonary pressures.

Suggested Reading

1. Attie F, Rosas M, Rijlaarsdam M et al. The adult patient with Ebstein anomaly. Outcome in 72 unoperated patients. Medicine (Baltimore) 2000; 79:27–36.
2. Oechslin E, Buchholz S, Jenni R. Ebstein's anomaly in adults: Doppler-echocardiographic evaluation. Thorac Cardiovasc Surg 2000; 48:209–13.

Case 6-4
Ebstein's Anomaly and Patent Foramen Ovale

This 55-year-old man, with Ebstein's anomaly of the tricuspid valve and no prior heart surgery, presented with progressive right heart failure symptoms, atrial fibrillation, worsening hypoxia (oxygen saturation 85%) and severe peripheral edema. Echocardiography demonstrated a patent foramen ovale with right-to-left shunting, Ebstein's anomaly with severe right atrial and ventricular enlargement and moderately reduced right ventricular systolic function. At right heart catheterization, pulmonary pressures were 22/9 (mean 15) mmHg . After careful discussion, he was referred for surgical intervention.

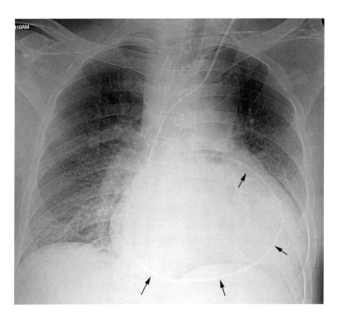

Fig 6-21. The preoperative chest radiograph shows the Swan-Ganz catheter (**arrows**) in the severely enlarged right heart.

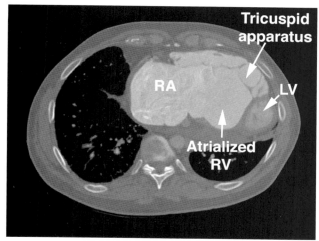

Fig 6-22. Chest CT demonstrated the enlarged right atrium (**RA**), the apically displaced tricuspid valve apparatus and the atrialized segment of the right ventricle (**RV**). For comparison, note the size of the left ventricle (**LV**).

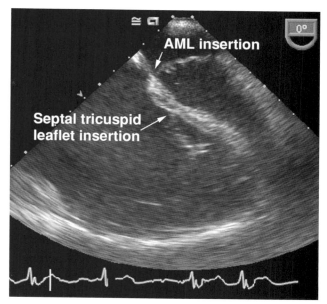

Fig 6-23. TEE imaging in a four-chamber view shows severe right heart enlargement with apical displacement of the septal leaflet of the tricuspid valve, compared with the anterior mitral leaflet (**AML**).

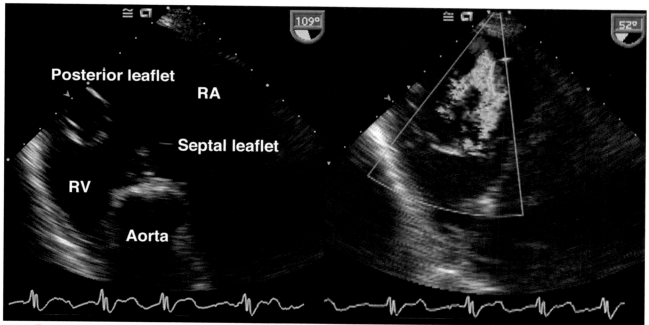

Fig 6-24. From a transgastric view, a long-axis view of the right heart shows the apically displaced tricuspid valve leaflets, with color flow indicating at least moderate tricuspid regurgitation.

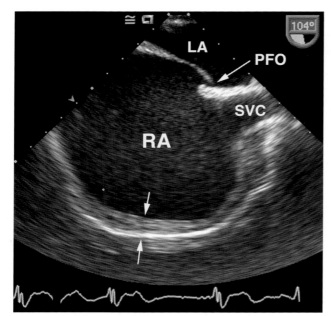

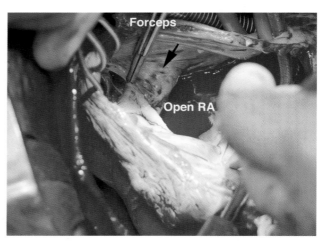

Fig 6-27. At surgery, the atrialized segment of the right ventricle is seen (**arrow**) with ventricular trabeculation on the atrial side of the tricuspid valve. The forceps are seen grasping a tricuspid leaflet.

Fig 6-25. The TEE right atrial view shows the increased thickness of the right atrial wall (**arrows**) and a patent foramen ovale (**PFO**) in the atrial septum.

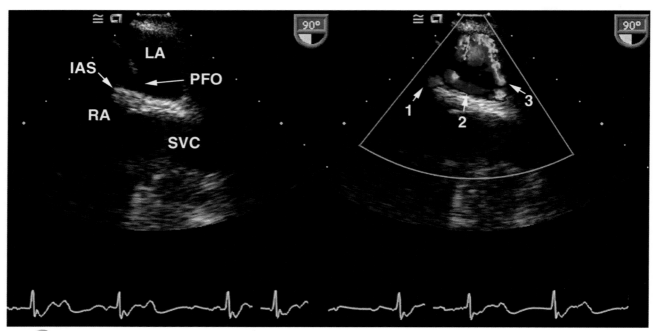

DVD **Fig 6-26.** Color flow through the PFO is demonstrated. **Arrow 1** indicates flow going from the right atrium through the defect and into the left atrium (red); **arrow 2** indicates flow hugging the left atrial side of the interatrial septum (**IAS**) (blue); **arrow 3** indicates flow heading towards the dome of the left atrium (red and aliased).

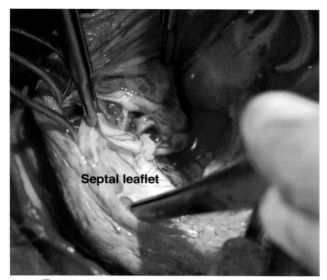

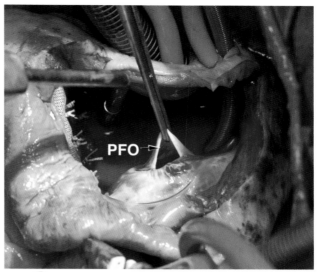

DVD **Fig 6-28.** The elongated, apically displaced septal leaflet of the tricuspid valve.

DVD **Fig 6-29.** The patent foramen ovale can be stretched easily, as shown.

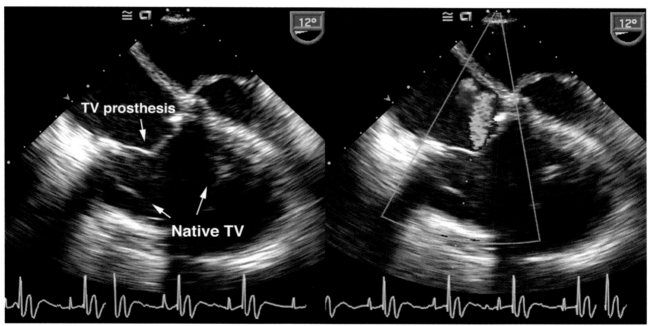

DVD **Fig 6-30.** After tricuspid valve replacement and PFO closure, the prosthesis is seen at the annulus level with residual native valve leaflets apically (*left*). Color Doppler demonstrates a small amount of central regurgitation (*right*). There is no flow across the interatrial septum.

Comments

This patient tolerated severe tricuspid regurgitation due to Ebstein's anomaly for many years, without symptoms of heart failure. Eventually, volume overload resulted in right atrial enlargement with stretching of the patent foramen ovale. Right atrial pressure exceeded left atrial pressure (due to the tricuspid regurgitation), with consequent right-to-left shunting across the PFO and arterial oxygen desaturation.

Although repair of the tricuspid valve is often possible in pediatric patients, repair is less likely to be successful in adult patients due to fibrosis of the valve structures and adherence of the apically displaced leaflets to the underlying ventricular wall.

Suggested Reading

1. Frescura C, Angelini A, Daliento L et al. Morphological aspects of Ebstein's anomaly in adults. Thorac Cardiovasc Surg 2000; 48:203–8.

Case 6-5
Tricuspid Valve Prolapse

This 33-year-old man with myxomatous mitral valve disease and a partial flail posterior leaflet with severe mitral regurgitation was referred for mitral valve repair.

The tricuspid valve was evaluated intraoperatively because of the concern for myxomatous involvement of the tricuspid valve.

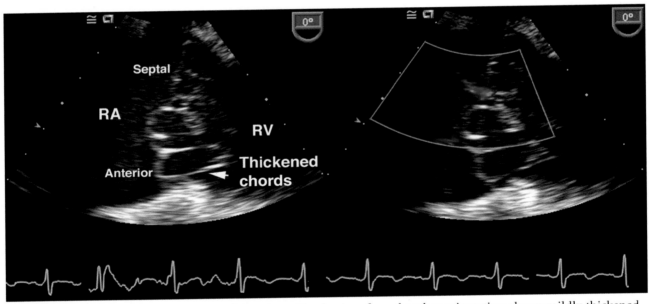

Fig 6-31. The low TEE view of the tricuspid valve in a four-chamber orientation shows mildly thickened, redundant leaflets with prolapse of the anterior and septal leaflets and prominent thickened chords. Color Doppler (*right*) demonstrates only a small jet of regurgitation.

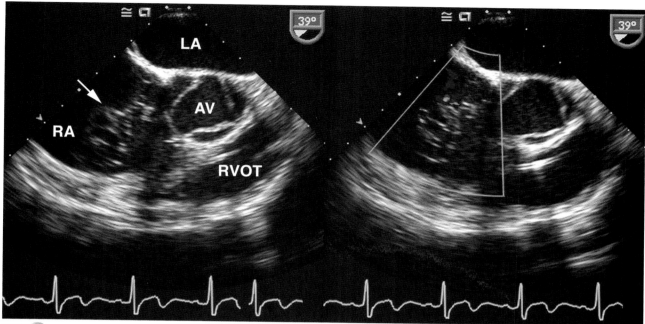

Fig 6-32. With the image plane rotated to 39 degrees, the redundant tricuspid valve leaflets are seen (**arrow**) in an orientation similar to a transthoracic short-axis view at the aortic valve level. Again, only mild regurgitation is demonstrated.

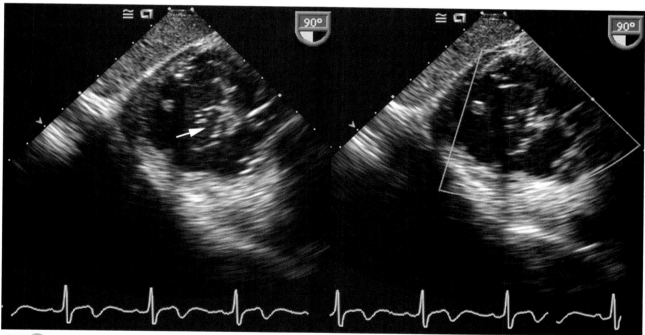

Fig 6-33. A transgastric short-axis view of the tricuspid leaflets (**arrow**) again shows the redundant valve.

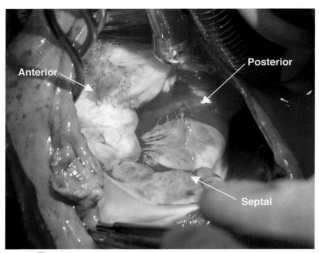

DVD **Fig 6-34.** Intraoperative inspection of the valve demonstrates the myxomatous appearance of the valve leaflets with redundancy and prolapse of all three leaflets.

Comments

Myxomatous valve disease most often affects the mitral valve, but other valves can also be affected. In patients with mitral valve prolapse, about one-third have tricuspid valve prolapse, although valve dysfunction is often only mild. The pulmonic valve can also occasionally be affected in patients with mitral valve prolapse.

Suggested Reading

1. Waller BF, Howard J, Fess S. Pathology of tricuspid valve stenosis and pure tricuspid regurgitation. Clin Cardiol 1995: 18:225–30.

Case 6-6
Flail Tricuspid Valve Leaflet with Valve Replacement

This 68-year-old man presented with increased shortness of breath 35 years after endocardial cushion defect repair (ventricular septal defect closure and repair of a cleft mitral valve). He had a permanent atrial and ventricular pacer with previous implantation of a second ventricular lead due to lead malfunction. He was referred for tricuspid valve repair or replacement.

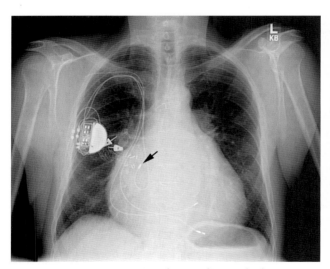

Fig 6-35. Posteroanterior chest radiograph shows three pacing leads, one with the tip in the right atrium (**arrow**) and two with the tips in the right ventricle. The cardiac silhouette is enlarged with evidence for right atrial and left atrial enlargement.

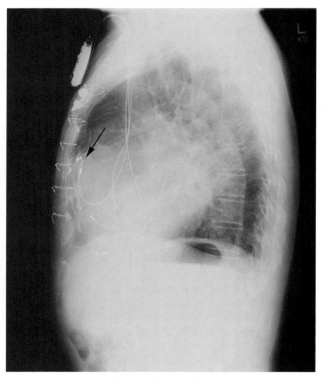

Fig 6-36. Lateral chest radiography shows cardiomegaly with right ventricular and left atrial enlargement. The pacing leads are again seen, with the right atrial lead indicated by the **arrow**.

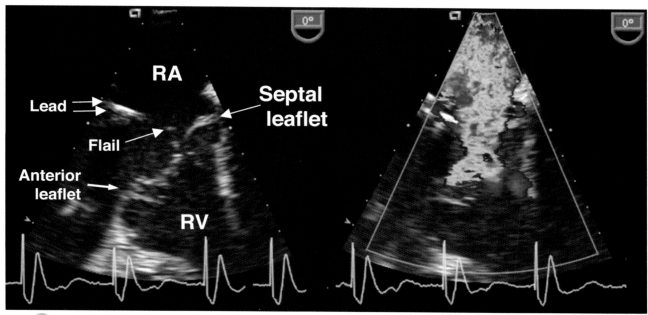

DVD **Fig 6-37.** In a low TEE view of the tricuspid valve, the anterior leaflet of the tricuspid valve shows a small area of flail leaflet, with prolapse into the right atrium in systole and independent motion. The flail segment is adjacent to one of the pacer leads, where it transverses the valve. Color Doppler (*right*) demonstrates a large area of regurgitation with a vena contracta of 10 mm.

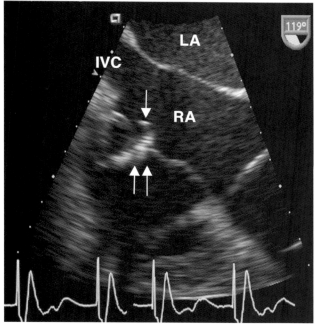

DVD **Fig 6-38.** Rotation of the image plane to 119 degrees to obtain a bicaval view provides another view of the flail segment of the tricuspid leaflet in systole (**arrows**).

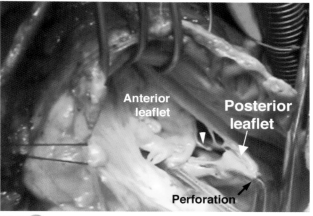

DVD **Fig 6-39.** Intraoperative inspection of the tricuspid valve showed that one of the pacer wires had perforated the valve leaflet (**arrow**). The pacer wire had also resulted in tethering of the posterior leaflet with impaired valve mobility. A torn chord of the anterior leaflet is seen (**arrowhead**).

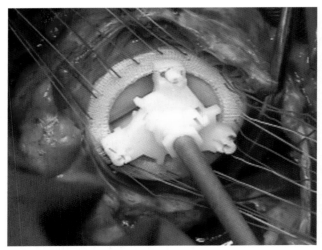

Fig 6-40. A bioprosthetic tricuspid valve replacement was performed showing positioning of the valve with placement of the periannular sutures.

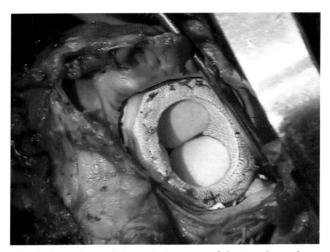

Fig 6-41. View of the atrial aspect of the implanted bioprosthetic valve.

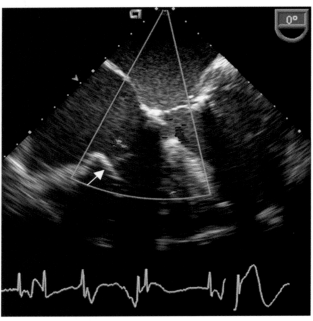

Fig 6-42. After weaning from cardiopulmonary bypass, the tricuspid valve prosthesis (**arrow**) was imaged in the four-chamber view, showing normal leaflet motion and no significant regurgitation.

with only mild or moderate disease. Measurement of vena contracta width is the most accurate approach; a vena contracta width >0.7 cm has a sensitivity of 89% and specificity of 93% for detection of severe regurgitation. Of course, as with left-sided regurgitation, evaluation in the operating room may underestimate severity compared to when the patient is awake and active. The density of the CW Doppler curve, relative to antegrade flow, and the presence of holosystolic flow reversal in the hepatic veins are other useful measures of tricuspid regurgitant severity.

Comments

Pacer wires traversing the tricuspid valve rarely result in significant valve dysfunction although cases of pacer lead-associated thrombus interfering with valve closure have been reported. Trauma to the tricuspid valve from repeated endomyocardial biopsies in post-transplant patients has also been reported.

Evaluation of tricuspid regurgitant severity can be difficult, as jet areas often appear relatively large, even

Suggested Reading

1. Ellenbogen KA, Hellkamp AS, Wilkoff BL et al. Complications arising after implantation of DDD pacemakers: the MOST experience. Am J Cardiol 2003; 92:740–1.

2. Leibowitz DW, Rosenheck S, Pollak A et al. Transvenous pacemaker leads do not worsen tricuspid regurgitation: a prospective echocardiographic study. Cardiology 2000; 93:74–7.

3. Messika-Zeitoun D, Thomson H, Bellamy M et al. Medical and surgical outcome of tricuspid regurgitation caused by flail leaflets. J Thorac Cardioavasc Surg 2004; 128: 196–302.

Case 6-7
Carcinoid Valve Disease

This 26-year-old woman had a carcinoid tumor originating in the small intestine with metastases to the liver and peritoneum. She was referred to cardiac surgery for tricuspid and pulmonic valve replacement.

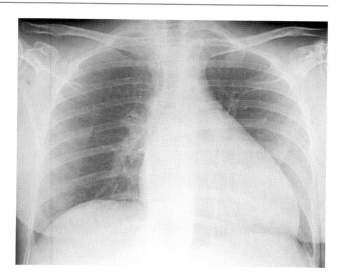

Fig 6-43. Posteroanterior chest radiograph shows cardiomegaly without evidence for pulmonary edema.

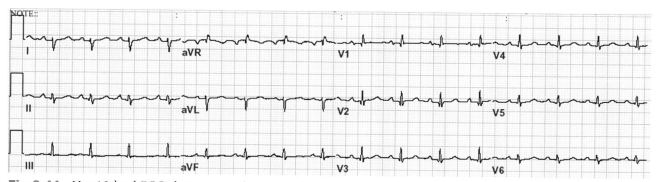

Fig 6-44. Her 12-lead ECG shows normal sinus rhythm with right axis deviation and diffusely low voltage.

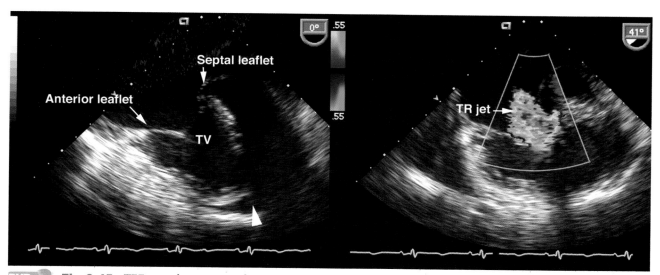

DVD **Fig 6-45.** TEE at 0 degrees in a four-chamber orientation demonstrates marked thickening and retraction of the tricuspid valve leaflets. Color Doppler at 40 degrees rotation (*right*) shows a very broad jet of tricuspid regurgitation (**TR**) with a vena contracta width of 20 mm due to reduced mobility of the shortened valve leaflets. A small pericardial effusion is also seen (**arrowhead**).

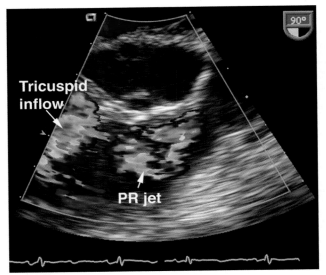

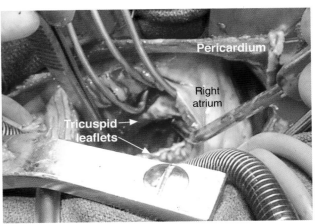

Fig 6-48. Intraoperative view of the tricuspid valve shows the thickened and retracted leaflets.

DVD ▶ **Fig 6-46.** Rotation to 90 degrees with lateral turning of the probe shows both the tricuspid inflow and pulmonic regurgitation (**PR**) signals in diastole.

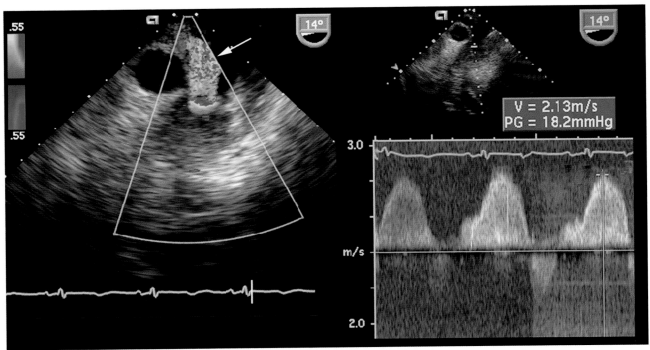

DVD ▶ **Fig 6-47.** From a high TEE view of the pulmonary artery looking down towards the pulmonic valve, the antegrade flow through the pulmonic valve (**arrow**) is seen on color Doppler (*left*) and continuous wave Doppler (*right*). The maximum velocity (**V**) is 2.1 m/s, which is consistent with mild stenosis. PG = pressure gradient.

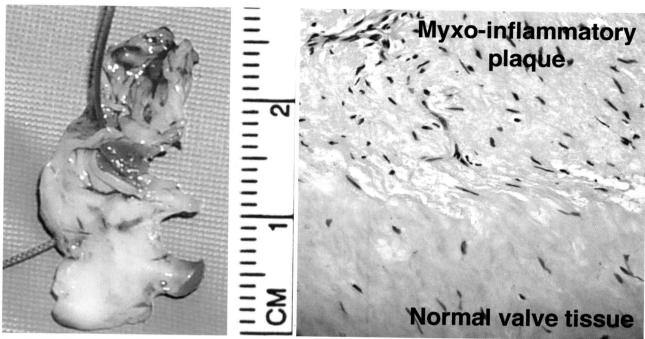

Fig 6-49. The explanted tricuspid valve with diffuse thickening and shortening of the leaflets. The histologic section in the right-hand panel demonstrates normal tricuspid valve tissue with superficial plaques of myxo-inflammatory material consistent with carcinoid heart disease.

Comments

Carcinoid valve disease is rare, but has a pathognomonic appearance on echocardiography with thickening, shortening and retraction of the tricuspid valve leaflets. Carcinoid valve disease is seen in patients with carcinoid tumor metastatic to the liver and is thought to be due to elevated levels of vasoactive substances such as serotonin (5-hydroxytryptamine), 5-hydroxytryptophan, histamine, bradykinin, tachykinins and prostaglandin. With cardiac involvement, over 90% have severe tricuspid regurgitation and most also have pulmonic valve involvement with combined stenosis and regurgitation. Left-sided involvement is unusual and is typically associated with a patent foramen ovale or lung metastases, as otherwise the vasoactive agents are inactivated in the lungs.

Suggested Reading

1. Pellikka PA, Tajik AJ, Khandheria BK et al. Carcinoid heart disease. Clinical and echocardiographic spectrum in 74 patients. Circulation 1993; 87:1188–96.

2. Robiolio PA, Rigolin VH, Wilson JS et al. Carcinoid heart disease. Correlation of high serotonin levels with valvular abnormalities detected by cardiac catheterization and echocardiography. Circulation 1995; 92:790.

3. Denney WD, Kemp WE Jr, Anthony LB et al. Echocardiographic and biochemical evaluation of the development and progression of carcinoid heart disease. J Am Coll Cardiol 1998; 32:1017.

4. Moller JE, Connolly HM, Rubin J et al. Factors associated with progression of carcinoid heart disease. N Engl J Med 2003; 348:1005.

Case 6-8
Pulmonic Valve Mass

This 73-year-old woman was referred for closure of a sinus venosus septal defect and a tricuspid valve annuloplasty for symptoms of congestive heart failure with progressive right ventricular dilation and tricuspid regurgitation.

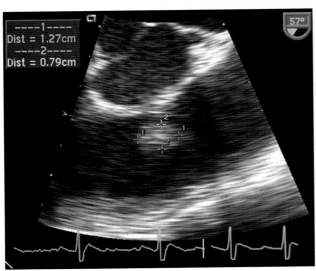

DVD **Fig 6-50.** An incidental finding on intraoperative TEE was a mass in the region of the pulmonic valve measuring 1.3 × 0.8 cm in diameter.

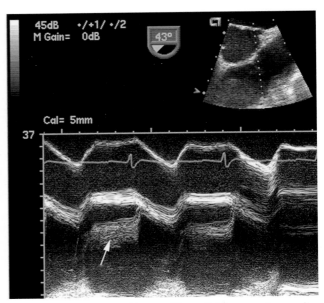

Fig 6-51. An M-mode recording of this mass (**arrow**) shows motion that parallels the motion of the pulmonic valve.

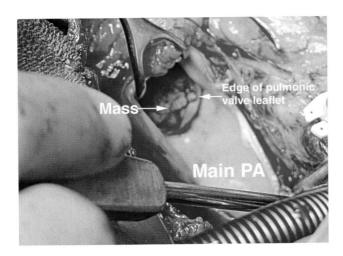

DVD **Fig 6-52.** Surgical inspection of the pulmonic valve showed a discrete mass on the leaflet that was carefully excised without damage to the valve leaflet.

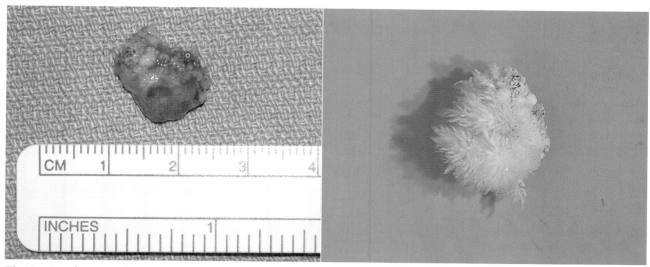

Fig 6-53. The excised mass on histologic examination was consistent with a papillary fibroelastoma (*left*). Often the frond-like in-vivo appearance of these tumors can only be demonstrated on the excised tissue by suspending the mass in water (*right*).

Comments

The differential diagnosis of a mass of the pulmonic valve includes a valvular vegetation, a thrombus or a tumor. The most common valve tumor is a benign papillary fibroelastoma. Although more often seen on left-sided valves, about 8% of papillary fibroelastomas are located on the pulmonic valve. The prevalence of papillary fibroelastomas increases with age and many are found as incidental findings in patients undergoing echocardiography for other indications. (see Chapter 11).

Suggested Reading

1. Gowda RM, Khan IA, Nair CK et al. Cardiac papillary fibroelastoma: a comprehensive analysis of 725 cases. Am Heart J 2003; 146:404–10.

2. Odim J, Reehal V, Laks H et al. Surgical pathology of cardiac tumors. Two decades at an urban institution. Cardiovasc Pathol 2003; 12:267–70.

Case 6-9
Subpulmonic Stenosis

This 24-year-old woman with Down's syndrome presented with a loud systolic murmur and mild functional impairment. She had undergone ventricular septal defect repair at age 4 years. On examination she had a 4/6 systolic ejection murmur at the upper left sternal border and a right ventricular heave. Echocardiography showed severe subpulmonic stenosis, which was confirmed by catheterization, and she was referred for surgical intervention.

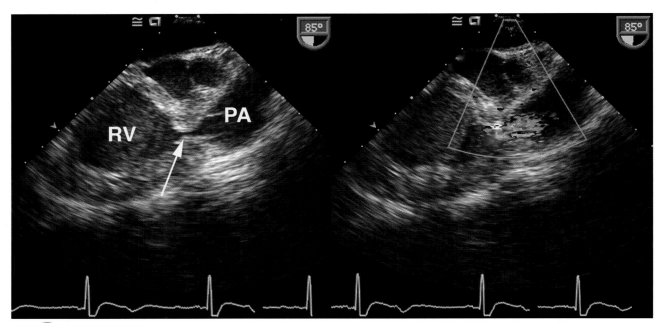

DVD **Fig 6-54.** In the RVOT view, from a high TEE probe position with the transducer rotated to 85 degrees (*left*), right ventricular hypertrophy and a narrowed RVOT are seen (*left*). Color Doppler *(right)* demonstrates evidence for an increased velocity; however, the intercept angle does not allow accurate recording of blood flow velocity from this view.

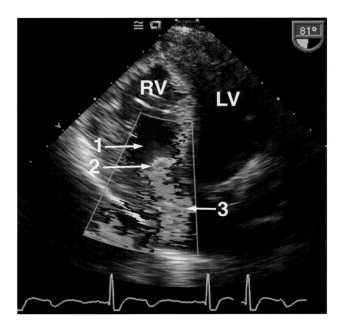

DVD **Fig 6-55.** In a transgastric apical view, the enlarged and hypertrophied right ventricle is seen. The color flow shows an increase in velocity from the uniform low-velocity flow in the ventricular chamber (**1**), with the increase in velocity at the stenotic area proximal to the pulmonic valve (**2**), and the flow disturbance in the pulmonary artery (**3**).

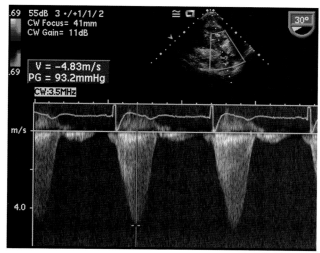

Fig 6-56. CW Doppler of right ventricular outflow from a transgastric view shows a velocity of at least 4.8 m/s, corresponding to a maximum pressure gradient of 93 mmHg. Although this may represent an underestimation of the pressure gradient, if the intercept angle between the ultrasound beam and jet is not parallel, it is still consistent with severe stenosis.

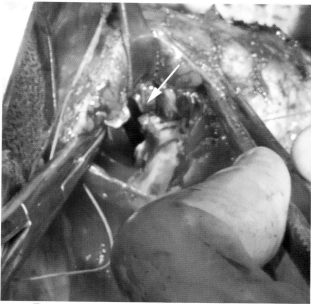

DVD **Fig 6-58.** With the RVOT opened longitudinally, the muscular subvalvular obstruction is seen (**arrow**).

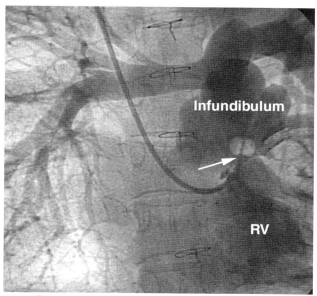

DVD **Fig 6-57.** Angiography demonstrated a trabeculated right ventricle with a subvalvular obstruction (**arrow**) and a large infundibular chamber.

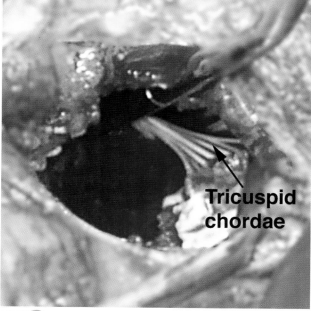

DVD **Fig 6-59.** After resection of the subvalvular muscular tissue, the tricuspid valve is seen through the enlarged outflow tract.

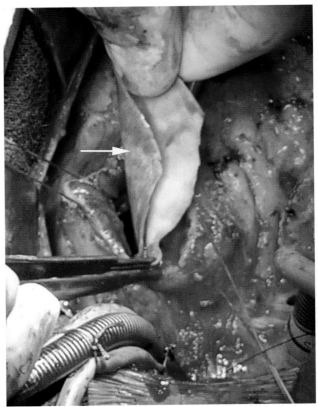

DVD **Fig 6-60.** An oval pericardial patch (**arrow**) was used to further enlarge the outflow tract.

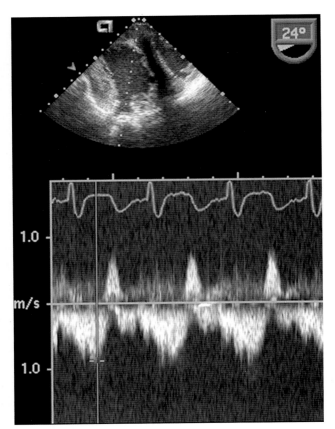

Fig 6-61. After the procedure, the maximum velocity in the RVOT is 0.9 m/s, using the same view as preoperatively (see **Fig 6-56**) at a similar blood pressure, although heart rate has increased.

Comments

Pulmonic stenosis is usually congenital, often in association with other cardiac abnormalities, and can be localized to the subvalvular, valvular or supra-valvular level. Most patients with significant pulmonic stenosis are diagnosed and treated in childhood. Some adults with mild isolated pulmonic stenosis are seen, but it is rare for severe stenosis to be diagnosed in an adult. Stenosis at the valve level may be amenable to percutaneous interventions, whereas muscular sub-valvular obstruction, as in this case, continues to require an open surgical approach.

The pulmonic valve and RVOT can be challenging to image by TEE due to the normal anterior location of the valve. However, with a careful and diligent search, diagnostic images can often be obtained. Usually the severity of stenosis will have been evaluated prior to surgery. If confirmation of stenosis severity is needed, a reasonably parallel intercept angle can often be obtained from a very high transesophageal position "looking" straight towards the pulmonic valve from the pulmonary artery bifurcation. The transgastric view, as in this case, may also provide a parallel intercept angle.

Suggested Reading

1. Almeda FQ, Kavinsky CJ, Pophal SG, Klein LW. Pulmonic valvular stenosis in adults: diagnosis and treatment. Catheter Cardiovasc Interv 2003; 60:546–57.

Case 6-10
Severe Pulmonic Regurgitation

This 26-year-old man had undergone surgical repair for tetralogy of Fallot as a child, with closure of a ventricular septal defect and pulmonary valvotomy. He presented now with increasing shortness of breath and atrial flutter. Echocardiography showed severe pulmonic regurgitation with severe right ventricular enlargement but only mildly reduced right ventricular systolic function. Pulmonary pressures were normal by echocardiography and at catheterization, with no evidence of branch pulmonary stenosis. He was referred for pulmonary valve replacement.

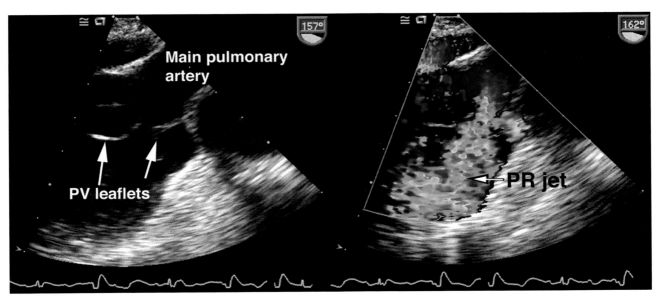

Fig 6-62. A high TEE view of the pulmonic valve in long axis with the image plane rotated to 157 degrees shows the pulmonic valve (**PV**) leaflets with severe thinning and prolapse of one leaflet (*left*). Color flow shows severe pulmonic regurgitation with the regurgitant jet nearly filling the RVOT.

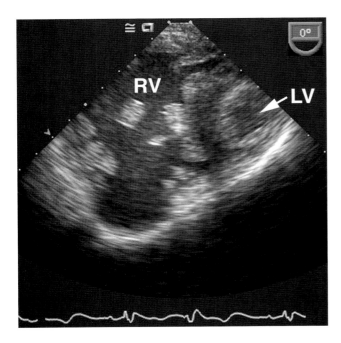

Fig 6-63. A transgastric view demonstrated the severe right ventricular dilation. Although pulmonary pressures were normal, the right ventricular wall appears hypertrophied. Notice the relatively much smaller left ventricle.

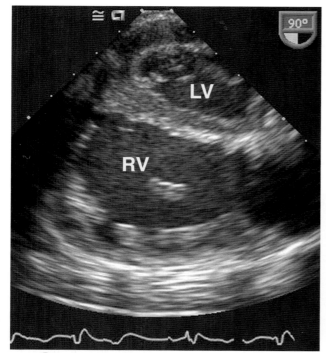

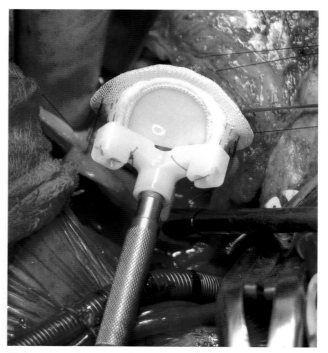

DVD **Fig 6-64.** This 90-degree basal transgastric image looks more like 0 degrees because of the abnormal orientation of the heart; this latter phenomenon is related to the mismatch in right and left chamber sizes. Right ventricular hypertrophy is again noted. On the DVD, paradoxical motion of the interventricular septum and septal diastolic flattening related to right ventricular volume overload are seen.

Fig 6-65. The stented tissue prosthetic valve is prepared for implantation.

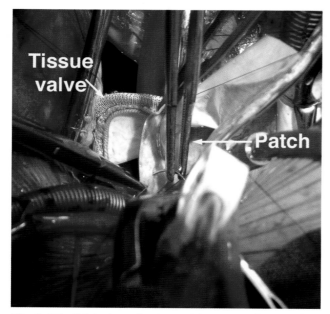

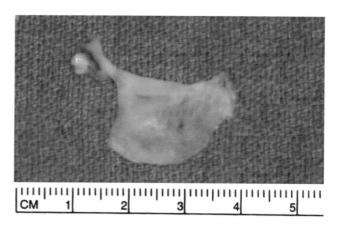

DVD **Fig 6-67.** The excised valve leaflet is dysmorphic and thin. Only one leaflet was identified. Of the other two leaflets, only blighted remnants were seen.

Fig 6-66. With the valve in position, a patch is used to enlarge the pulmonic annulus.

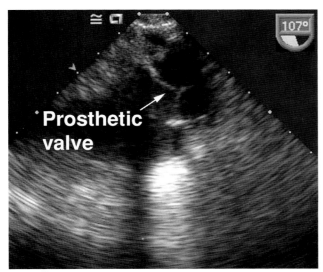

DVD **Fig 6-68.** The tissue prosthetic valve on TEE images after the procedure shows thin leaflets with normal motion. There was no regurgitation.

Comments

Pulmonic regurgitation late after repair of tetralogy of Fallot is common, with moderate-to-severe regurgitation in up to 50% of patients. The consequent right ventricular volume overload results in progressive right ventricular enlargement and eventual systolic dysfunction. However, evaluation of the severity of pulmonic regurgitation can be problematic. The width of the diastolic flow stream by color Doppler is helpful, with a narrow jet consistent with mild regurgitation and a jet that fills the RVOT consistent with severe regurgitation. Because the velocity of pulmonic regurgitation is low, when pulmonary pressures are normal, regurgitation may be missed by color Doppler unless the examiner is aware of this possibility. Other helpful parameters are the intensity of the continuous wave Doppler regurgitant signal, relative to antegrade flow, and the slope (or pressure half-time) of the diastolic signal. Holodiastolic flow reversal in the main pulmonary artery, due to severe pulmonic regurgitation, should be distinguished from diastolic flow due to patent ductus arteriosus.

Suggested Reading

1. Silversides CK, Veldtman GR, Crossin J et al. Pressure half-time predicts hemodynamically significant pulmonary regurgitation in adult patients with repaired tetralogy of Fallot. J Am Soc Echocardiogr 2003; 16:1057–62.

2. Li W, Davlouros PA, Kilner PJ et al. Doppler-echocardiographic assessment of pulmonary regurgitation in adults with repaired tetralogy of Fallot: comparison with cardiovascular magnetic resonance imaging. Am Heart J 2004; 147:165–72.

7

Adult Congenital Heart Disease

Atrial Septal Defects

Case 7-1
Patent Foramen Ovale

Intraoperative transesophageal echocardiography (TEE) in a patient undergoing coronary artery bypass grafting demonstrated a patent foramen ovale (PFO).

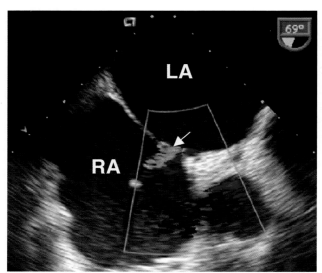

DVD ▶ Fig 7-1. A view of the left atrium (**LA**) and right atrium (**RA**) from a high esophageal position at 69 degrees rotation demonstrates the PFO at the limbus of the fossa ovalis with color Doppler showing a small jet of flow from left to right (**arrow**).

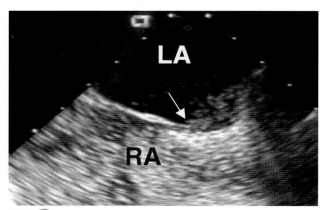

DVD ▶ Fig 7-2. Injection of agitated saline in a peripheral vein opacifies the right heart due to the effect of microbubbles. The microbubbles in hand-agitated saline do not pass through the pulmonary capillaries, leaving the left heart unopacified in the absence of an intracardiac shunt. In this case, a magnified image at about 70 degrees rotation shows the passage of contrast from right to left across the patent foramen ovale (**arrow**).

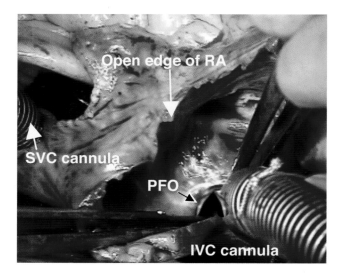

Fig 7-3. An intraoperative view, with the right atrium (**RA**) opened, demonstrated the PFO in the interatrial septum.

Comments

A PFO can be demonstrated on TEE in 20–25% of adults. The PFO typically is best seen from a high esophageal view of the atrial septum, with the transducer rotated between 60 and 90 degrees. The PFO is seen at the junction of the secundum septum (covering the fossa ovalis) and the primum septum. In most patients the PFO is small and functions as a "flap valve," with no flow across the septum when atrial pressures are low and left atrial pressure is slightly higher than right atrial pressure. With a transient elevation in right atrial pressure, for example with Valsalva maneuver, the flap valve opens and blood can flow from right to left. With chronic elevation in atrial pressure, the PFO may become stretched with a defect between the right and left atrium allowing flow, even at rest. A small PFO is typically a benign incidental finding without associated clinical symptoms or signs.

However, there is an association between the presence of a PFO and cryptogenic stroke, with studies in progress testing the hypothesis that closing the PFO will decrease the risk of recurrent stroke.

Suggested Reading

1. Stewart MJ. Contrast echocardiography. Heart 2003; 89:342–48.

2. Hara H, Virmani R, Ladich E et al. Patent foramen ovale: current pathology, pathophysiology, and clinical status. J Am Coll Cardiol 2005; 46:1768–76.

3. Woods TD, Patel A. A critical review of patent foramen ovale detection using saline contrast echocardiography: when bubbles lie. J Am Soc Echocardiogr 2006; 19:215–22.

4. Homma S, Sacco RL. Patent foramen ovale and stroke. Circulation 2005; 112:1063–72.

5. Meier B, Lock JE. Contemporary management of patent foramen ovale. Circulation 2003; 107:5–9.

Case 7-2
Atrial Septal Aneurysm

This 48-year-old woman with recurrent neurologic events was found to have an atrial septal aneurysm with evidence of right-to-left shunting on intracardiac echocardiography with agitated saline used for right heart contrast.

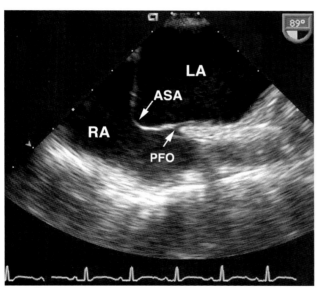

Fig 7-4. In a high TEE view at about 90 degree of rotation the bulging of the atrial septum into the RA is seen. The curvature of the atrial septum exceeds 1.5 cm and persists in both systole and diastole, consistent with the diagnosis of an atrial septal aneurysm (**ASA**). There also is a small patent foramen ovale.

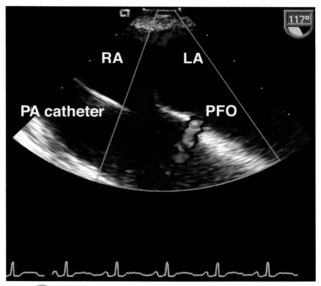

Fig 7-5. Color Doppler demonstrates left-to-right flow across the PFO.

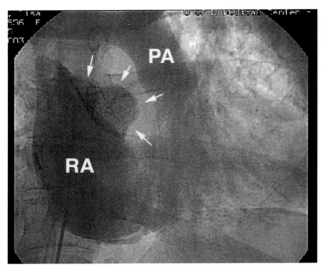

DVD **Fig 7-6.** Right atrial angiography shows the opacified right atrium with the septum bulging into the left atrium. With the elevation of right atrial pressure during the angiogram, the septal curvature reverses (**arrows**) (see **Fig 7-4**).

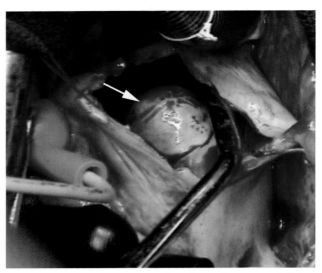

Fig 7-7. An intraoperative view from the opened right atrium shows the central septum (**arrow**) bulging into the right atrium (see DVD for Fig 7-8).

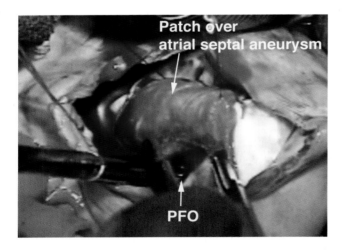

DVD **Fig 7-8.** At surgery, with the right atrium open, the large atrial septal aneurysm and small atrial septal defect were plicated and closed using a pericardial patch.

Comments

In addition to a PFO, this patient has an atrial septal aneurysm, defined as transient bulging of the fossa ovalis region greater than 1.5 cm in the absence of chronically elevated left or right atrial pressures. The presence of an atrial septal aneurysm is associated with a higher risk of embolic stroke than a PFO alone, most likely related to the high (>90%) prevalence of fenestrations of the septum in patients with a septal aneurysm. In patients with recurrent neurologic events despite adequate medical therapy, PFO closure is recommended, either surgically or using a percutaneously inserted closure device.

Suggested Reading

1. Kerut EK, Norfleet WT, Plotnick GD et al. Patent foramen ovale: a review of associated conditions and the impact of physiological size. J Am Coll Cardiol 2001; 38:613–23.

Case 7-3
Secundum Atrial Septal Defect

This 50-year-old man presented with increasing shortness of breath on exertion. After a negative pulmonary evaluation, he underwent echocardiography that demonstrated a secundum atrial septal defect (ASD).

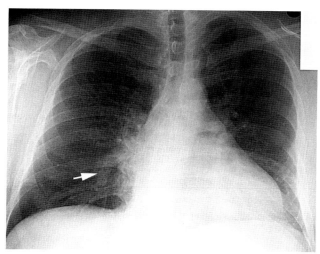

Fig 7-9. The PA chest radiograph shows cardiomegaly with prominent right atrial border and enlarged right pulmonary artery (**arrow**).

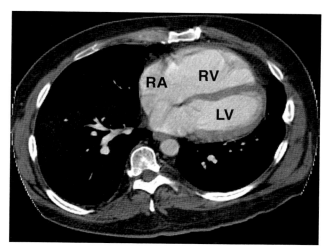

Fig 7-11. Chest CT demonstrates severe right ventricular and right atrial enlargement.

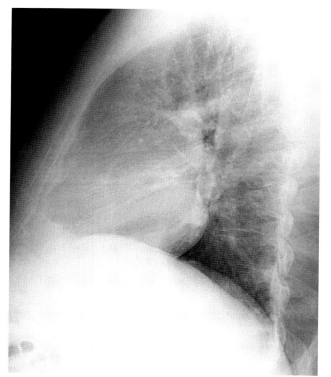

Fig 7-10. On the lateral chest radiograph, the right ventricular enlargement is evident with opacification of the retrosternal space by the enlarged right ventricle.

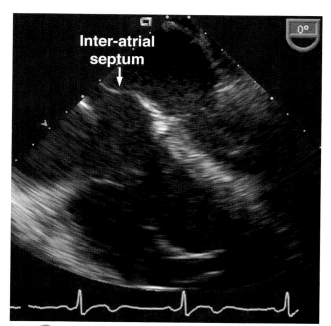

Fig 7-12. The TEE four-chamber view shows an enlarged right ventricle and atrium, although the atrial septum appears intact in this image plane.

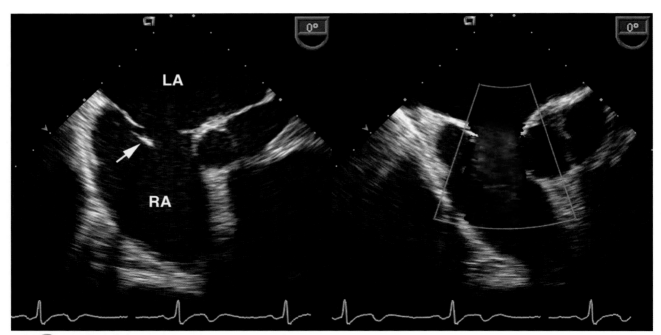

DVD **Fig 7-13.** Slight anteflexion of the probe, with the image plane now including the aortic valve, demonstrates the ASD with left-to-right flow and a defect diameter of 18 mm. The arrow indicates a pulmonary artery catheter in the right atrium.

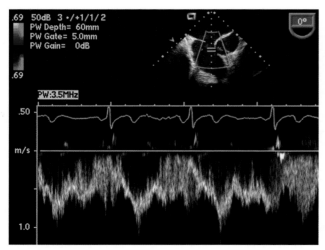

Fig 7-14. Pulsed Doppler confirms left-to-right flow in both systole and diastole.

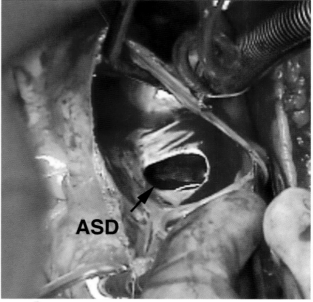

DVD **Fig 7-15.** Following sternotomy, the right atrial appendage was noted to be more red than usual, consistent with the shunting of oxygenated left atrial blood. Through an open right atrium, a 2 × 1 cm ASD was identified.

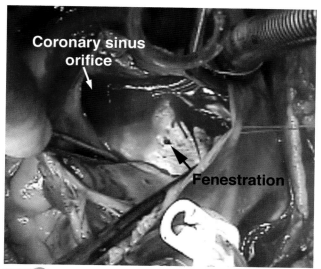

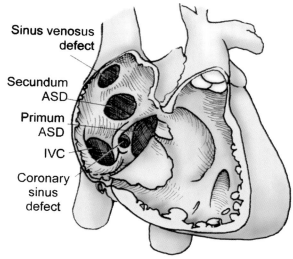

Fig 7-16. In addition, a smaller but separate defect was noted adjacent to the tendon of Todaro (at the origin of the coronary sinus).

Fig 7-18. This schematic shows the relative anatomy of the different kinds of ASD. (Reproduced with permission from Linker D. Practical Echocardiography of Congenital Heart Disease. Philadelphia: Churchill Livingstone, 2000. ©Elsevier Inc.)

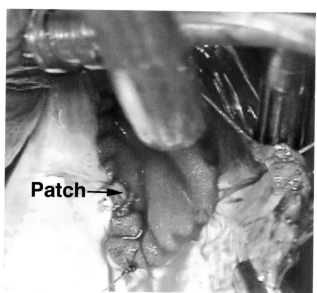

Fig 7-17. Both defects were closed with a single pericardial patch, with the postoperative image demonstrating the patch across the defect. The man had atrial flutter 5 days postoperatively and was easily cardioverted back into sinus rhythm. However, he subsequently had recurrent atrial flutter that was treated with radiofrequency catheter ablation of the caval tricuspid isthmus.

Comments

The most common type of atrial septal defect (ASD) is a secundum ASD, with the defect located centrally in the septum typically measuring ≥1 cm diameter.

Although most ASDs are diagnosed and treated in childhood, a substantial number are not recognized until young adulthood, with a few diagnosed only later in life, as in this case.

The TEE features of an atrial septal defect are the consequence of right-sided volume overload. Blood flows left to right across the atrial defect so that the right heart pumps a larger stroke volume than the left heart. The severity of shunting is measured as the pulmonary flow (Qp) to systemic flow (Qs) ratio, where 1 is normal. A Qp:Qs ratio >1.5:1 is associated with progressive right atrial and right ventricular enlargement. In addition, septal curvature is reversed with "paradoxical" septal motion. Pulmonary hypertension is unusual with a secundum ASD. TTE may demonstrate the atrial defect itself with color Doppler showing left-to-right flow. A contrast study can be performed when right heart enlargement is present and images of the atrial septum are suboptimal.

TEE provides better images of the interatrial septum and is helpful when percutaneous closure is planned, to measure the size of the defect and evaluate the rim of tissue that will anchor the device.

Suggested Reading

1. Brickner ME, Hillis LD, Lange RA. Congenital heart disease in adults. First of two parts. N Engl J Med 2000; 342:256–63.
2. Brickner ME, Hillis LD, Lange RA. Congenital heart disease in adults. Second of two parts. N Engl J Med 2000; 342:334–42.

Case 7-4
Primum Atrial Septal Defect

This 34-year-old asymptomatic woman was incidentally noted to have a murmur which prompted echocardiography. This study revealed a large primum ASD with left-to-right flow and a Qp:Qs of 2.5:1. In addition, a cleft anterior leaflet of the mitral valve with moderate mitral regurgitation was demonstrated.

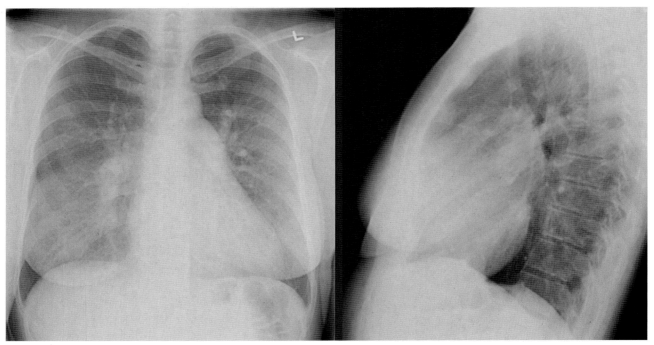

Fig 7-19. Chest radiography shows enlargement of the right and left atrium, right ventricle and pulmonary artery, with increased pulmonary blood flow.

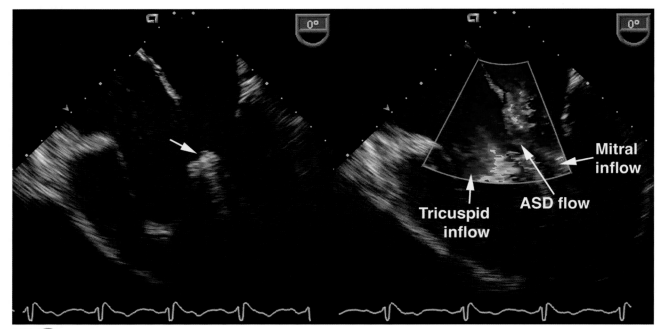

DVD **Fig 7-20.** In a four-chamber view in diastole on 2D (*left*) and color (*right*) the crest of the ventricle septum is seen (**arrow**) with the open tricuspid and mitral valve on either side. With the mitral and tricuspid valves open and the large atrial defect, all four cardiac chambers have equal pressures in diastole.

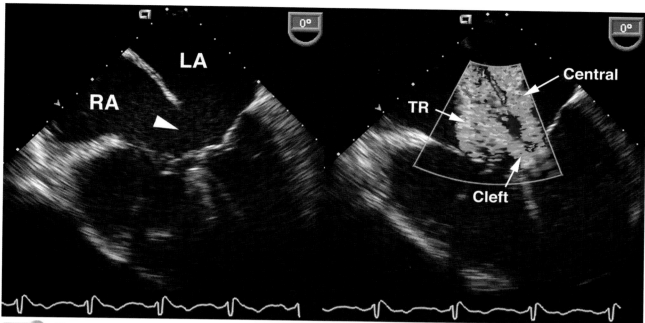

DVD **Fig 7-21.** In the same view in systole, the tricuspid and mitral valve are closed. The arrowhead indicates the ASD. Moderate-to-severe mitral regurgitation is seen, in part due to the cleft anterior mitral valve leaflet.

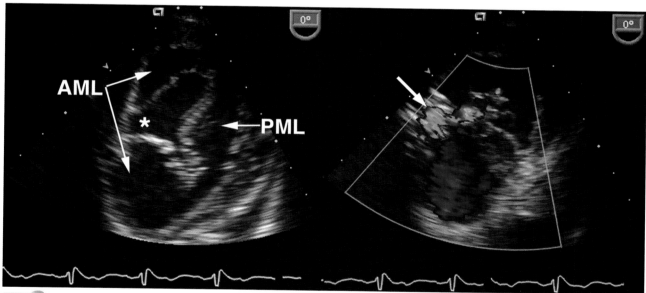

DVD **Fig 7-22.** A short-axis view of the mitral valve obtained with the probe retroflexed just distal to the gastroesophageal junction, demonstrates the cleft (**asterisk**) in the anterior mitral leaflet (**AML**). On the right, regurgitant flow is seen through the cleft (**arrow**).

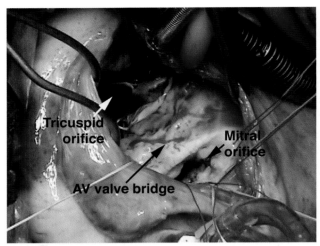

DVD ▶ **Fig 7-23.** At surgery, opening the right atrium reveals the absence of the primum septum, and the two atrioventricular (**AV**) valves.

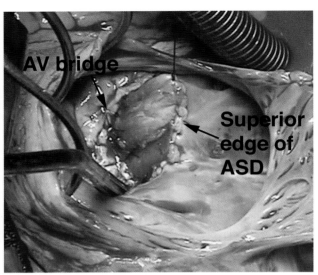

DVD ▶ **Fig 7-25.** At surgery, the ostium primum defect was closed with a pericardial patch.

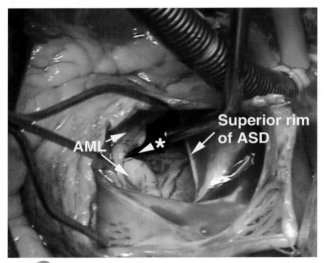

DVD ▶ **Fig 7-24.** The cleft in the anterior mitral leaflet is demonstrated (**asterisk**).

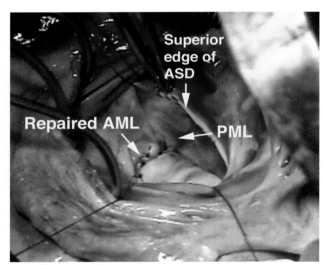

DVD ▶ **Fig 7-26.** The anterior mitral leaflet (**AML**) was repaired by suturing the cleft leaflet and placing a 30 mm annular ring.

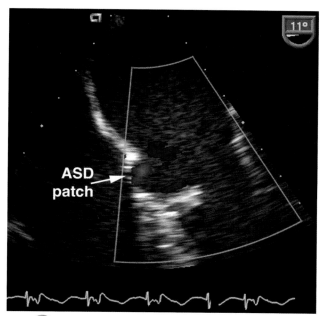

Fig 7-27. A post-procedure four-chamber view shows the ASD patch with no residual flow.

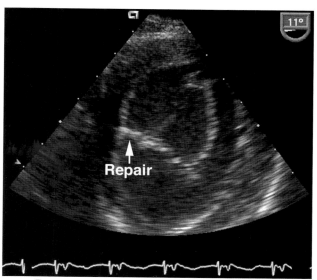

Fig 7-28. A post-procedure short-axis view of the mitral valve, in the same orientation as **Fig 7-22**, shows the repair of the cleft leaflet, with some residual central mitral regurgitation.

Comments

A primum ASD is seen in the base of the septum, adjacent to the atrioventricular valve plane and, in effect, is a partial atrioventricular canal defect. The defect is best seen in a four-chamber view, both on 2D imaging and with color Doppler. These defects are large, typically requiring surgical closure with placement of a patch. Many patients have associated abnormalities of the atrioventricular valve, most commonly a cleft anterior mitral valve leaflet. Some cleft leaflets can be repaired by approximation of the two segments, but others require replacement if the valve is deformed or if there is excessive tension when the segments are sutured together. The echocardiographer should also carefully evaluate for a ventricular septal defect (VSD) in patients with a primum ASD.

Suggested Reading

1. Masani ND. Transoesophageal echocardiography in adult congenital heart disease. Heart 2001; 86(Suppl 2):II30–40.

2. Randolph GR, Hagler DJ, Connolly HM et al. Intraoperative transesophageal echocardiography during surgery for congenital heart defects. J Thorac Cardiovasc Surg 2002; 124:1176–82.

Case 7-5
Sinus Venosus Atrial Septal Defect

This 34-year-old man presented with increasing fatigue, shortness of breath and palpitations. After an episode of atrial fibrillation, he underwent echocardiography which showed a probable ASD with moderate right ventricular and right atrial enlarge-ment. TEE demonstrated the anatomy of the sinus venosus defect, with a maximum diameter of 2.4 cm. Right heart catheterization showed normal right heart pressures with a Qp:Qs ratio of 2.5:1.

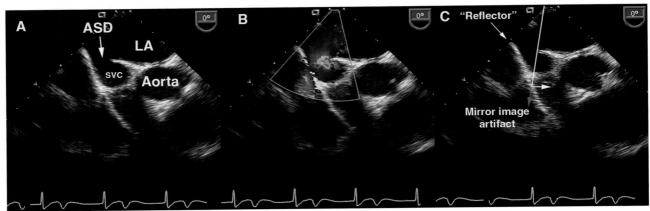

DVD **Fig 7-29.** From a high TEE position at 0 degrees, the communication (**arrow**, **ASD**) between the superior vena cava (**SVC**) and left atrium (**LA**) is seen (*A*). Color flow demonstrates low-velocity flow through this region (*B*). The strong reflective property of the lateral SVC border leads to a mirror image artefact (*C*). See Comment for explanation.

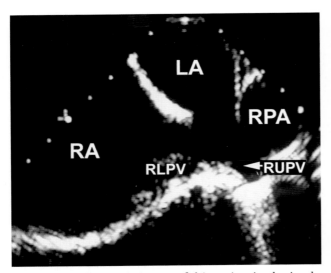

Fig 7-30. A long-axis image of this region is obtained by rotating the image plane to 117 degrees. The ASD between the left atrium (**LA**) and right atrium (**RA**) is seen in immediate proximity to the right upper pulmonary vein (**RUPV**) and right lower pulmonary vein (**RLPV**) which enters the atrium on the right side of the septum. The right pulmonary artery (**RPA**) is seen superiorly.

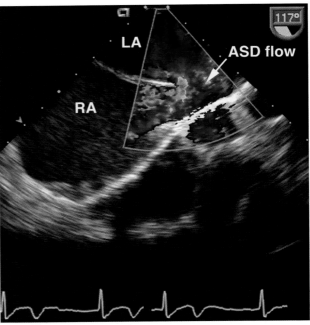

DVD **Fig 7-31.** Color flow demonstrates flow between the two atria at the superior aspect of the atrial septum.

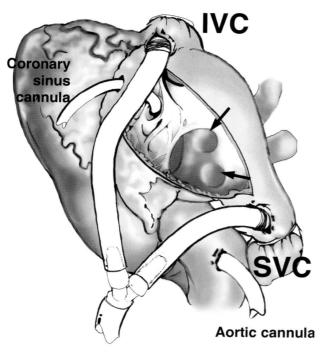

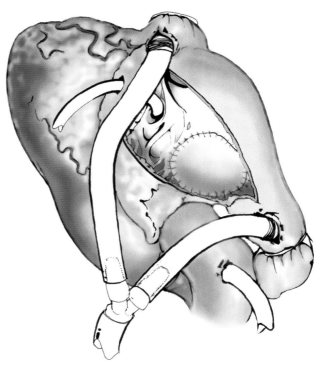

Fig 7-32. Schematic drawing of the surgical findings with the ASD straddling the right upper and lower pulmonary veins (**arrows**). Cannulas are present in the superior and inferior vena cava and in the ascending aorta for cardiopulmonary bypass. (Courtesy of Starr Kaplan.)

Fig 7-34. As shown in this schematic, the defect was closed using a double-patch repair technique, including repositioning the pulmonary venous drainage to the left side of the septum. (Courtesy of Starr Kaplan.)

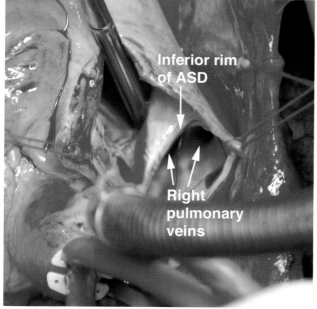

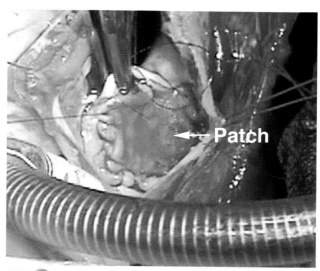

Fig 7-35. Intraoperative photograph of the patch repair of the ASD, corresponding to **Fig 7-34**.

Fig 7-33. Intraoperative photograph corresponding to **Fig 7-32**.

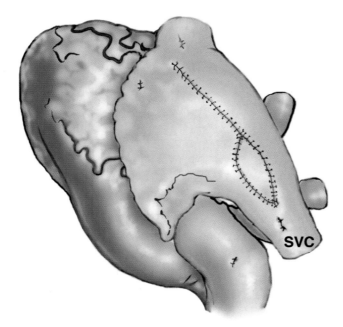

Fig 7-36. The heart is decannulated. The closure of the right atrium extends to include the distal part of the superior vena cava (**SVC**). (Courtesy of Starr Kaplan.)

Comments

Sinus venosus defects are most often located at the superior aspect of the atrial septum near the junction with the superior vena cava, although some are found near the junction of the inferior vena cava and right atrium. Diagnosis can be difficult on transthoracic echocardiography (TEE) because the atrial septum appears intact in most views. Often the diagnosis is suspected based on the presence of right heart enlargement and a positive contrast study, with the defect itself only visualized on TEE. Even with TEE imaging, these defects can be missed unless care is taken to examine the entire atrial septum, including the segments at the entrance of the superior and inferior vena cava. Sinus venous defects may be associated with anomalous entry of one or more pulmonary veins into the right atrium, as in this case. On TEE, the examiner should take time to identify all four pulmonary veins entering the left atrium.

In Fig 7-29C, emitted ultrasound strikes the lateral border of the SVC and is reflected to the right, thereby imaging part of the right atrium (white arrow). The red arrow shows the path the ultrasound would have taken, so that the portion of the right atrium is also artificially represented as a 'mirror image'.

Suggested Reading

1. Ettedgui JA, Siewers RD, Anderson RH et al. Diagnostic echocardiographic features of the sinus venosus defect. Br Heart J 1990; 64:329–31.

2. Kronzon I, Tunick PA, Freedberg RS et al. Transesophageal echocardiography is superior to transthoracic echocardiography in the diagnosis of sinus venosus atrial septal defect. J Am Coll Cardiol 1991; 17:537–42.

3. Kremkau FW, Taylor KJ. Artifacts in ultrasound imaging. J Ultrasound Med 1986; 5(4):227–37.

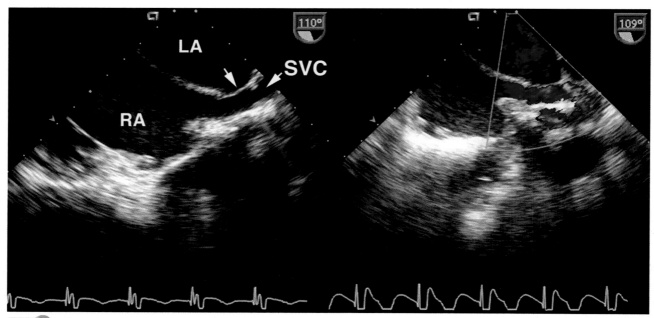

DVD **Fig 7-37.** A postoperative TEE image at 110 degrees shows the patch repair of the defect (**arrow**) with no residual interatrial flow (*right*) on color Doppler.

Ventricular Septal Defects

Case 7-6
Membranous (infracristal) VSD

This 41-year-old man with diabetes and hypertension had a known small VSD since childhood. After a scrape on his ankle became infected, he developed *Staphylococcus aureus* endocarditis with vegetations involving the right side of the VSD. His clinical course was complicated by septic shock, septic pulmonary emboli, adult respiratory distress syndrome and acute ST-elevation myocardial injury, with a normal coronary angiogram. He fully recovered and was referred for closure of the VSD.

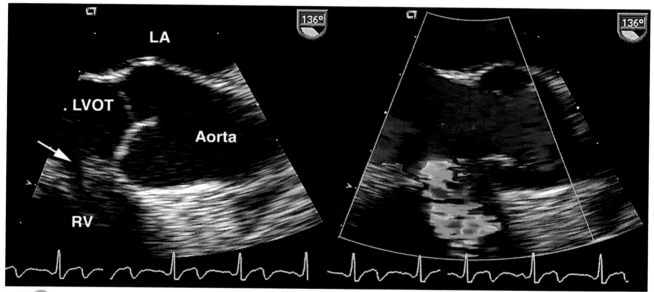

DVD **Fig 7-38.** In a long-axis view (at 135 degrees) of the left ventricular outflow tract (**LVOT**), apparent loss of continuity is seen in the region of the membranous ventricular septum (**arrow**). There is a mobile sock-like aneurysm on the right ventricular side.

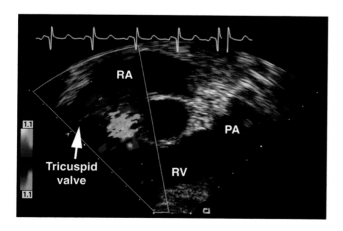

Fig 7-39. In a transthoracic study, reoriented to simulate a TEE orientation, the VSD flow is seen to enter the RV adjacent to the tricuspid valve.

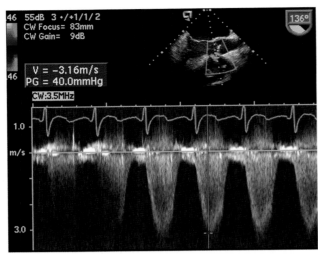

Fig 7-40. Continuous wave Doppler of this flow indicates a systolic ejection-type velocity of at least 3.2 m/s. This is consistent with flow from the left to the right ventricle (estimated pressure difference by Doppler of 40 mmHg), although the pressure difference may be underestimated due to a non-parallel intercept angle between the ultrasound beam and direction of blood flow.

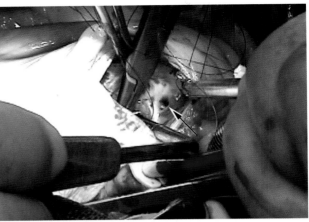

Fig 7-42. The VSD (**arrow**) was inspected first via an incision in the pulmonary artery. The defect was 8 mm in diameter, with no evidence of active infection.

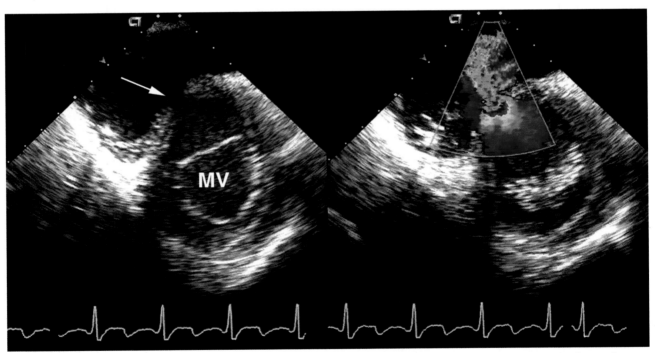

Fig 7-41. Epicardial images were acquired by the surgeon, with the ultrasound transducer in a sterile sleeve, for further evaluation of the anatomy of the defect. There is a discontinuity (**arrow**) in the septum just apical to the aortic valve (note the anterior mitral leaflet in this view) and color flow demonstrates left-to-right flow across this defect.

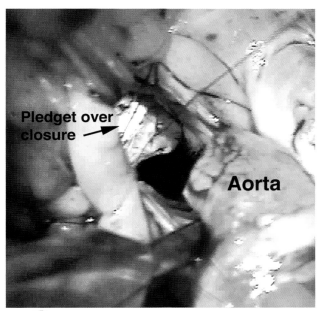

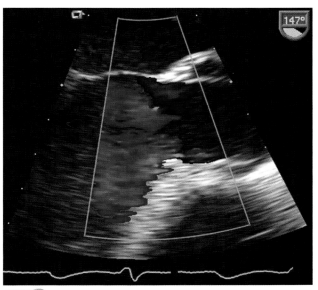

Fig 7-44. Post-procedure echocardiographic images showed no residual defect.

Fig 7-43. Next, an aortotomy was performed and the defect was visualized from the left side of the septum. Again, there was no evidence of active infection. Because of the small size of the defect, it was repaired with a primary closure.

Comments

In adults, a small membranous VSD is typically asymptomatic. Diagnosis is based on the presence of a loud systolic murmur, with echocardiographic confirmation of the diagnosis. Many membranous defects are partially closed by thin tissue, possibly related to the triscuspid valve apparatus, with an echocardiographic appearance described as a ventricular septal "aneurysm", even though this tissue is normal. Most small membranous VSDs are not closed, as these defects are well tolerated hemodynamically with no data to suggest adverse cardiovascular outcomes. However, patients with a VSD are at increased risk of endocarditis and should receive antibiotic prophylaxis. When endocarditis occurs, vegetations are typically located in the area of jet turbulence, on the right ventricular side of the defect and the tricuspid valve. Once endocarditis occurs, closure of the defect is often recommended to prevent recurrent infection.

Suggested Reading

1. Walpot J, Peerenboom P, van Wylick A et al. Aneurysm of the membranous septum with ventricular septal defect and infective endocarditis. Eur J Echocardiogr 2004; 5:391–3.
2. Neumayer U, Stone S, Somerville J. Small ventricular septal defects in adults. Eur Heart J 1998; 19:1573–82.
3. Yilmaz AT, Ozal E, Arslan M et al. Aneurysm of the membranous septum in adult patients with perimembranous ventricular septal defect. Eur J Cardiothorac Surg 1997; 11:307–11.

Case 7-7
Muscular VSD

This 32-week premature infant was noted to have a systolic murmur.

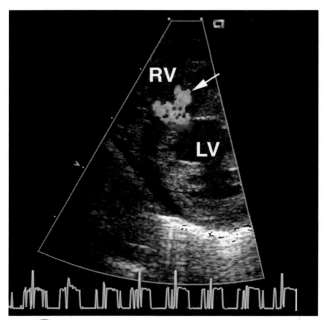

DVD ▶ **Fig 7-45.** Transthoracic short-axis view demonstrates a small VSD in the mid-segment of the septum with left-to-right flow in systole (**arrow**).

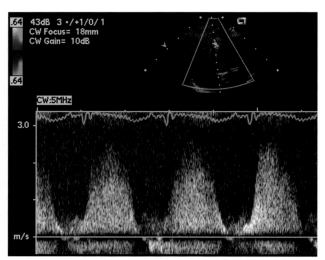

Fig 7-47. Continuous wave Doppler shows a high-velocity signal, although the maximum velocity is probably underestimated due to a non-parallel intercept angle.

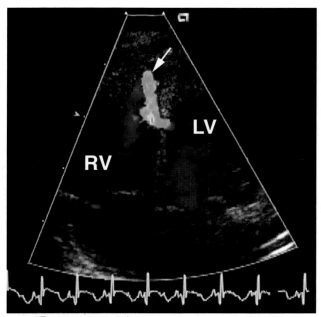

DVD ▶ **Fig 7-46.** In a four-chamber transthoracic view, the VSD is again seen, with a localized area of left-to-right flow (**arrow**).

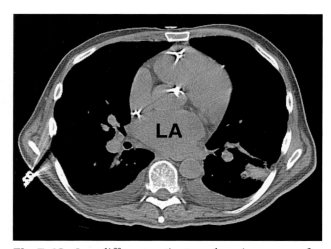

Fig 7-48. In a different patient, undergoing surgery for aortic stenosis, preoperative CT showed a large left atrium.

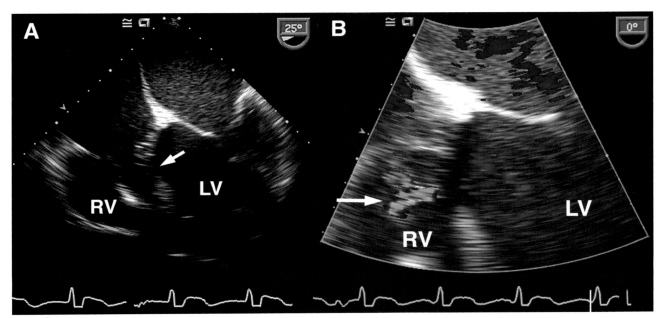

DVD **Fig 7-49.** In this patient, a small muscular VSD was found on 2D imaging (*A*, **arrow**), confirmed by color Doppler (*B*, **arrow**), and closed through the aortic root at the time of aortic valve replacement.

Comments

Most muscular VSDs are small and many close spontaneously in childhood. In this infant, the murmur resolved by 18 months of age. Occasionally, a small congenital muscular VSD is seen in an adult. However, most defects of the muscular septum in adults are acquired as a result of endocarditis or ventricular septal rupture after myocardial infarction.

Suggested Reading

1. Tee SD, Shiota T, Weintraub R et al. Evaluation of ventricular septal defect by transesophageal echocardiography: intraoperative assessment. Am Heart J 1994; 127:585–92.

Case 7-8
Supracristal VSD

This 51-year-old man with a VSD and enlargement of the sinuses of Valsalva was referred for repair of the VSD and aortic root replacement.

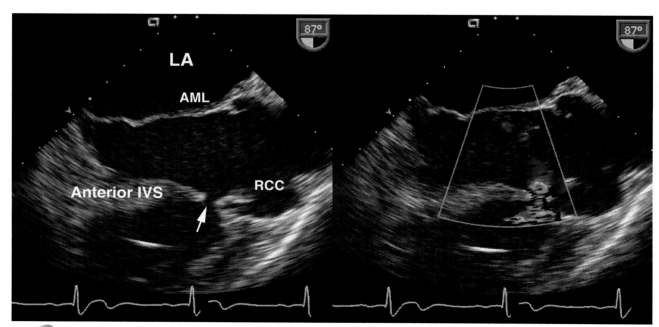

DVD ▶ **Fig 7-50.** In a long-axis view of the aortic valve, a small defect in the anterior interventricular septum (**IVS**) is seen immediately adjacent to the right coronary cusp (**RCC**) of the aortic valve, with color Doppler (*right*) demonstrating left-to-right flow through this region. Compare this image with **Fig 7-38** and note the position of the defect relative to the aortic valve. The sinuses of the Valsalva diameter is 53 mm in this view.

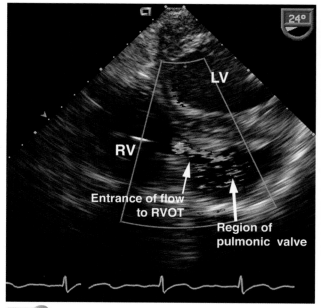

DVD ▶ **Fig 7-51.** In a transgastric view of the RVOT, the entrance of the VSD flow just proximal to the pulmonic valve is seen.

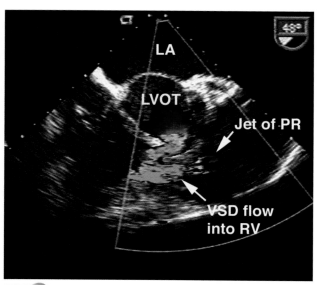

DVD ▶ **Fig 7-52.** In a short-axis view, the VSD is seen to empty into the right ventricle just below the pulmonic valve.

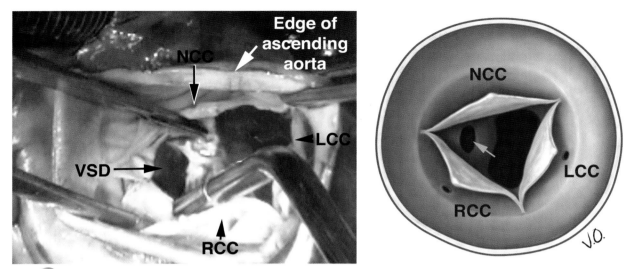

DVD **Fig 7-53.** At surgery, and in the corresponding drawing (**arrow**), the VSD is seen via an aortotomy incision immediately adjacent to the aortic valve.

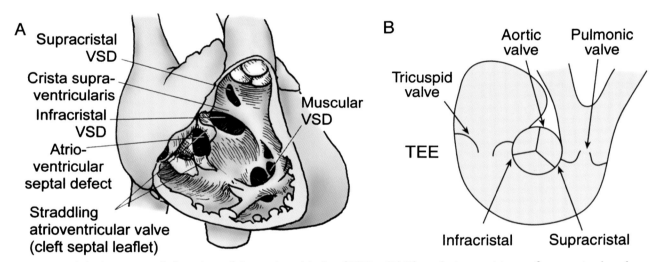

Fig 7-54. (*A*) The anatomic location of the various kinds of VSDs. (*B*) The relative positions of supracristal and infracristal (membranous) VSDs in transesophageal orientation. (Reproduced with permission from Linker D. Practical Echocardiography of Congenital Heart Disease. Philadelphia: Churchill Livingstone, 2000. ©Elsevier Inc.)

Comments

Supracristal VSDs are uncommon compared with membranous VSDs in adults. A supracristal VSD is located just inferior to the pulmonic valve and, as in this case, is often associated with abnormal anatomy of the aortic sinuses and/or dysfunction of the aortic valve due to lack of support of the aortic annulus. A short-axis view of the aortic valve is very helpful in differentiating the types of VSDs. In the short-axis view, a membranous VSD is seen immediately adja-

cent to the right coronary cusp (near the tricuspid valve). In contrast, a supracristal VSD is closer to the left coronary cusp, adjacent to the pulmonic valve (see **Fig 7-54**).

Suggested Reading

1. Sheil ML, Baines DB. Intraoperative transoesophageal echocardiography for paediatric cardiac surgery—an audit of 200 cases. Anaesth Intensive Care 1999; 27:591–5.

Abnormalities of the Great Vessels

Case 7-9
Patent Ductus Arteriosus

A continuous murmur was noted in this premature infant, and echocardiography was requested.

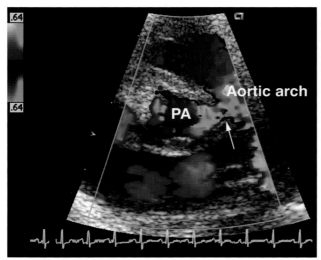

DVD **Fig 7-55.** In this neonate, a high esophageal view of the pulmonary artery in the short axis and the aortic arch in the long axis demonstrate a discontinuity (**arrow**) between the descending thoracic aorta and pulmonary artery (**PA**), with color Doppler demonstrating flow from the aorta into the PA in diastole across the patent ductus.

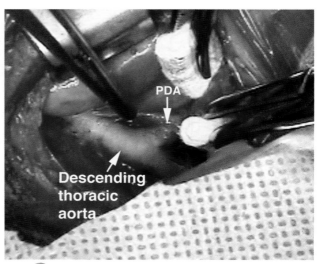

DVD **Fig 7-56.** At surgery the patent ductus arteriosus (**PDA**) was identified and ligated.

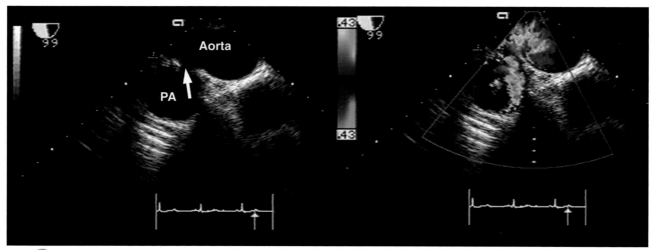

DVD **Fig 7-57.** In an adult with a patent ductus, a high esophageal view shows discontinuity (**arrow**) between the descending thoracic aorta and pulmonary artery (**PA**), which is confirmed by color Doppler (*right*).

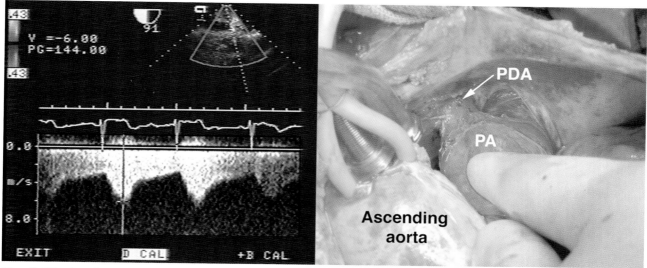

Fig. 7-58. On the *left*, continuous wave Doppler shows the high velocity continuous (systolic and diastolic) flow signal in the pulmonary artery. On the *right*, in an image obtained from the right side of the operating table and looking cephalad, the patent ductus (**PDA**) is seen coming into the PA.

Comments

The diagnosis of a PDA on echocardiography is based on the finding of an abnormal flow signal in the pulmonary artery that is most prominent in diastole but persists into systole, reflecting flow from the higher-pressure descending thoracic aorta into the pulmonary artery. The jet may be directed centrally into the main pulmonary artery or may deviate towards the wall of the vessel. In the cases shown here, color flow also demonstrated flow in the ductus itself, although this is not always possible.

In adults with a previously undiagnosed PDA, the first clue on echocardiography may be the presence of holodiastolic flow reversal in the descending thoracic aorta. In the absence of significant aortic regurgitation, the finding of holodiastolic retrograde flow in the aorta should prompt further evaluation for a PDA.

Suggested Reading

1. Kronzon I, Tunick PA, Rosenzweig BP. Quantification of left-to-right shunt in patent ductus arteriosus with the PISA method. J Am Soc Echocardiogr 2002; 15:376–8.

2. Chang ST, Hung KC, Hsieh IC et al. Evaluation of shunt flow by multiplane transesophageal echocardiography in adult patients with isolated patent ductus arteriosus. J Am Soc Echocardiogr 2002; 15:1367–73.

Case 7-10
Aortic Coarctation (Postductal)

This 57-year-old woman with a long history of a mild aortic coarctation, presented with symptoms of lower extremity claudication and difficulty controlling her hypertension. She also had a systolic murmur on auscultation.

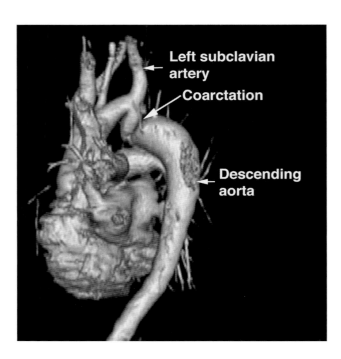

DVD ▶ **Fig 7-59.** 3D reconstruction of the aorta from contrast CT images showing the small aortic arch, with an aortic coarctation distal to the left subclavian artery. The proximal descending thoracic aorta is dilated.

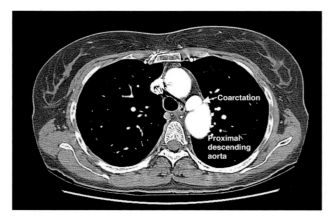

Fig 7-60. The CT image plane at the level of the coarctation shows the small distal arch and the larger proximal descending thoracic aorta, connected by the area of coarctation.

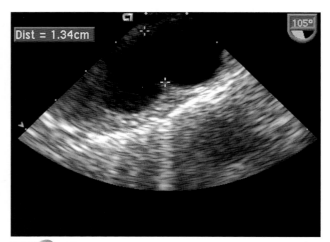

DVD ▶ **Fig 7-61.** On intraoperative TEE images of the descending thoracic aorta just distal to the left subclavian, the narrowing at the coarctation site can be demonstrated. An oblique image plane may result in over- or underestimation of aortic diameter, so that this approach should not be used for the definitive diagnosis.

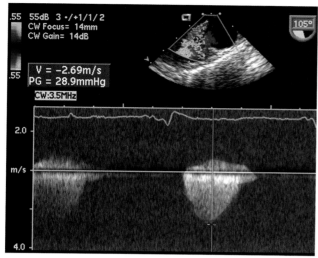

Fig 7-62. The velocity of flow through the coarctation is elevated at 2.7 m/s, which is consistent with a maximum gradient of 29 mmHg. The velocity and pressure gradient may be underestimated as it may not be possible to obtain a parallel intercept angle between the ultrasound beam and direction of blood flow. However, a severe coarctation is typically accompanied by diastolic "run-off" or persistent antegrade flow in diastole due to the high pressure on the upstream side of the narrowing, compared with downstream.

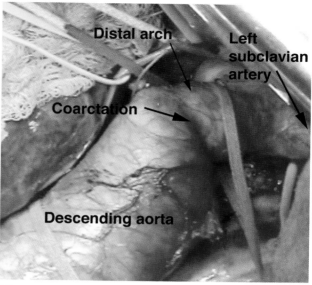

Fig 7-63. This intraoperative view from the patient's left side shows the coarctation just distal to the arch and left subclavian artery. The descending thoracic aorta is dilated. The segment of the aorta containing the coarctation was resected and replaced with a 26 mm Dacron tubular graft.

Comments

Patients with an aortic coarctation have elevated upper body blood pressure, with the severity of hypertension proportional to the severity of the aortic obstruction. However, even with a previous coarctation repair, recurrent hypertension is common, related either to recurrent stenosis or to long-term neurohormonal changes. Claudication is due to inadequate lower extremity blood flow with exercise due to the narrowed aorta. Although the severity of the coarctation may be evaluated on physical examination (comparison of upper- and lower-extremity blood pressures) or by 3D chest CT, the initial diagnosis is often made on echocardiography, and Doppler data may be used in patient follow-up.

The diagnosis of aortic coarctation on transthoracic echocardiography is based on the characteristic Doppler findings with an increased antegrade velocity in the descending thoracic aorta and persistent antegrade flow in diastole. Even with transthoracic imaging, the pressure gradient may be underestimated because the high-velocity jet is often eccentric compared with the suprasternal position of the transducer. On TEE imaging, accurate evaluation of the pressure gradient is rarely possible due to the intercept angle using this transducer position. However, TEE has the advantage that the coarctation can be visualized on 2D imaging, with color Doppler showing the site of the increase in flow velocity.

Suggested Reading

1. Panten RR, Harrison JK, Warner J et al. Aortic dissection after angioplasty and stenting of an aortic coarctation: detection by intravascular ultrasonography but not transesophageal echocardiography. J Am Soc Echocardiogr 2001; 14:73–6.

Case 7-11
Coarctation (in association with a bicuspid aortic valve)

This 29-year-old man, with a history of coarctation repair at age 5 years, presented with hypertension and was found to have a recurrent coarctation.

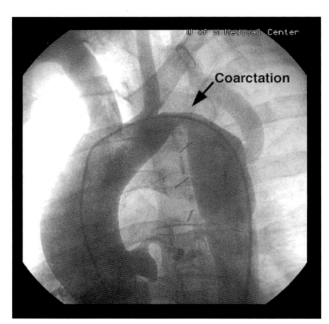

Fig 7-64. A contrast aortogram shows a severe coarctation of the aorta in the distal arch.

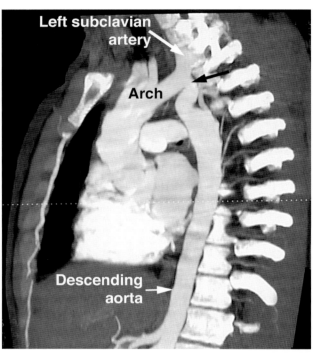

Fig 7-65. A sagittal CT image shows the coarctation (**arrow**) just distal to the left subclavian artery.

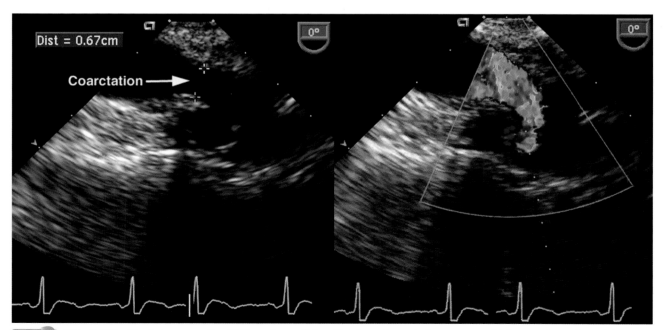

DVD **Fig 7-66.** On intraoperative TEE, a view of the distal aortic arch from a very high esophageal position shows the narrowing (*left*) and increased flow velocity (*right*) at the coarctation site.

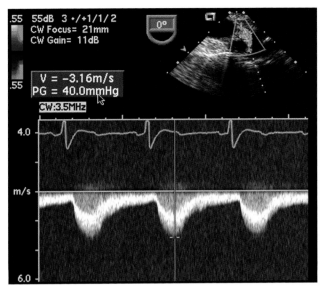

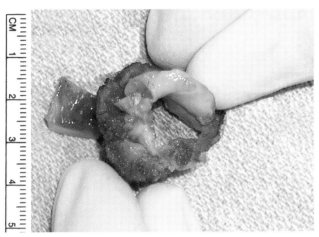

Fig 7-69. At surgery, the narrowed segment of the aorta was resected and the aorta was reconstructed with a Dacron tube graft.

Fig 7-67. Continuous wave Doppler of this region shows a high-velocity signal with a persistent decrescendo velocity pattern in diastole, consistent with severe coarctation. The antegrade velocity peak likely is an underestimate.

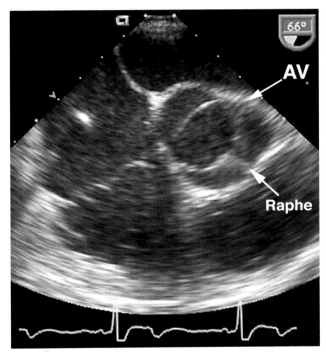

Fig 7-68. The short-axis image of the aortic valve demonstrates a bicuspid valve with an anterior–posterior orientation of the leaflets and a raphe in the larger leaflet (corresponding to fusion of the right and left coronary cusps).

Comments

In patients with an aortic coarctation, 50% have a bicuspid aortic valve. Conversely, about 10% of patients with a bicuspid aortic valve also have an aortic coarctation. In patients with Turner's syndrome, there is a high prevalence of both bicuspid aortic valve and aortic coarctation. Although the exact mechanism of this association is not known, because both conditions are inherited, it is assumed that this phenotype represents an underlying developmental disorder of the aortic valve and aorta. Similar to other patients with a bicuspid aortic valve, those with an associated aortic coarctation are also at risk for progressive dilation of the aorta. The clinical implication of this association is that aortic valve anatomy should be assessed in patients with an aortic coarctation. In addition, echocardiographic examination in patients with a bicuspid aortic valve should include recording of the velocity signal in the descending thoracic aorta, as well as measurement of upper- and lower-extremity blood pressures.

Suggested Reading

1. Gopal AS, Arora NS, Vardanian S et al. Utility of transesophageal echocardiography for the characterization of cardiovascular anomalies associated with Turner's syndrome. J Am Soc Echocardiogr 2001; 14:60–2.

Case 7-12
Persistent Left Superior Vena Cava

This 49-year-old woman was referred for evaluation of hypertension and a cardiac murmur. A blood pressure difference of 40 mmHg was noted between the arm and leg, and transthoracic echocardiography showed an aortic coarctation. At surgery, the coarctation was located between the left carotid and left subclavian arteries. The coarctation was repaired using a patch repair. Incidentally, a persistent left superior vena cava was noted.

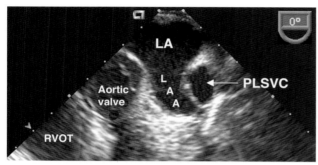

Fig 7-70. A high esophageal view at 0 degrees shows an echo-free circular structure, a persistent left superior vena cava (**PLSVC**) lateral to the left atrial appendage (**LAA**).

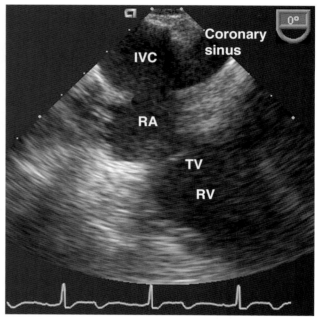

Fig 7-71. A low esophageal view shows the entrance of an enlarged coronary sinus into the right atrium.

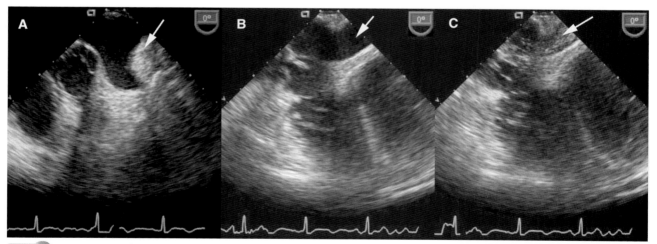

Fig 7-72. The injection of contrast via the left arm shows appearance of contrast in the structure (**arrow**) lateral to the left atrial appendage (A) and contrast entering the right atrium via the coronary sinus (**arrows**) (B and C). These findings are consistent with a persistent left superior vena cava.

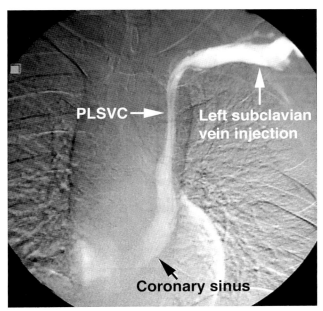

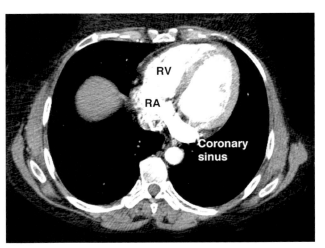

Fig 7-75. A CT scan at the heart level shows a dilated coronary sinus.

Fig 7-73. A venogram with injection of contrast into the left subclavian vein shows the left-sided superior vena cava entering the coronary sinus.

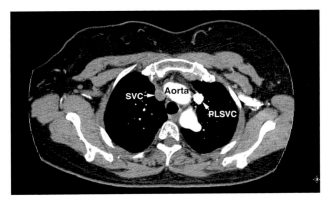

Fig 7-74. A CT scan with contrast at the level of the ascending aorta shows opacification of the left SVC but not the right SVC, as contrast was injected via the left arm.

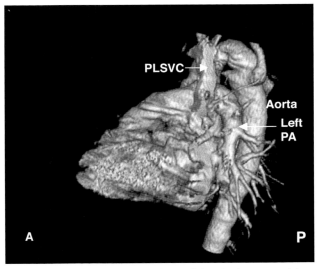

Fig 7-76. A 3D reconstruction of the CT images with the heart rotated to the left shows the PLSVC.

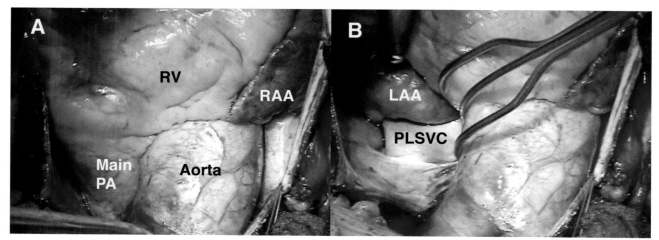

Fig 7-77. Intraoperative findings show the normal position of the aorta and pulmonary artery (*A*). When the great arteries are retracted gently, the PLSVC and LAA can be seen (*B*).

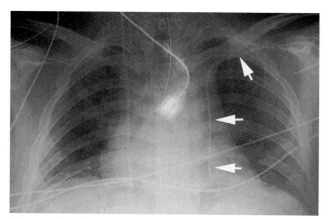

Fig 7-78. Chest radiograph showing a central venous catheter in the PLSVC (**arrows**).

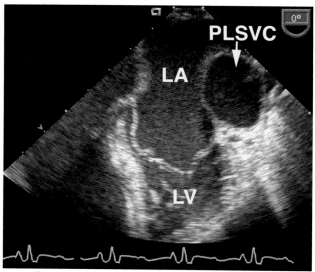

DVD **Fig 7-79.** This next patient, a 22-year-old female, had previously undergone repair of tetralogy of Fallot as a child, and now presented for tricuspid and pulmonic valve replacements for valvular regurgitation. This mid-esophageal four-chamber view shows the large PLSVC lateral to the LA.

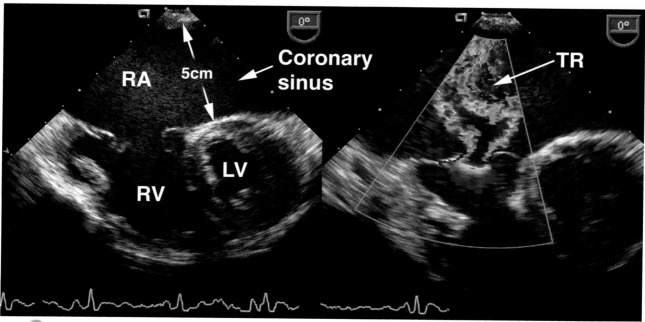

Fig 7-80. In this low esophageal view, there is non-coaptation of the tricuspid leaflets, resulting in severe TR. The coronary sinus measures 5 cm in diameter.

Comments

About 0.5% of adults have both a normal superior vena cava entering the right atrium from the right side of the mediastinum, and also have a persistent left-sided superior vena cava. This PLSVC typically drains into the coronary sinus and, from there, into the right atrium. Because the pattern of blood flow is normal, there are no clinical symptoms or signs associated with a PLSVC. Most of these patients are diagnosed when they become ill, if echocardiography is performed or if a central venous catheter enters the right atrium from a left mediastinal position.

On echocardiography, a PLSVC is recognized based on the finding of an enlarged coronary sinus. The coronary sinus is seen in short axis in a left ventricular long-axis view. From the standard four-chamber view, the transducer can be advanced in the esophagus to visualize the coronary sinus along its long axis. This view shows the entrance of the coronary sinus into the right atrium. Typically, the size of the dilated coronary sinus is 1–2 cm. The massive enlargement of the

coronary sinus in the second case is most likely due to the severely elevated right atrial pressure.

If the diagnosis of a PLSVC is in doubt, a contrast injection in a left arm vein will demonstrate contrast in the coronary sinus before contrast is seen in the right atrium. Chest CT or MR also can be used to define the caval anatomy in more detail.

During open heart surgery, the presence of a PLSVC with coronary sinus enlargement will negate the effectiveness of retrograde cardioplegia.

Suggested Reading

1. Garduno C, Chew S, Forbess J et al. Persistent left superior vena cava and partial anomalous pulmonary venous connection: incidental diagnosis by transesophageal echocardiography during coronary artery bypass surgery. J Am Soc Echocardiogr 1999; 12:682–5.

2. Gonzalez-Juanatey C, Testa A, Vidan J et al. Persistent left superior vena cava draining into the coronary sinus: report of 10 cases and literature review. Clin Cardiol 2004; 27:515–18.

Complex Congenital Heart Disease

Case 7-13
Tetralogy of Fallot

This 35-year-old woman presented with reduced exercise tolerance and cyanosis and was diagnosed with uncorrected tetralogy of Fallot.

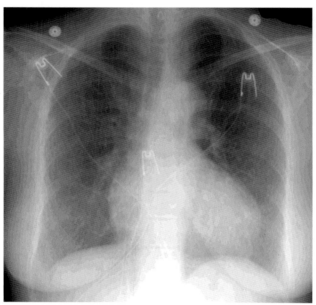

Fig 7-81. The PA chest radiograph shows the typical "boot-shaped" heart with a prominent left ventricle.

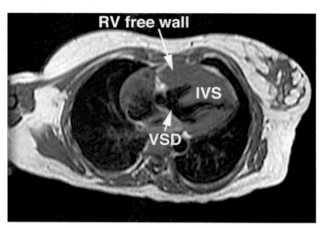

Fig 7-82. A CT image at the level of the ventricle shows the large ventricular septal defect (**VSD**) with the interventricular septum (**IVS**) and the hypertrophy of the right ventricular (**RV**) free wall.

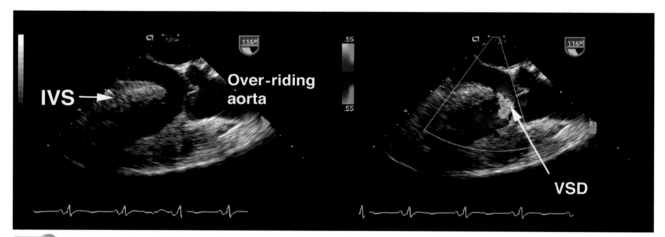

Fig 7-83. In a TEE long-axis view at 116 degrees, the large aorta that "over-rides" or "straddles" the ventricular septum and the large VSD are seen. Color flow Doppler (*right*) confirms the low-velocity flow across the defect.

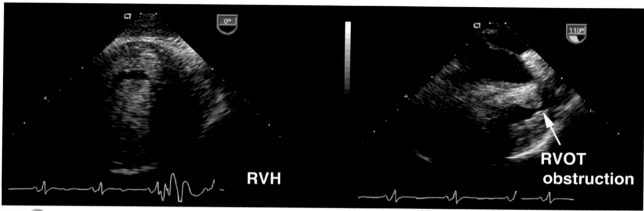

DVD **Fig 7-84.** In a transgastric short-axis view (*left*) and a long-axis view turned towards the right heart (*right*) the subpulmonic muscular obstruction and severe right ventricular hypertrophy (**RVH**) are seen.

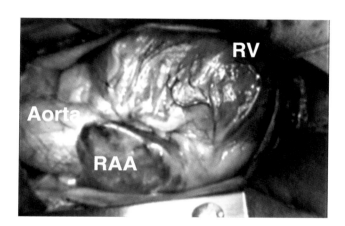

DVD **Fig 7-85.** At surgery, the cyanotic heart with an enlarged and hypertrophied right ventricle is seen. In this DVD of the operation, taken from the surgeon's perspective from the right side of the patient, the right ventricle is initially opened, a myomectomy of the outflow tract is performed, the VSD is closed with a synthetic patch, and a right-sided homograft is placed.

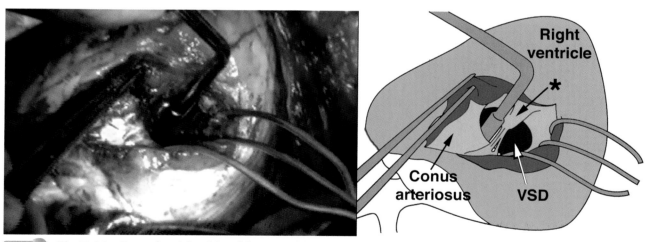

DVD **Fig 7-86.** From the right side of the OR table, the right ventricular wall has been incised, and the edges reflected. Behind the septal papillary muscle (**asterisk**) of the tricuspid valve, the VSD is seen.

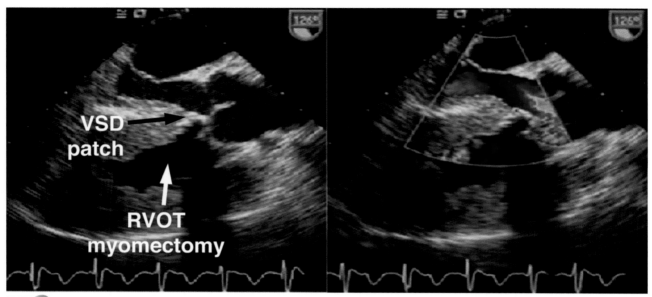

Fig 7-87. Post-repair, the VSD is closed, and the RVOT enlarged on these long-axis images (*left*). Color flow Doppler reveals an intact repair (*right*).

Comments

Tetralogy of Fallot is the most common type of complex congenital heart disease. Diagnosis is based on the presence of:

- a VSD
- an enlarged aorta that is positioned over the crest of the ventricular septum, often referred to as an "over-riding aorta"
- right ventricular outflow obstruction at the subvalvular, valvular or supravalvular level
- compensatory right ventricular hypertrophy.

Most patients with tetralogy of Fallot are diagnosed and undergo surgical repair in childhood. However, a few patients remain undiagnosed until later in life.

Despite the presence of a large VSD, pulmonary pressures remain low because the pulmonary bed is "protected" by the right ventricular outflow obstruction. Surgical repair includes patch closure of the VSD and relief of right ventricular outflow obstruction by a surgical repair or placement of a right ventricular to pulmonary artery valved conduit.

Suggested Reading

1. Therrien J, Marx GR, Gatzoulis MA. Late problems in tetralogy of Fallot—recognition, management, and prevention. Cardiol Clin 2002; 20:395–404.

2. Joyce JJ, Hwang EY, Wiles HB et al. Reliability of intraoperative transesophageal echocardiography during Tetralogy of Fallot repair. Echocardiography 2000; 17:319–27.

Case 7-14
Subaortic Membrane

This 25-year-old woman presented during pregnancy with increasing exertional dyspnea. Examination revealed a 4/6 systolic murmur at the base radiating to the carotids. Transthoracic echocardiography demonstrated a subaortic membrane with an antegrade velocity of 5.4 m/s.

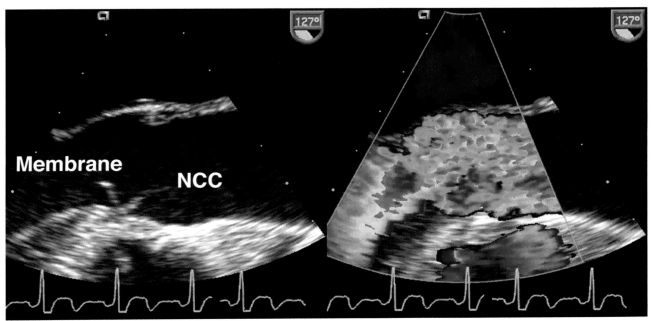

DVD **Fig 7-88.** In a long-axis TEE view at 127 degrees, a linear echo consistent with a subaortic membrane is seen adjacent to the right coronary cusp of the aortic valve. Color Doppler (*right*) shows aliasing at the level of the membrane, suggesting an increased velocity due to obstruction to blood flow. On the DVD, a small amount of aortic regurgitation is appreciated.

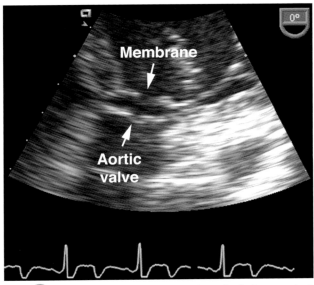

DVD **Fig 7-89.** In a transgastric apical view angled anteriorly to image the aortic valve, the linear membrane is seen about 0.5 cm proximal to the aortic valve plane.

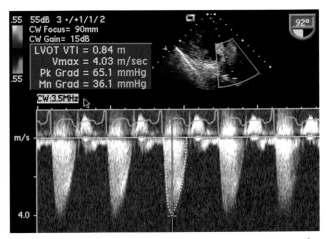

Fig 7-90. Continuous wave Doppler interrogation of the aortic valve from a transgastric long-axis view yields a maximum velocity of at least 4.0 m/s, with a mean gradient of 36 mmHg.

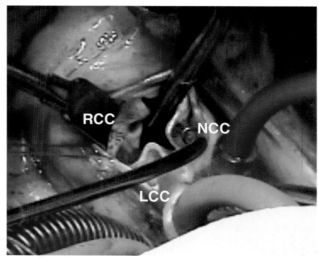

DVD ● **Fig 7-91.** Intraoperative photograph of the aortic valve with the non (**NCC**), right (**RCC**) and left coronary cusps (**LCC**).

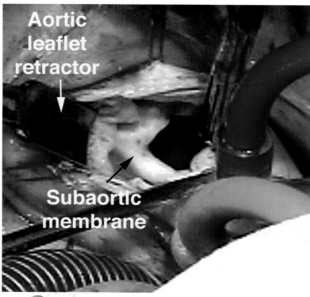

DVD ● **Fig 7-92.** With the aortic leaflets retracted, the white subaortic membrane is seen. The membrane was uneventfully resected.

Comments

The symptoms and physical examination findings of subaortic membranes are similar to valvular aortic stenosis, and this diagnosis should be considered in younger patients with evidence of left ventricular outflow obstruction. The membrane itself may be difficult to visualize on transthoracic imaging. However, color and pulsed Doppler evidence for acceleration

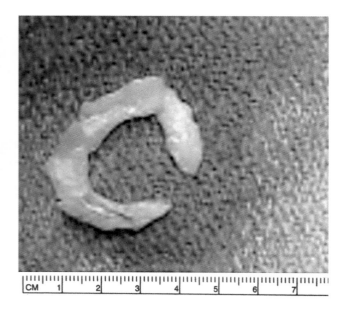

Fig 7-93. The resected membrane showing the C-shaped membrane that nearly encircled the outflow tract. Echocardiography 1 month after surgery showed only a small area of increased echogenicity along the ventricular septum in the subaortic region with no evidence for significant obstruction to flow.

of flow proximal to the aortic valve suggests this possibility. Aortic regurgitation may be present if turbulence from the subaortic stenosis has damaged the valve leaflets. TEE imaging both confirms the diagnosis and allows delineation of the anatomy of the membrane. Aspects important in surgical planning are the type of subaortic obstruction (muscular versus membranous), the distance between the membrane and the aortic valve, the presence of severity of aortic regurgitation and any evidence for attachments between the membrane and the valve leaflets. When aortic valve function is normal, the subaortic membrane typically can be resected with preservation of the aortic valve, as in this case.

Suggested Reading

1. Ge S, Warner JG Jr, Fowle KM et al. Morphology and dynamic change of discrete subaortic stenosis can be imaged and quantified with three-dimensional transesophageal echocardiography. J Am Soc Echocardiogr 1997; 10:713–16.

2. Movsowitz C, Jacobs LE, Eisenberg S et al. Discrete subaortic valvular stenosis: the clinical utility and limitations of transesophageal echocardiography. Echocardiography 1993; 10:485–7.

Case 7-15
Supravalvular Aortic Membrane (Williams Syndrome), Cor Triatriatum

This 53-year-old woman was transferred from another hospital for congestive heart failure, after a 6-week course of IV antibiotics for enterococcal bacteremia. Echocardiography showed a trileaflet aortic valve that was thickened with systolic doming and with a linear echo at the sinotubular junction, suggestive of a supravalvular membrane. The antegrade Doppler velocity was 4.9 m/s with a mean transaortic gradient of 56 mmHg and a continuity equation valve area of 0.6 cm^2. The left ventricle showed moderate concentric hypertrophy, with an ejection fraction of 73%. She was referred for surgical intervention.

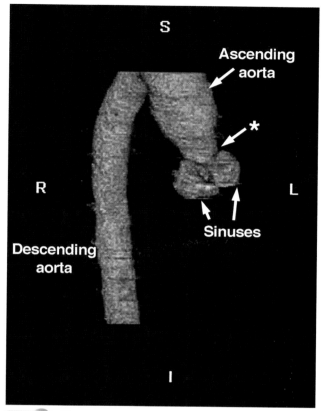

Fig 7-95. 3D reconstructed CT reveals a narrowing (**asterisk**) above the sinuses of Valsalva.

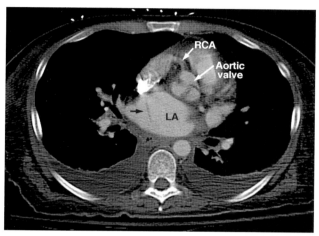

Fig 7-94. CT scan shows a thickened aortic valve. Note is made of the right coronary artery (**RCA**). Within the left atrium (**LA**), a linear density is seen (**black arrow**), suggestive of cor triatriatum.

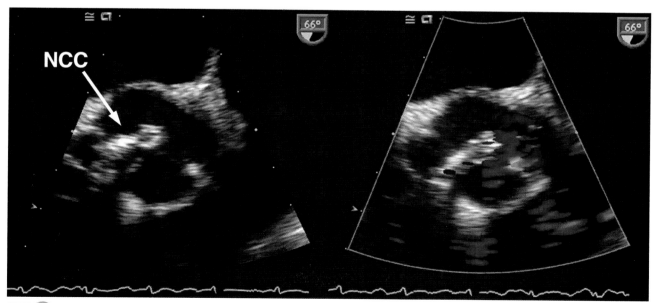

Fig 7-96. TEE of the aortic valve in short-axis view shows a thickened NCC, which is consistent with the patient's previous history of endocarditis.

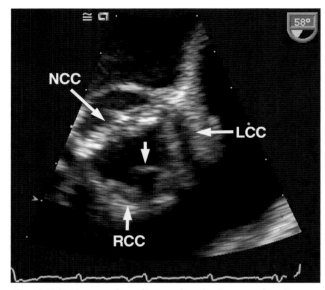

Fig 7-97. In systole, a linear density is seen, but its proximity to the aortic valve cannot be determined in this plane.

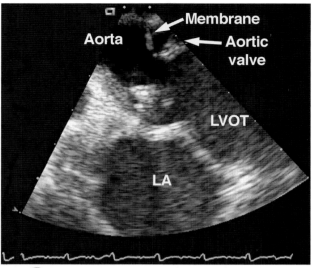

DVD **Fig 7-99.** Epiaortic scan confirmed the TEE findings.

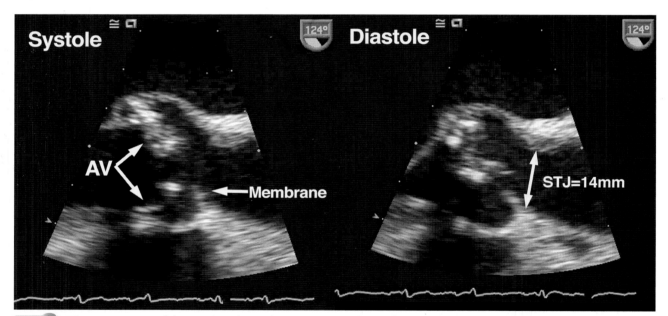

DVD **Fig 7-98.** TEE of the aortic valve in long-axis view shows the abnormal valve, a very narrowed sinotubular junction (**STJ**) and a linear density attached to the anterior aspect of the STJ. In real time, the density is thick and immobile.

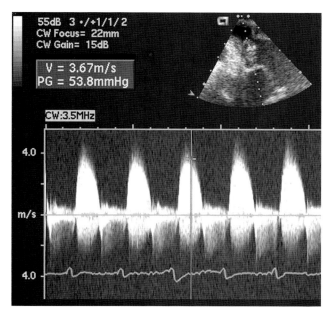

Fig 7-100. With epiaortic scanning, CW Doppler through the valve shows an intense signal with a peak gradient of 54 mmHg, and a mean gradient of 34 mmHg.

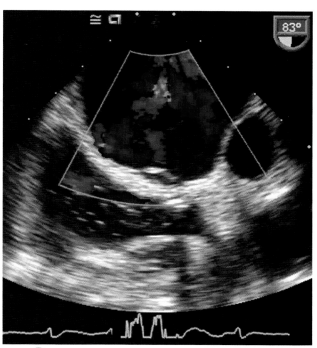

DVD **Fig 7-102.** Color flow Doppler shows free communication across the cor triatriatum, in a view in the same orientation as the right-hand panel of **Fig 7-101**.

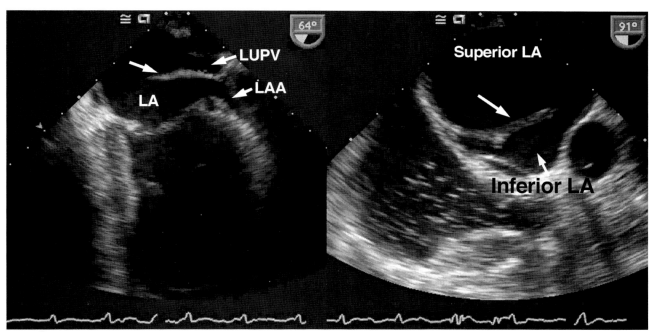

DVD **Fig 7-101.** Incidental note was made of a non-obstructive cor triatriatum (**arrow**), seen in the right-hand panel arising from the fossa ovalis, and in the left-hand panel attaching to the ridge between the left atrial appendage (**LAA**) and left upper pulmonary vein (**LUPV**).

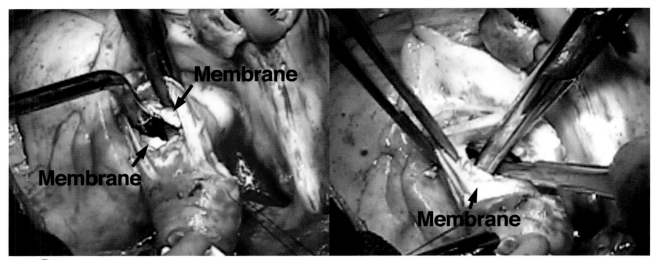

DVD **Fig 7-103.** Following aortotomy, two components of the rigid membrane were seen above the aortic valve, attached to the STJ. In the right-hand panel, an instrument is placed under the membrane, and identifies the ostium of the left main coronary artery. The aortic valve was resected, and the membrane excised.

Comments

Obstruction to ventricular outflow at the supravalvular level is uncommon and is usually diagnosed in childhood. In addition to a supravalvular membrane, Williams syndrome includes developmental delay, "elfin" facial features and hypercalcemia and is due to deletion of the elastin gene located at chromosome 7q11.23. Other causes of supravalvular aortic stenosis include an autosomal dominant inherited form (without Williams syndrome), sporadic cases and patients with homozygous familial hypercholesterolemia. Supravalvular aortic stenosis may be associated with other cardiac abnormalities, including aortic valve leaflet deformity (as in this case), pulmonary stenosis, coronary artery anomalies and aortic coarctation.

The clinical presentation and management of supravalvular aortic stenosis are similar to that of valvular aortic stenosis. Echocardiographic diagnosis and evaluation of disease severity is similar to native valve stenosis, with the exception that the level of obstruction is supravalvular, instead of at the valve level. As in this case, TEE is often needed to adequately visualize the anatomy.

Cor triatriatum is a cardiac malformation in which a fibromuscular membrane divides the left atrium into two chambers: a superior posterior chamber that receives the pulmonary venous inflow and an inferior anterior chamber or true left atrium that contains the LAA and mitral valve orifice. Communication between the two chambers usually occurs through one or more defects in the membrane, and is most often asymptomatic. In rare cases in which the communication is limited, pulmonary venous hypertension results.

Case 7-16
Corrected Transposition of the Great Arteries (Ventricular Inversion)

This 19-year-old women with congenitally corrected transposition of the great vessels was referred for systemic atrioventricular (AV) valve replacement for severe regurgitation with worsening systemic ventricular function and progressive heart failure symptoms.

Physical examination showed a blood pressure of 103/55 mmHg, regular heart rate at 118 bpm, weight of 106 lb, a hyperdynamic precordium and a 3/6 holosystolic murmur heard throughout the precordium.

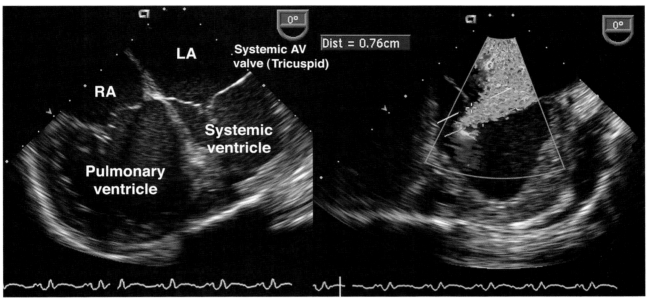

DVD **Fig 7-104.** The TEE four-chamber view (*left*) demonstrates dilated systemic and pulmonary ventricles. The systemic ventricle is an anatomic right ventricle that ejects into the aorta. The pulmonary ventricle is an anatomic left ventricle that ejects into the pulmonary artery. The pulmonary ventricle is severely dilated, with severely reduced systolic function. The systemic ventricle is mildly dilated, with moderate global hypokinesis. Color Doppler (*right*) demonstrates severe regurgitation of the systemic AV valve (anatomic tricuspid valve) with a vena contracta width of 0.7 cm.

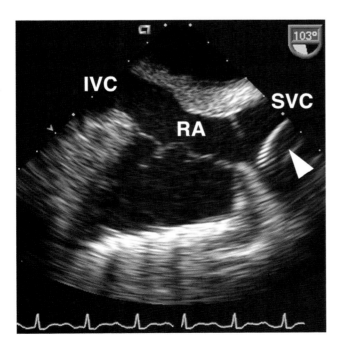

Fig 7-105. The bicaval view shows the superior vena cava and inferior vena cava (**SVC, IVC**) entering the right atrium (**RA**). A venous drainage cannula (**arrowhead**) is seen in the SVC.

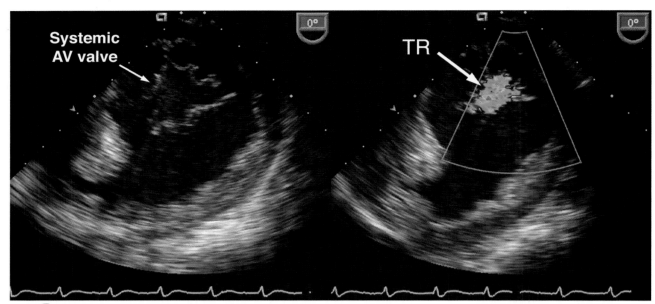

DVD▶ **Fig 7-106.** A transgastric short-axis view in diastole (*left*) demonstrates the tricuspid valve in the systemic ventricle. In systole (*right*), a central regurgitant jet is appreciated.

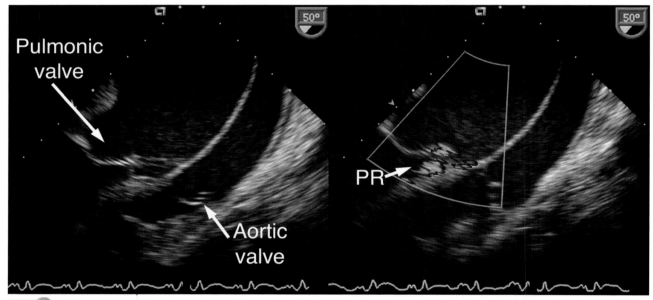

DVD▶ **Fig 7-107.** A long-axis view of the aorta shows that the aortic and pulmonic valves are seen in long axis in the same image plane and the great vessels are parallel to each other. The pulmonary artery is markedly dilated compared with the smaller aorta. Color Doppler (*right*) shows mild pulmonic regurgitation (**PR**).

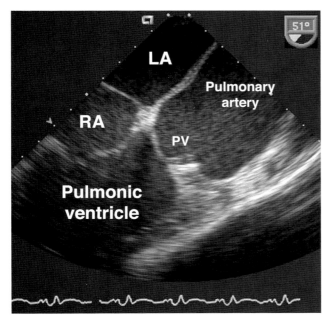

DVD ▸ **Fig 7-108.** Changing the angle of interrogation to 51 degrees, with slight rightward turning of the probe, gives a view of the right atrium (**RA**), the pulmonic ventricle, the pulmonic valve (**PV**) and the pulmonary artery, similar to a long-axis view.

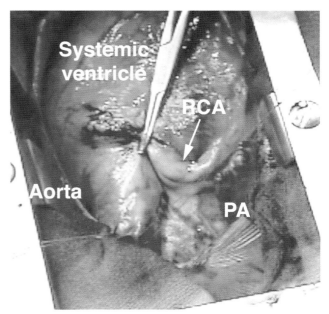

Fig 7-110. An intraoperative photograph shows the side-by-side great vessels with an anterior aorta (note the right coronary artery arising from the aorta).

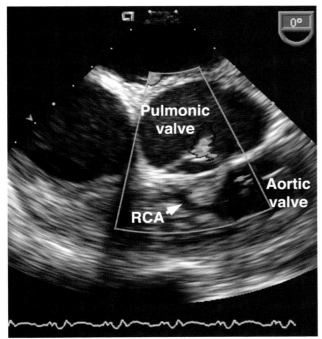

DVD ▸ **Fig 7-109.** A short-axis view shows the aortic and pulmonic valves in the same image plane. The origin of the right coronary artery (**RCA**) is also seen.

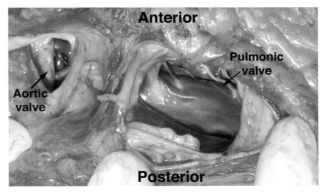

Fig 7-111. In another patient with similar anatomy who underwent heart transplantation, a photograph of the explanted heart with the great vessels removed shows the side-by-side pulmonic and aortic valves.

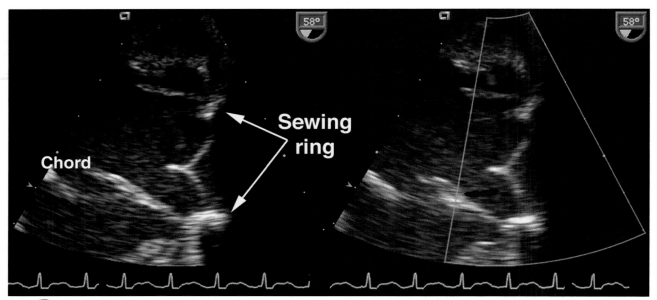

DVD **Fig 7-112.** A tissue prosthesis in the systemic AV position is seen in a transgastric two-chamber view in systole. Some of the valve chords were retained to help preserve ventricular function. Color Doppler (*right*) demonstrated no regurgitation.

Comments

With complex congenital heart disease, the echo-cardiographer should seek to define the pathway of blood flow and identify each cardiac chamber and valve. With congenitally corrected transposition of the great vessels, systemic venous blood returns to the right atrium, flows through the mitral valve into the left ventricle and is then ejected into the pulmonary artery, across the pulmonic valve. The pulmonary veins drain into the left atrium, oxygenated blood crosses the tricuspid valve into the right ventricle and is then ejected across the aortic valve into the aorta. Thus, the movement of oxygenated blood is normal, only the ventricles are reversed; therefore, this condition is sometimes called "ventricular inversion." These patients typically come to medical attention because of associated defects such as tricuspid (systemic AV valve) regurgitation, VSD, pulmonic stenosis and heart block.

The identification of the right atrium is based on the entrance of the IVC and SVC into this chamber. The pulmonary veins usually drain into the left atrium.

Shape and wall thickness cannot be used to distinguish the right and left ventricles when there is transposition of the great vessels, as dilation and hypertrophy alter the geometry of both ventricles. However, the AV valves stay with the corresponding ventricular chamber, so that the mitral valve identifies the anatomic left ventricle and the tricuspid valve the anatomic right ventricle, although it is important to distinguish a cleft mitral valve from a trileaflet tricuspid

valve. Other features that identify the anatomic right ventricle include:

- the annular plane of the tricuspid valve is slightly more apical than the mitral annulus (see **Fig 7-104**)
- the right ventricle has a moderator band and more prominent trabeculation.

Great vessel anatomy is determined by following the vessels distally. The pulmonary artery is identified based on bifurcation into branches that supply the pulmonary vasculature. The aorta is identified by the arch and head and neck vessels. The semilunar valves are positioned in the corresponding great vessel: e.g. aortic valve in the aorta, pulmonic valve in the pulmonary artery. Unlike the normal perpendicular orientation of aortic and pulmonic valve planes, both valves are in the same plane with transposition of the great vessels. The aorta and pulmonary artery are side by side (with the aorta anterior) unlike the normal criss-cross relationship with the pulmonary artery anteriorly.

Suggested Reading

1. Caso P, Ascione L, Lange A et al. Diagnostic value of transesophageal echocardiography in the assessment of congenitally corrected transposition of the great arteries in adult patients. Am Heart J 1998; 135:43–50.

Case 7-17
Tricuspid Atresia with Fontan Physiology

This 42-year-old man with tricuspid atresia underwent surgical palliation as a child with connection of the right atrium to the pulmonary artery. Thus, all the systemic venous return was directed to the pulmonary artery without an intervening ventricle (e.g. Fontan physiology). The pulmonary artery was oversewn just distal to the pulmonic valve so that the entire ventricular output was directed to the systemic vasculature. He did well for many years, leading an active life, including bicycling. He was able to complete a college education followed by a full-time professional career.

His major cardiac limitation was due to recurrent atrial arrhythmias, which were treated with medication, a pacemaker and several ablation procedures. However, progressive right atrial enlargement was associated with worsening arrhythmias, symptoms and signs of right heart failure and evidence of a protein-losing enteropathy. He was referred for right atrial reduction with surgical revision of the Fontan conduit.

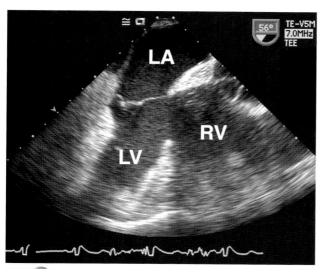

DVD **Fig 7-113.** A TEE view at 56 degrees demonstrates the left atrium, mitral valve and left ventricle. A large ventricular septal defect is present so that the left and right ventricles function as a common chamber.

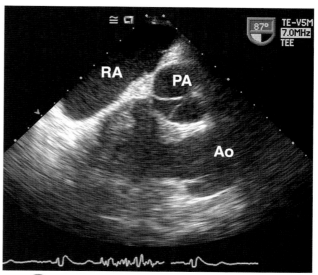

DVD **Fig 7-114.** With the image plane rotated further to 87 degrees, the pulmonary artery (**PA**) and aorta (**Ao**) are seen. In this patient, the pulmonary artery had been oversewn just distal to the pulmonic valve. Although there is some motion of the bicuspid pulmonic valve, there is no significant antegrade flow. Both the pulmonic and aortic valve arise from the common ventricular chamber.

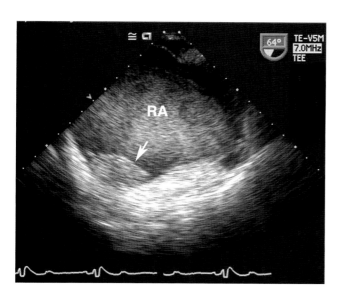

DVD **Fig 7-115.** With the transducer turned towards the patient's right side at an image plane of 64 degrees, the severe enlarged right atrium (**RA**) with marked spontaneous contrast and a mural thrombus (**arrow**) is seen.

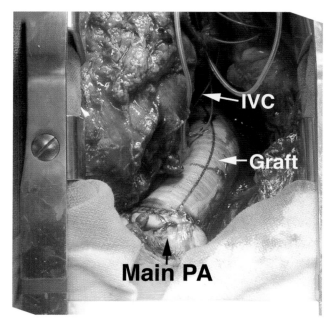

Fig 7-116. At surgery, the right atrial size was reduced and a common atrium formed with the right and left chambers. A Dacron non-valved conduit was placed from the IVC to the main PA, as seen in this photograph. The SVC was connected directly to the right PA.

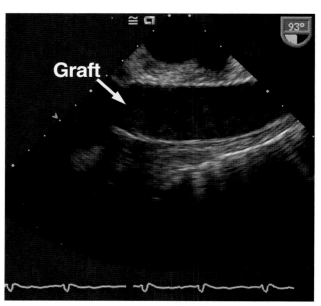

Fig 7-117. The graft is visualized on TEE using a 93-degree image plane with the transducer turned towards the patient's right side.

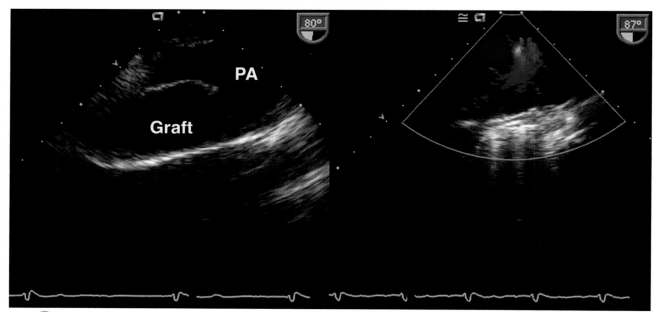

Fig 7-118. The transducer is moved cephalad to image more superior segments of the graft and the connection to the PA. Color Doppler shows no obstruction to flow at the distal anastomosis of the graft.

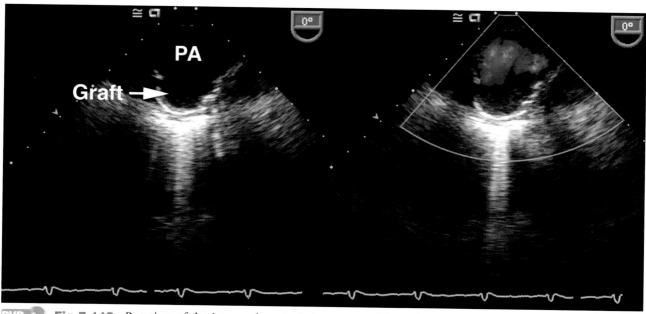

Fig 7-119. Rotation of the image plane to 0 degrees provides a short-axis view of the graft at the entrance into the PA.

Comments

In complex congenital heart disease with only one functional ventricle, as in this patient with tricuspid atresia, one surgical option is to direct the systemic venous return into the pulmonary vasculature without an intervening ventricle. Thus, pulmonary blood flow is not pulsatile, and adequate forward flow depends on systemic venous pressure being higher than left atrial pressure, a pattern of pulmonary flow often termed Fontan physiology. Early in the history of this procedure, the vena caval connections were left intact and the right atrium was connected to the pulmonary artery. However, as these patients grew to adulthood, the right atrium progressively enlarged, leading to refractory atrial arrhythmias, elevated systemic venous pressures and compression of the pulmonary veins. The current surgical approach is to connect the SVC and IVC more directly to the pulmonary artery, to avoid progressive right atrial enlargement. In patients with the earlier procedure, as in this patient, revision of the Fontan procedure to eliminate the right atrium may be considered when arrhythmias are refractory or for progressive right heart failure symptoms.

Suggested Reading

1. Kawahito S, Kitahata H, Tanaka K et al. Intraoperative evaluation of pulmonary artery flow during the Fontan procedure by transesophageal Doppler echocardiography. Anesth Analg 2000; 91:1375–80.
2. Mavroudis C, Deal BJ, Backer CL. The beneficial effects of total cavopulmonary conversion and arrhythmia surgery for the failed Fontan. Semin Thorac Cardiovasc Surg Pediatr Card Surg Annu 2002; 5:12–24.

8

Hypertrophic Cardiomyopathy

Case 8-1
Transplant for Hypertrophic Cardiomyopathy

This 26-year-old woman with hypertrophic cardiomyopathy and prolonged QT syndrome was referred for heart transplantation for low-output heart failure with clinical symptoms of fatigue and marked exercise intolerance with New York Heart Association (NYHA) class III symptoms despite maximal medical therapy. Right heart catheterization documented a pulmonary artery pressure of 24/9 mmHg with a pulmonary wedge pressure of 10 mmHg. Cardiac output was 5.8 L/min, with a cardiac index of 2.9 L/min.

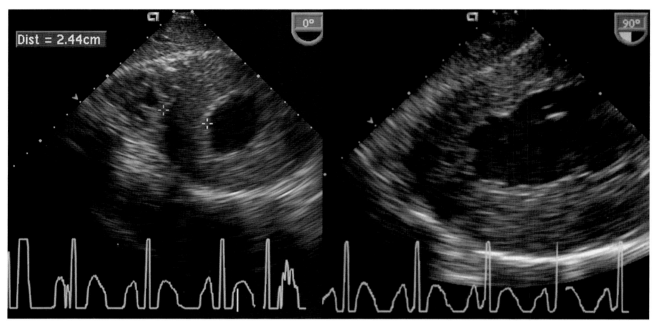

Fig 8-1. Transgastric short-axis view shows severe hypertrophy of the left ventricle with a septal thickness of 2.4 cm (*right*). Transgastric long-axis view also shows severe hypertrophy of the left ventricle. The DVD shows the short-axis (*left*) and two-chamber (*right*) transgastric views.

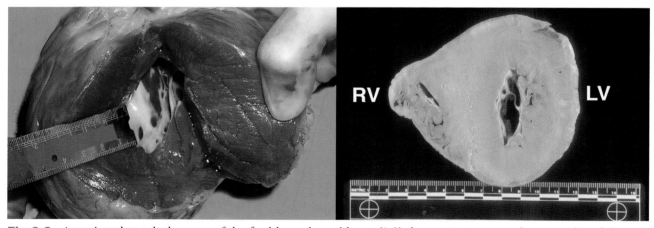

Fig 8-2. A section through the apex of the freshly explanted heart (*left*) demonstrates severe hypertrophy of the ventricular myocardium. At pathologic examination (*right*), the heart was severely hypertrophied (cardiac mass = 655 g), with a pattern typical for hypertrophic cardiomyopathy; the left ventricular cavity was extremely small.

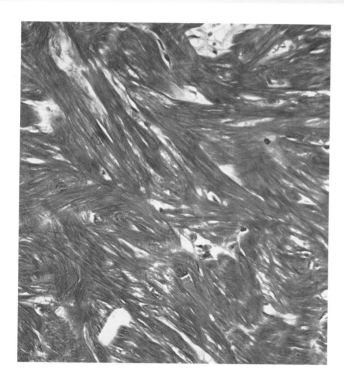

Fig 8-3. Histologic examination revealed severe cardiomyocyte disarray, with mild-to-moderate interstitial fibrosis.

Case 8-2
Myectomy for Dynamic Left Ventricular Outflow Tract Obstruction

This 64-year-old man was referred for surgical intervention for hypertrophic cardiomyopathy with severe dynamic subaortic obstruction. He had an 8-month history of increasing exertional dyspnea, chest pain and syncope. Echocardiography showed hypertrophic cardiomyopathy with severe outflow obstruction and severe mitral regurgitation. Coronary angiography showed no significant epicardial coronary artery disease.

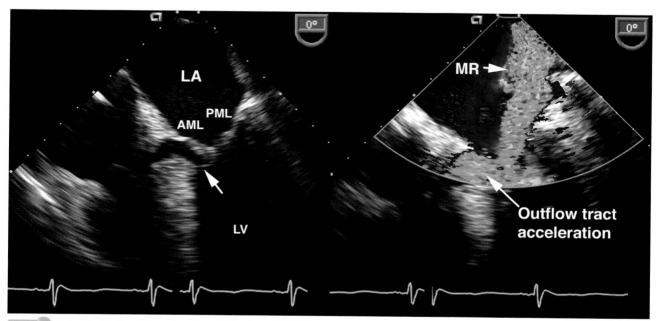

Fig 8-4. The four-chamber TEE view (*left*) demonstrates systolic anterior motion of the mitral valve leaflet (**arrow**). Color Doppler (*right*) shows both an increased outflow tract velocity (the green color indicates variance due to a high flow velocity with signal aliasing) and severe mitral regurgitation (**MR**).

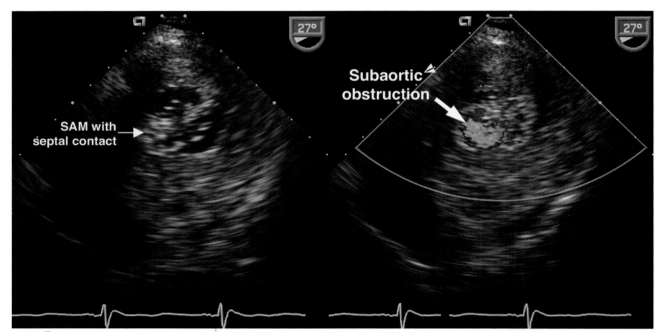

Fig 8-5. The transgastric short-axis view at the mitral valve level shows the severely hypertrophied left ventricle; there is systolic anterior motion (**SAM**) of the anterior mitral leaflet with interventricular septal contact (*left*) and color flow (*right*) demonstrating the subaortic obstruction.

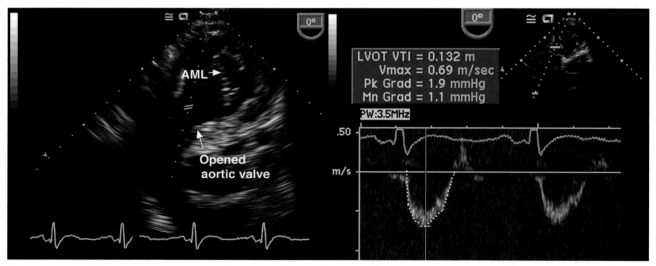

Fig 8-6. In a different patient without hypertrophic cardiomyopathy, an example of using the transgastric apical view for evaluation of left ventricular outflow is shown. The image plane is angulated anteriorly from the deep transgastric four-chamber view to show the aortic valve (*left*). Then, pulsed or continuous wave Doppler examination of flow is recorded: in this case, showing a normal velocity of 0.7 m/s (*right*). The maximal velocity may be underestimated by this approach, as it is not always possible to obtain a parallel intercept angle between the ultrasound beam and direction of blood flow. However, the actual velocity is at least as high as the recorded velocity.

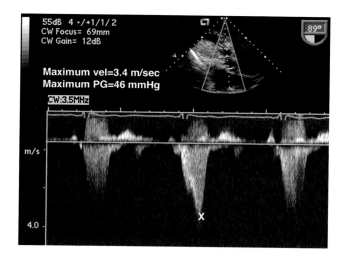

Fig 8-7. In this patient with hypertrophic cardiomyopathy, continuous wave Doppler from the transgastric apical view demonstrates a late-peaking high-velocity systolic signal with a maximum velocity of 3.4 m/s, corresponding to a maximum pressure gradient (**PG**) of 46 mmHg. The PG may be even higher when the patient is awake and active.

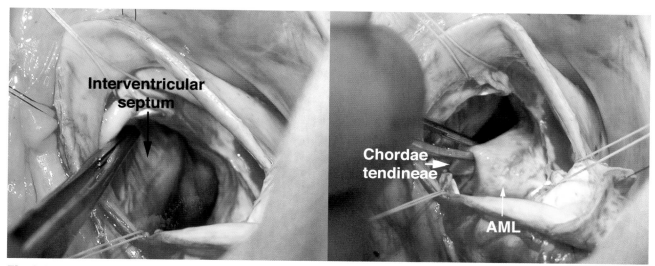

Fig 8-8. At surgery, the left ventricular outflow tract is approached via the ascending aorta, and through the passively opened aortic valve. In a normal example in which the aortic valve has been removed, the structures visible in the LVOT are: anteriorly, the interventricular septum (*left*); posteriorly, the AML (*right*).

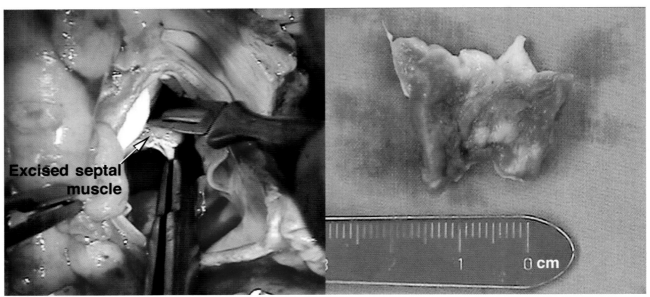

Fig 8-9. In this patient with hypertrophic cardiomyopathy, a trough of septal myocardium was removed anteriorly with a depth and length of approximately 1 cm, taking care to avoid creating a VSD. Because of severe subaortic obstruction with systolic anterior motion of the AML, the mitral valve was replaced with a low-profile mechanical valve. Both anterior and posterior chords were preserved, but the anterior leaflet was partly excised, with the remnants of the AML incorporated into the medial and lateral suture lines.

Comments

Hypertrophic cardiomyopathy is an autosomal dominant inherited disease that is characterized by asymmetric hypertrophy of the left ventricle, diastolic dysfunction and, in a subset of patients, dynamic subaortic obstruction. There are several different patterns of left ventricular hypertrophy but all have in common relative sparing the basal segment of the inferior–posterior left ventricular wall. In some cases, symptoms are predominantly a result of diastolic dysfunction, as in the first case above. Typically, relaxation is decreased early in the disease, with decreased compliance occurring late in the disease. Diastolic dysfunction is associated with elevated filling pressures and a reduced forward cardiac output, resulting in symptoms of exertional fatigue and dyspnea.

The dynamic outflow obstruction that occurs in some patients is related to systolic anterior motion of the mitral leaflets and an anatomically abnormal mitral valve. There is often coexisting mitral regurgitation due to malcoaptation of the leaflets at the site of systolic anterior motion. Symptoms of angina, dyspnea and syncope occur in some, but not all, patients with outflow obstruction. Outflow obstruction is dynamic in that it varies during the ejection period, with the maximal obstruction in late systole.

In addition, the degree of outflow obstruction varies with loading conditions: typically, it increases with a decrease in ventricular volume (e.g. hypovolemia), a decrease in systemic vascular resistance (e.g. with vasodilators) or an increase in contractility (e.g. with exercise).

Treatment options include medical therapy, percutaneous ablation of the septal myocardium in selected patients, and surgical myotomy/myectomy, sometimes with concurrent mitral valve replacement.

Suggested Reading

1. Woo A, Wigle ED, Rakowski H. Echocardiography in the evaluation and management of patients with hypertrophic cardiomyopathy. In: Otto CM, ed. The Practice of Clinical Echocardiography, 2nd edn. Philadelphia: WB Saunders, 2002: 588–612.

2. Maron BJ. Hypertrophic cardiomyopathy: a systematic review. JAMA 2002; 287:1308–20.

3. Hagueh SR, Ommen SR, Lakkis NM et al. Comparison of ethanol septal reduction therapy with surgical myectomy for the treatment of hypertrophic obstructive cardiomyopathy. J Am Coll Cardiol 2001; 38:1701–6.

4. Nishimura RA, Holmes DR Jr. Clinical practice. Hypertrophic obstructive cardiomyopathy. N Engl J Med 2004; 350:1320–7.

9

Pericardial Disease

Pericardial effusion

Pericardial constriction

Pericardial Effusion

Examples of pericardial effusions seen on intra-operative TEE in several different patients are shown.

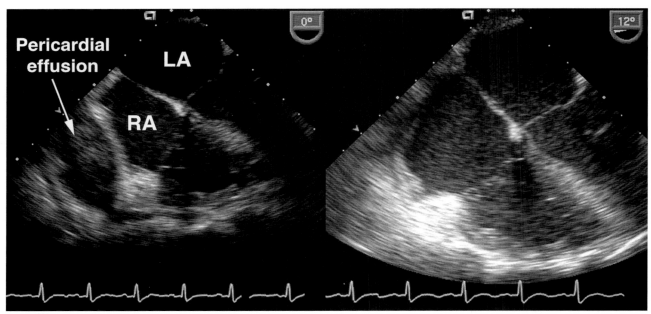

DVD **Fig 9-1.** From a high transesophageal position, an echo-free space is seen adjacent to the right atrium in a four-chamber view (*left*). At the end of the surgical procedure, the pericardial effusion is no longer present (*right*).

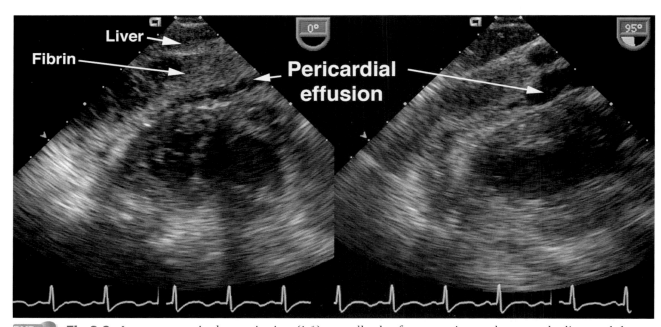

DVD **Fig 9-2.** In a transgastric short-axis view (*left*) a small echo-free space is seen between the liver and the epicardial surface of the heart, consistent with a pericardial effusion. With rotation of the image plane to 95 degrees, in a two-chamber view of the left ventricle, the effusion is seen. There is fibrinous material within the effusion, consistent with a subacute process.

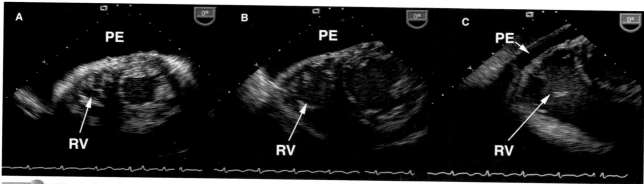

Fig 9-3. This series of transgastric images in a short-axis view from left to right shows a pericardial effusion (**PE**) of diminishing size as the fluid is removed by percutaneous needle pericardiocentesis. Note that the size of the left and right ventricles increases as the pericardial fluid is removed, suggesting that high intrapericardial pressures prevented normal diastolic ventricular filling, e.g. pericardial tamponade physiology.

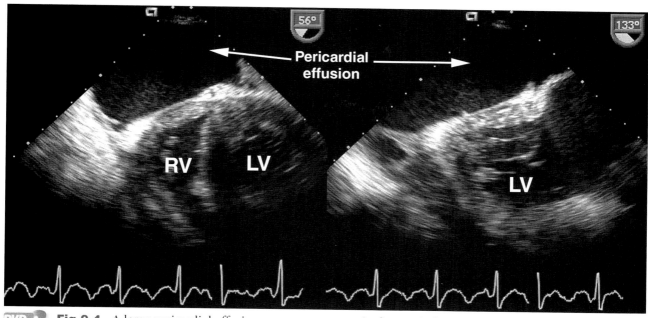

Fig 9-4. A large pericardial effusion seen on transgastric short-axis (*left*) and two-chamber (*right*) views.

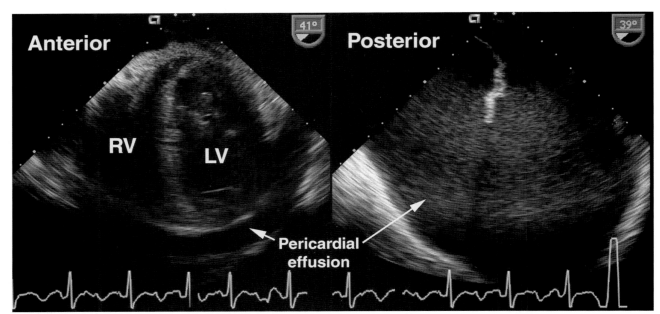

Fig 9-5. From a basal transgastric position rotated to 41 degrees, an echo-free space consistent with an effusion is seen anterior to the left ventricle. In this view, the amount of fluid appears only moderate. However, when the image plane is angulated posteriorly (*right*) a large echo-free space consistent with effusion is seen. This space is most consistent with pericardial rather than pleural fluid, because in real time it is seen to be continuous with the pericardial fluid collection seen initially.

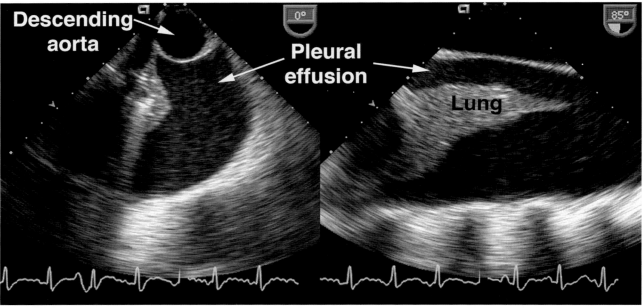

Fig 9-6. With the transducer turned laterally to image the descending thoracic aorta, a large echo-free space consistent with a pleural effusion is seen in both short- and long-axis views of the descending aorta. Note that the pleural effusion, unlike a pericardial effusion, is posterior to the descending aorta. In addition, lung tissue is seen within the fluid-filled space.

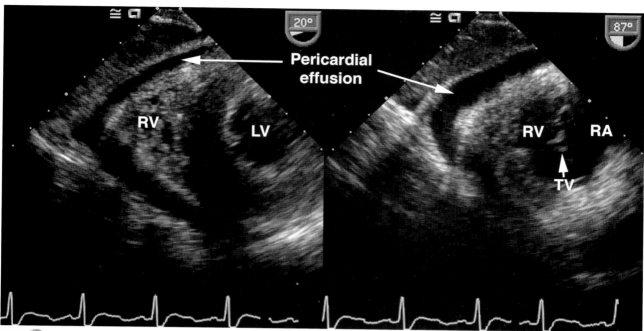

Fig 9-7. This patient presented with ascending aortic dissection, and signs of pericardial tamponade. In the transgastric short-axis view (*left*) and long-axis view (*right*), both the right atrium (**RA**) and right ventricle (**RV**) are seen to be compressed by the pericardial effusion. TV = tricuspid valve.

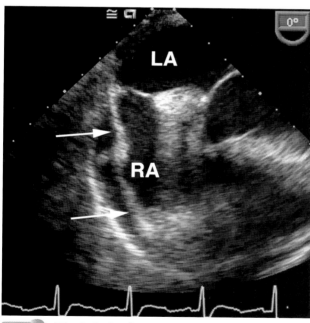

Fig 9-8. In the same patient as **Fig 9-7**, right atrial collapse is seen (**arrows**).

Comments

A pericardial effusion is diagnosed based on the echocardiographic finding of an echolucent area around the heart. Pericardial effusions are usually circumferential, with fluid filling the entire pericardial space around the right and left ventricles, although pericardial effusions may also be asymmetric due to adhesions resulting in areas of loculated fluid, especially in patients with prior cardiac surgical procedures.

The pericardial space extends to the origin of the great vessels, with the narrow transverse sinus of the pericardium extending posterior to the aorta and pulmonary artery. Fluid in the transverse sinus is rarely seen. The pericardial space encloses the right atrium, with pericardial reflections at the junctions of the SVC and IVC with the right atrium, so that fluid adjacent to the right atrium is commonly seen. A small pocket of pericardial fluid also may be seen posterior to the left atrium, where the oblique sinus of the pericardium extends into the region between the four pulmonary veins.

A pericardial effusion is distinguished from a pleural effusion by its location. Pericardial fluid posterior to the left ventricle and left atrium is anterior to the descending thoracic aorta, whereas pleural fluid extends posterior to the descending aorta. Fluid adjacent to the right atrium may be either pleural or pericardial, with the latter inferred from the presence of a pericardial effusion in other views. The presence of a compressed lung in the echolucent space helps confirm a diagnosis of pleural effusion.

Pericardial fluid may be well tolerated if the pressure within the pericardial space is low, for example with a chronic effusion that has accumulated slowly. Even very large chronic effusions may be associated with normal hemodynamics. However, if the pressure in the pericardial space exceeds the diastolic pressure in the cardiac chambers, hemodynamic changes are seen. When pericardial pressure exceeds right atrial pressure, the free wall of the right atrium inverts or "collapses" and right atrial filling volumes are reduced. Similarly, the left atrium and right ventricle can be compressed when pericardial pressure exceeds the pressure in that cardiac chamber. Tamponade physiology can even occur with loculated effusions if there is compression of one of the cardiac chambers. The diagnosis of tamponade due to a loculated effusion can be challenging. In addition, chamber collapse may not be seen, even when pericardial pressures are high, if the wall of the chamber is thickened or fibrotic.

Along with chamber collapse, a high pericardial pressure restricts the total cardiac volume. Thus, as the right-sided chambers increase in size with inspiration, due to negative intrathoracic pressures and increased venous return, the left-sided chambers are compressed with a reduction in forward cardiac output. These reciprocal inspiratory changes in right and left ventricular diastolic filling result in the drop in blood pressure seen with inspiration, or pulsus paradoxus.

Suggested Reading

1. Munt BI, Kinnaird T, Thompson CR. Pericardial disease. In: Otto CM, ed. The Practice of Clinical Echocardiography, 2nd edn. Philadelphia: WB Saunders, 2002: 639–57.

2. Swanton BJ, Keane D, Vlahakes GJ, Streckenbach SC. Intraoperative transesophageal echocardiography in the early detection of acute tamponade after laser extraction of a defibrillator lead. Anesth Analg 2003; 97(3):654–6.

3. Spodick DH. Acute cardiac tamponade. N Engl J Med 2003; 349(7):684–90.

Pericardial Constriction

This 57-year-old man was referred for coronary artery bypass grafting surgery and pericardiectomy for pericardial constriction. About 4 years ago, he presented with exertional dyspnea and lower extremity edema. Echocardiography showed a thickened pericardium with increased central venous pressure and evidence for reciprocal respiratory changes in right and left ventricular diastolic filling. Left and right ventricular size and systolic function were normal, and estimated pulmonary systolic pressure was 30 mmHg. Cardiac catheterization confirmed equalization of right and left ventricular diastolic pressures, with a square-root sign ($\sqrt{}$) in the ventricular diastolic pressure curve. There was no etiology identified for his pericardial disease. Specifically, there was no history of pericarditis, chest surgery or trauma, radiation therapy, or rheumatologic disease. He denied a history of tuberculosis and a ppd was negative.

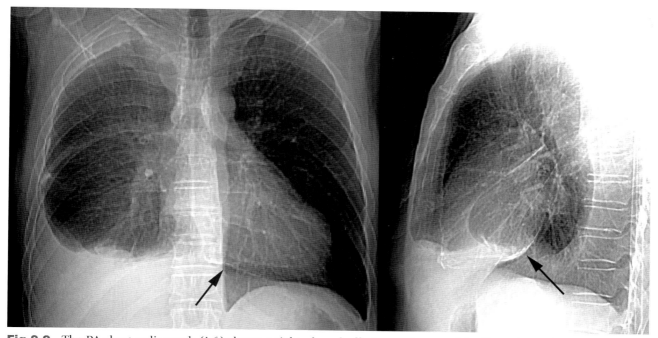

Fig 9-9. The PA chest radiograph (*left*) shows a right pleural effusion and a very faint line of calcification (**arrow**) at the inferior aspect of the left ventricle. The lateral chest radiograph (*right*) shows an area of dense pericardial calcification (**arrow**) along the posterior aspect of the left ventricle.

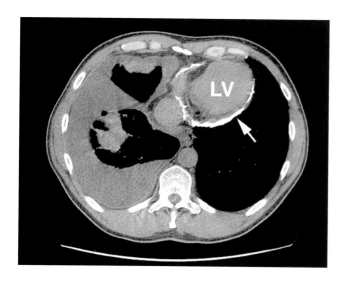

Fig 9-10. A chest CT scan shows marked thickening and increased density of the pericardium, consistent with pericardial thickening and calcification. There is a moderately sized right pleural effusion and some compressive right lower lobe atelectasis. The man's CT findings also included liver cirrhosis and splenomegaly, suggesting portal hypertension, probably related to his constrictive pericarditis.

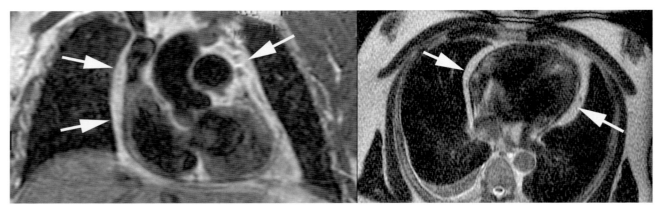

Fig 9-11. MRI demonstrates thickened pericardium (**arrows**) in both coronal (*left*) and axial (*right*) views.

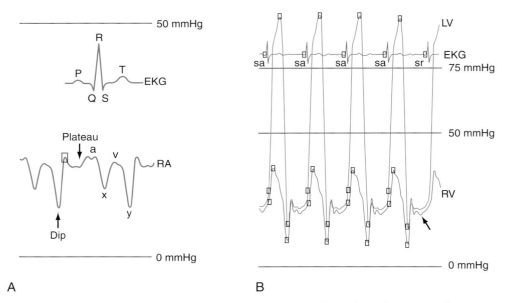

A   B

Fig 9-12. (*A*) Right atrial pressure tracing. The early diastolic dip and later diastolic plateau form the square-root sign (√), typical in constrictive pericarditis. (*B*) There is equalization of RV and LV diastolic pressure (**arrow**), also typical in constrictive pericarditis.

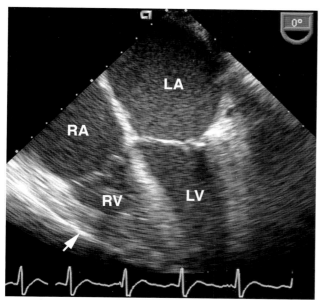

DVD **Fig 9-13.** In this four-chamber view, the atria are enlarged and the ventricular chambers are small, as expected with pericardial constriction. An area of pericardial thickening along the right ventricular free wall is seen (**arrow**).

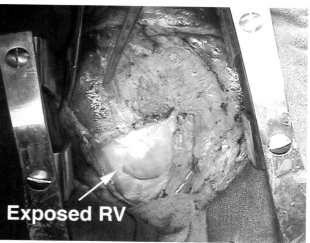

DVD **Fig 9-15.** At surgery, the pericardium was severely thickened and calcified. The pericardium was stripped from phrenic nerve to phrenic nerve laterally.

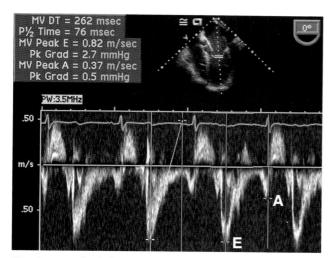

Fig 9-14. The left ventricular diastolic filling pattern shows a high E/A ratio and a steep deceleration slope. This pattern of diastolic filling is consistent with rapid early diastolic filling, with impaired late diastolic filling due, in this case, to pericardial constriction. This pattern of diastolic filling is also seen with severe left ventricular diastolic dysfunction due to decreased compliance.

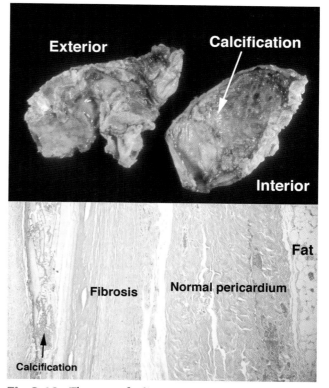

Fig 9-16. The gross findings on pathology were segments of fibrotic pericardium, with a thickness ranging from 0.3 to 1.4 cm. Microscopic examination showed fibrosis, calcification and patchy chronic inflammation consistent with constrictive pericarditis.

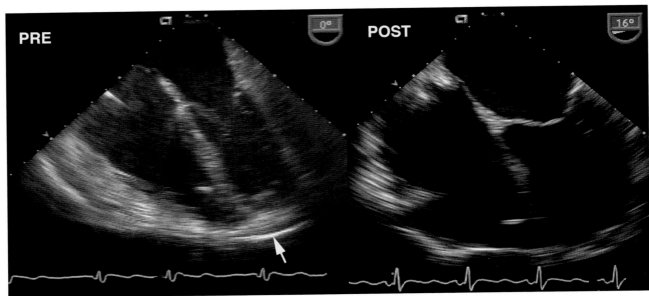

Fig 9-17. Comparison of the preoperative (*left*) and post-pericardiectomy (*right*) four-chamber views using the small depth scale shows the increased size of the ventricular chambers after relief of constrictive physiology. The arrow indicates thickened pericardium.

Comments

Constrictive pericarditis may be due to prior infectious pericarditis (tuberculous or viral), trauma or cardiac surgery, rheumatologic disorders, neoplasia, or mediastinal radiation, but in many cases a cause is not found. The basic pathophysiology of constriction is that the adherence, thickening and fibrosis of the pericardium result in the ventricles being unable to fill adequately in diastole. The primary problem in clinical diagnosis is distinguishing pericardial constriction from a restrictive cardiomyopathy. Both are characterized by small ventricles with normal systolic function, abnormal diastolic filling patterns, biatrial enlargement and an elevated central venous pressure. However, with restrictive cardiomyopathy, pulmonary pressures are often elevated, the pericardium is normal in thickness and the diastolic pressures in the right and left ventricles are not equal.

The hallmark of pericardial constriction is a thickened pericardium, as in this case. Although echocardiography often first suggests the diagnosis of constriction, evaluation of the presence and severity of pericardial thickening by echocardiography is limited. Both CT and MRI provide better definition of pericardial anatomy and should be considered when echocardiography suggests this diagnosis.

With both pericardial constriction and restrictive cardiomyopathy, the pattern of ventricle filling on a single cardiac cycle is characterized by a rapid early diastolic filling phase, and a reduced atrial contribution to filling. However, when multiple beats are examined, there are no significant respiratory changes in patients with restrictive cardiomyopathy. In contrast, in patients with pericardial constriction, there are marked reciprocal respiratory changes in left and right ventricular diastolic filling. The rigid adherent pericardium limits the total cardiac volume so that as right-sided filling increases with inspiration, the left ventricle is compressed and left-sided filling decreases. The opposite changes occur with expiration. Tissue Doppler evaluation is also helpful for diagnosis of constrictive pericarditis.

At cardiac catheterization, there is equalization of the diastolic pressures in the cardiac chambers with pericardial constriction. The demonstration that right and left ventricle diastolic pressures are equal (within 5 mmHg of each other) after volume loading is diagnostic for constriction. The diastolic pressure curve also classically shows an early diastolic dip, due to the initial high-pressure gradient from atrium to ventricle, followed by rapid equalization of pressures as the constricted ventricle quickly fills to capacity. The late diastolic plateau phase is flat, as there is no further ventricular filling and no change in ventricular pressure. This results in the pressure curve looking like the mathematical symbol for a square root ($\sqrt{\ }$).

Suggested Reading

1. Rajagopalan N, Garcia MJ, Rodriguez L et al. Comparison of new Doppler echocardiographic methods to differentiate constrictive pericardial heart disease and restrictive cardiomyopathy. Am J Cardiol 2001; 87(1):86–94.

2. Sengupta PP, Mohan JC, Mehta V et al. Accuracy and pitfalls of early diastolic motion of the mitral annulus for diagnosing constrictive pericarditis by tissue Doppler imaging. Am J Cardiol 2004; 93(7):886–90.

3. Rienmuller R, Groll R, Lipton MJ. CT and MR imaging of pericardial disease. Radiol Clin North Am 2004; 42(3):587–601, vi.

10

Diseases of the Great Vessels

Aneurysms

Case 10-1
Ascending Aortic Aneurysm

This 71-year-old female had undergone bileaflet mechanical aortic valve replacement for a bicuspid aortic valve 18 years previously. On periodic follow-up echocardiography, her valve prosthesis continued to function normally but she had progressive dilation of the ascending aorta. She was referred for surgical intervention for an ascending aortic aneurysm.

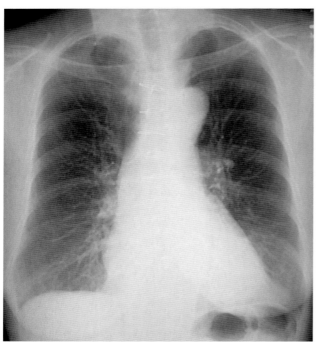

Fig 10-1. PA chest radiograph demonstrates slight prominence of the ascending aorta with a relatively normal arch.

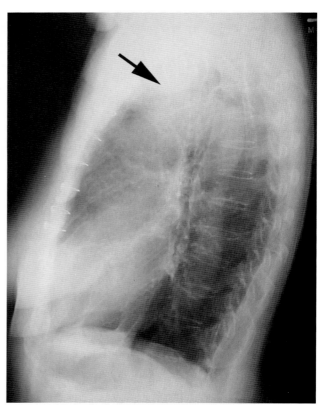

Fig 10-2. However, the lateral chest radiograph demonstrates the markedly enlarged ascending aorta, with the retrosternal space opacified by the enlarged aorta (**arrow**). Sternal wires are present from her previous valve surgery.

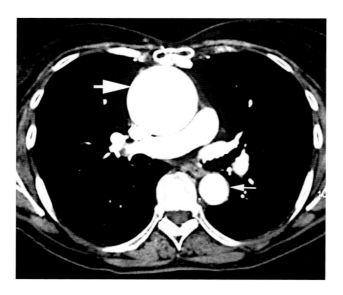

Fig 10-3. Contrast CT at the level of the ascending aorta demonstrated a large aneurysm of the ascending aorta (**large arrow**). The descending thoracic aorta diameter is normal at this level (**small arrow**).

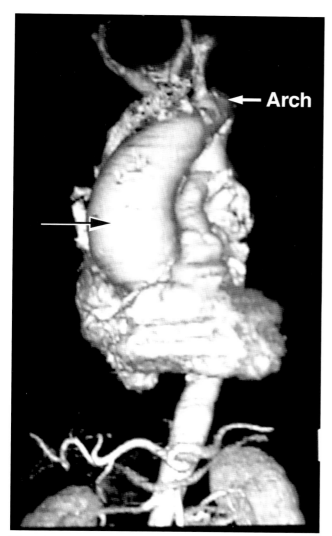

Fig 10-4. 3D reconstruction of the CT images shows the extent of the aortic aneurysm (**arrow**) with dilation maximal in the mid-ascending aorta, tapering to a normal diameter by the mid arch.

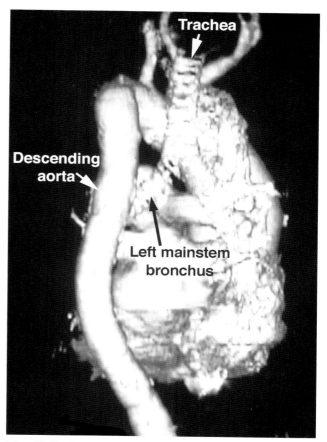

Fig 10-5. On rotation of the 3D image to show the posterior aspect of the mediastinum, the relatively normal descending thoracic aorta can be seen.

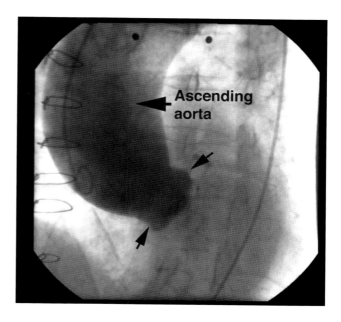

DVD Fig 10-6. Aortography demonstrates the dilated ascending aorta and sinuses of Valsalva (**arrow**). In real time, a small amount of aortic regurgitation is appreciated.

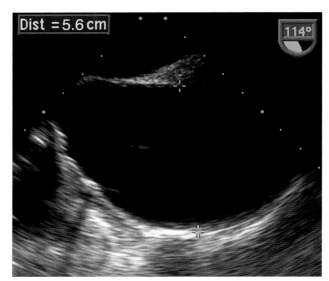

Fig 10-7. Intraoperative TEE from a high position in a long-axis view of the ascending aorta shows a maximum dimension of 5.6 cm.

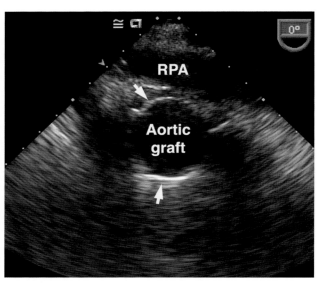

Fig 10-9. After the procedure, a short-axis TEE image of the ascending aorta demonstrates the tube graft, with the right pulmonary artery posteriorly. Note the bright echoes from the synthetic graft material (**arrows**).

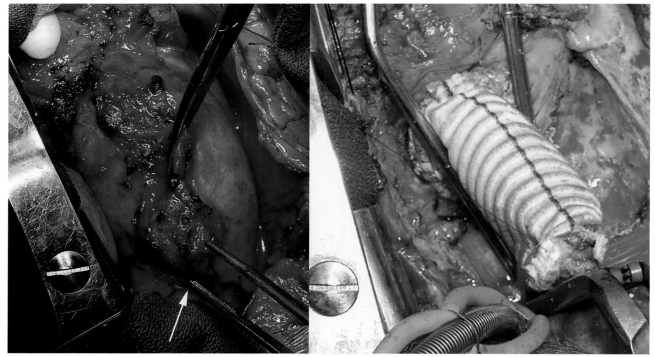

Fig 10-8. At surgery, the ascending aorta was severely dilated. However, the sinuses of Valsalva were relatively normal in size and there was substantial scarring at the previous aortotomy site. This view is from the anesthesiologist's perspective: the valve level is at the top of the photograph, with the arch at the bottom (by the open forceps, **arrow**) (*left*). The aneurysm was resected, beginning about 1 cm above the coronary orifices and extending to the proximal aortic arch. An interposition Dacron tube graft replacement of the ascending aorta was performed. (*right*).

Comments

The ascending aorta is best visualized on TEE in a long-axis view at about 120 degrees rotation. Long-axis images of more cephalad segments of the ascending aorta can be achieved by pulling the transducer back in the esophagus. Short-axis views of the sinuses and first few centimeters of the ascending aorta can be obtained at about 30 degrees rotation, but interposition of the air-filled trachea limits visualization of more cephalad segments of the aorta in a short-axis orientation. Another view of the ascending aorta can be obtained starting with a view of the descending thoracic aorta in short axis, turning the probe towards the patient's right side at the level of the arch and then angling the image plane inferiorly. However, even with careful adjustment of image planes, the junction of the ascending aorta with the aortic arch may not be visualized on TEE.

The normal morphology of the aorta is characterized by symmetric sinuses of Valsalva, with a well-defined junction between the sinuses and tubular segment of the ascending aorta, e.g. the sinotubular junction. The ascending aorta contour is smooth, with gradual tapering from the ascending aorta into the arch and descending thoracic aorta.

Because of the complex anatomy of the aorta, the diameter is typically measured at several places during a complete examination: the annulus, the sinuses, the sinotubular junction, the ascending aorta, the arch, the descending thoracic aorta and the proximal abdominal aorta. The term "aortic root" generally refers to the segment of the aorta from the annulus to the arch. The severity of an ascending aortic aneurysm is defined by the maximum aortic dimension at any point within the aortic root.

The presence of a bicuspid aortic valve is associated with dilation of the ascending aorta. In addition, the risk of aortic dissection is 8–9 times higher in patients with a bicuspid aortic valve than in subjects with a normal trileaflet aortic valve. After aortic valve surgery, the strongest risk factor for progressive aortic dilation is the previous diagnosis of a bicuspid aortic valve, as in this case.

Suggested Reading

1. Fedak PW, Verma S, David TE et al. Clinical and pathophysiological implications of a bicuspid aortic valve. Circulation 2002; 106:900–4.

2. Ryan EW, Bolger AF. Aortic dissection and trauma: value and limitations of echocardiography. In: Otto CM, ed. The Practice of Clinical Echocardiography. Philadelphia: Elsevier/Saunders, 2002.

Case 10-2
Thoracoabdominal Aortic Aneurysm

This 56-year-old man presented with numbness of the 4th and 5th digits of his left hand. Although he had a long history of cigarette smoking, he had no other medical problems and denied any other symptoms. Chest radiography revealed a widened mediastinal silhouette, so he was referred for further evaluation. Pulmonary function tests and a stress-imaging cardiac study were normal.

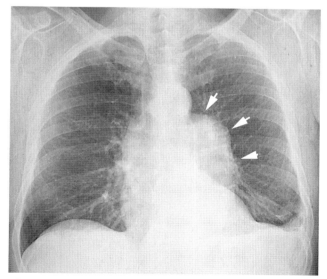

Fig 10-10. PA chest radiograph demonstrates a widened mediastinum with what appears to be a large mass that projects along the upper left heart border (**arrows**).

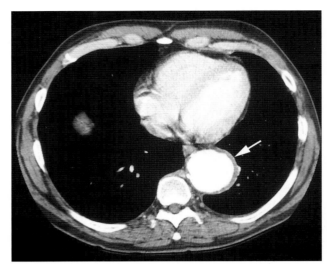

Fig 10-11. Chest CT with contrast at the level of the left ventricle shows the dilated descending thoracic aorta (**arrow**). The contrast-filled lumen is surrounded by lower-density tissue consistent with laminated thrombus within the aneurysm.

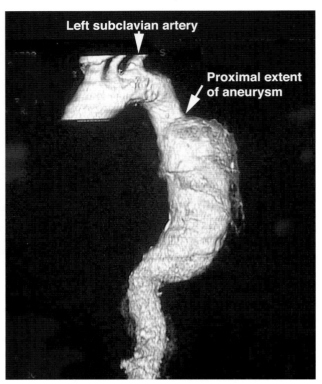

Fig 10-13. 3D reconstruction of the CT images shows the extent of the aneurysm from just beyond the left subclavian artery to the celiac artery.

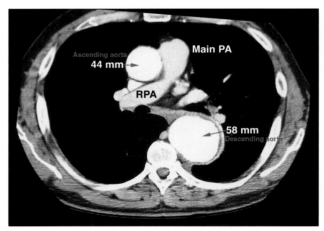

Fig 10-12. At the level of the right pulmonary artery (**PA**), the ascending aorta is mildly dilated at 44 mm but the descending thoracic aorta is severely dilated at 58 mm.

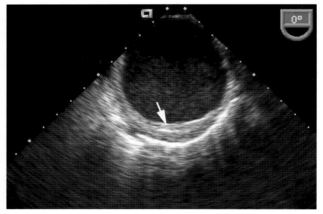

Fig 10-14. Intraoperative TEE, with the probe turned towards the descending thoracic aorta, shows the dilated aorta with laminated thrombus (**arrow**).

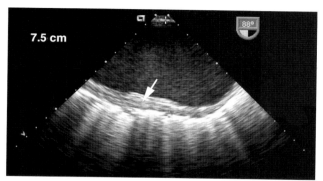

7.5 cm

Fig 10-15. A longitudinal view of the descending thoracic aorta shows the dilation and thrombus (**arrow**).

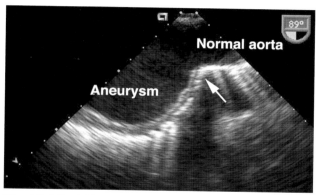

Normal aorta

Aneurysm

Fig 10-16. A TEE view with the probe moved superiorly in the esophagus shows the transition from a relatively normal-sized aortic arch to the dilated descending thoracic aorta (**arrow**).

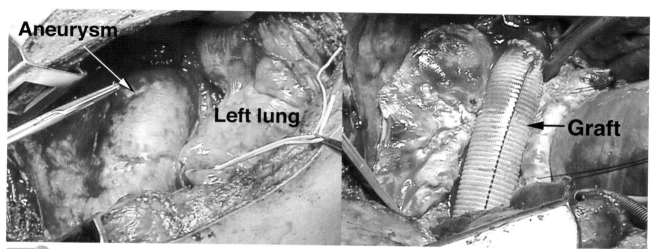

Aneurysm

Left lung

Graft

Fig 10-17. At surgery, in an image taken from the left side of the patient, a left thoracotomy approach was used to visualize the aneurysm. A 28 mm Hemashield graft was placed, using BioGlue to support the proximal and distal anastomoses. The native aorta was closed over the graft.

Comments

The descending thoracic aorta is imaged using TEE starting at the transgastric position, by turning the probe to the patient's left until the circular cross-sectional image is seen. After adjusting image depth and gain, the probe is slowly withdrawn in the esophagus, providing sequential serial views of the descending aorta. Imaging in a short-axis orientation as the probe is withdrawn is recommended so that the entire intimal surface of the aorta is included in the scan. However, long-axis views may be helpful when abnormalities are found, to better define the extent of disease.

Case 10-3
Aortic Pseudoaneurysm

This 41-year-old man with reactive arthritis underwent mechanical aortic valve replacement 9 years ago for aortic regurgitation. Four months ago he developed prosthetic valve endocarditis. He was treated with antibiotics and repeat aortic valve replacement, with that procedure complicated by a paravalvular abscess that required placement of a pericardial patch in the periannular region. Postoperatively, he had persistent paravalvular regurgitation, and repeat echocardiography showed "rocking" of the prosthesis and a possible pseudoaneurysm. A preoperative transesophageal echocardiogram demonstrated valve dehiscence with blood flow from the aorta into an anterior echo-free space that also communicated with the left ventricle. He was referred for surgery.

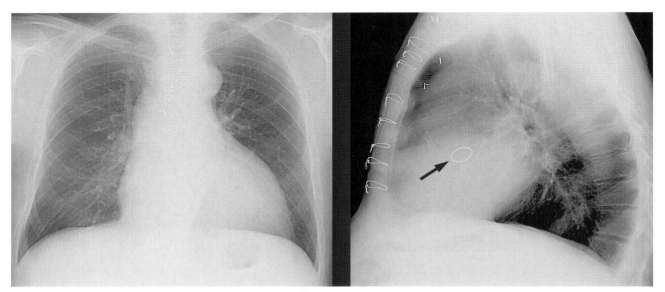

Fig 10-18. Chest radiography shows prominence of the ascending aorta. The lateral view demonstrates an enlarged ascending aorta with opacification of the retrosternal space, and the presence of the radiopaque ring of the prosthetic valve (**arrow**).

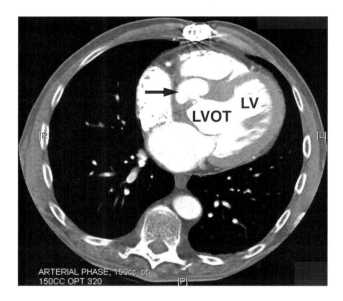

Fig 10-19. Chest CT with contrast at the level of the left ventricle (**LV**) shows an abnormal area (**arrow**) filled with contrast, anterior to the LV outflow tract (**LVOT**), that communicates with the LVOT.

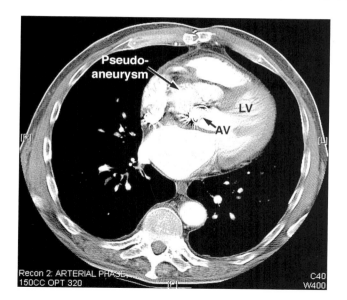

Recon 2: ARTERIAL PHASE
150CC OPT 320   C40
                                 W400

Fig 10-20. Chest CT with contrast at the level of the prosthetic aortic valve (**AV**). Anterior to the aortic valve replacement is a collection of contrast with irregular borders, which is extraluminal, measuring 2.3 × 4.2 cm. These findings are consistent with an aortic pseudoaneurysm.

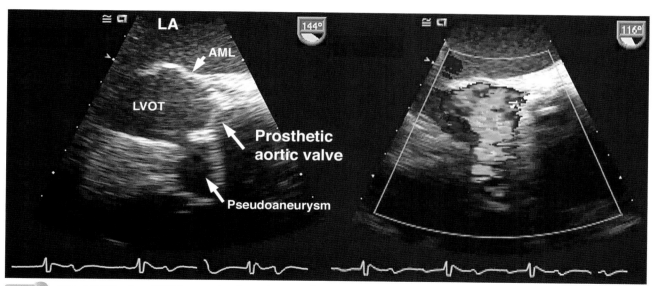

DVD **Fig 10-21.** In a TEE long-axis plane (at 144 degrees rotation) the pseudoaneurysm is seen anterior to the prosthetic aortic valve. Color Doppler (*right*) demonstrates flow in and out of the pseudoaneurysm from the LVOT.

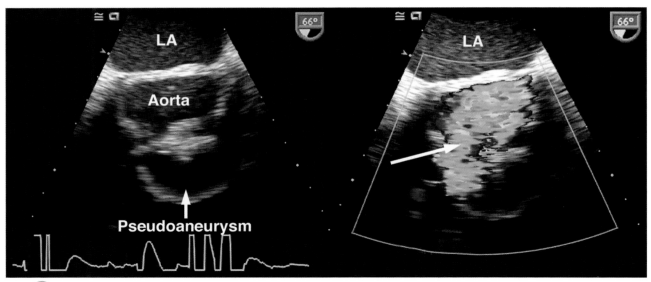

DVD **Fig 10-22.** In a short-axis TEE view at the level of the ascending aorta, a large echo-free space with irregular borders (**arrow**), consistent with a pseudoaneurysm, is seen. Color flow Doppler (*right*) demonstrates communication between the pseudoaneurysm and the patient's heart (**arrow**).

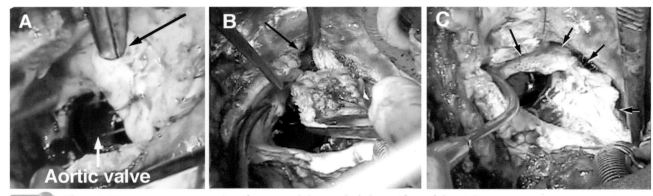

DVD **Fig 10-23.** At surgery, opening the aorta (*A*) revealed the orifice of the right coronary artery (**arrow**) just above the prosthetic aortic valve. (*B*) The anterior aortic wall has been retracted to reveal the entrance into the pseudoaneurysm (**arrow**). (*C*) After removal of the anterior aortic wall, a very large pseudoaneurysm was appreciated, originating from underneath the right main coronary artery and extending down to the middle of the non-coronary sinus.

In another example, this 43-year-old male originally presented 2 years prior to the current admission with an acute type A aortic dissection that originated above the aortic valve and extended to the iliac bifurcation. At that time, his ascending aorta was replaced with a tube graft on cardiopulmonary bypass. He was readmitted to our institution with chest pain and *Staphylococcus aureus* bacteremia. A CT scan revealed a large mediastinal hematoma; anterior and posterior pseudoaneurysms were seen at the proximal end of the aortic graft.

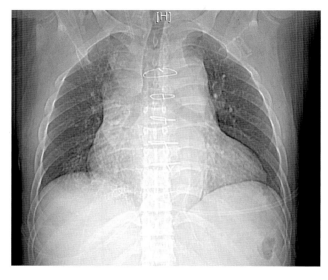

Fig 10-24. PA chest X-ray shows an enlarged mediastinum.

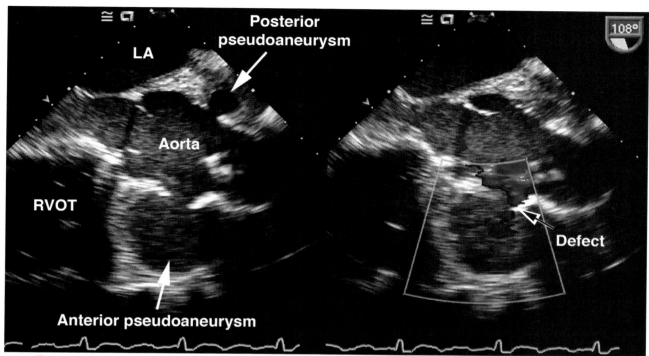

Fig 10-25. Long-axis view of the aortic valve and ascending aorta shows dehiscence of the proximal end of the aortic graft, and both anterior and posterior pseudoaneurysms. Color Doppler (*right*) reveals flow from the aorta, through the defect and into the anterior pseudoaneurysm.

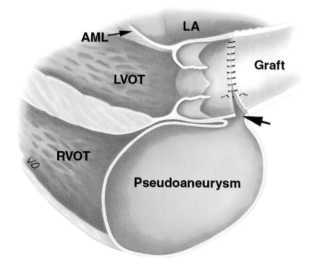

Fig 10-26. This drawing, corresponding to the long-axis TEE in **Fig 10-25**, demonstrates the origin (**arrow**) of the pseudoaneurysm.

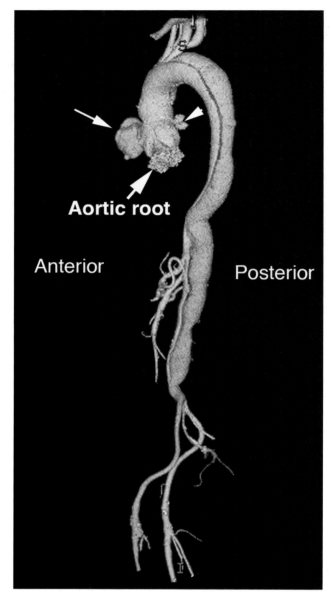

Fig 10-27. 3D CT reconstruction shows the pseudoaneurysms (**arrows**) in relation to the aortic root.

Comments

Paravalvular infection may result in rupture of the tissues around the valve. With a mitral paravalvular abscess, rupture occurs into the pericardial space and, like a post-myocardial infarction rupture of the LV, may be contained by pericardial adhesions, resulting in a left ventricular pseudoaneurysm. Similarly, with an aortic annular abscess, paravalvular infection may rupture externally, instead of into an adjacent cardiac chamber. At the site of rupture, adhesions and scarring limit the extravasation of blood resulting in a contained space or pseudoaneurysm. In the first patient, the valve dehiscence extended both above and below the valve plane so that blood entered the pseudoaneurysm from the aorta, and exited into the LV outflow tract,

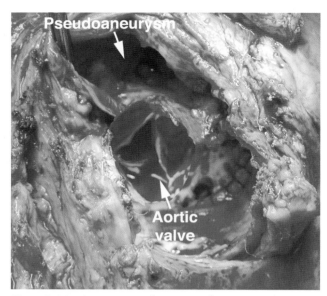

Fig 10-28. At surgery, a large pseudoaneurysm was seen anterior to the aortic root.

simulating aortic regurgitation. Surgical intervention is needed because the pseudoaneurysm will continue to expand and may rupture. In addition, an infection pseudoaneurysm, like an abscess, must be eliminated in order to control the infection.

With the complex anatomy of a pseudoaneurysm, integration of data from multiple imaging modalities is needed in the preoperative assessment of the patient. Echocardiography is ideal for evaluation of aortic valve hemodynamics and left ventricular function, and is often the initial test suggesting a pseudoaneurysm. Transesophageal imaging often can define the entrance into the pseudoaneurysm and the location relative to the other cardiac chambers. However, wider field of view tomographic images, obtained with CT or MR imaging provide better evaluation of the extent and size and the pseudoaneurysm.

Suggested Reading

1. Zoghbi WA. Echocardiographic recognition of unusual complications after surgery on the great vessels and cardiac valves. In: Otto CM, (Ed). The Practice of Clinical Echocardiography. Philadelphia: WB Saunders, 2002.

2. Baker WB, Klein MS, Reardon MJ, Zoghbi WA. Left ventricular pseudoaneurysm complicating mitral valve replacement: transesophageal echocardiographic diagnosis and impact on management. J Am Soc Echocardiogr 1993; 6:548–52.

3. Ronderos RE, Portis M, Stoermann W, Sarmiento C. Are all echocardiographic findings equally predictive for diagnosis in prosthetic endocarditis? J Am Soc Ecocardiogr 2004; 17:664–69.

4. Mohammadi S, Bonnet N, Leprince P et al. Reoperation for false aneurysm of the ascending aorta after its prosthetic replacement: surgical strategy. Ann Thorac Surg 2005; 79:147–52.

Dissection

Case 10-4
Aortic Arch Dissection

This 51-year-old man had a history of dissection of the ascending aorta with placement of an ascending aortic graft and valve resuspension 10 years previously. He now presents with epigastric pain and an aortic arch dissection diagnosed by CT imaging.

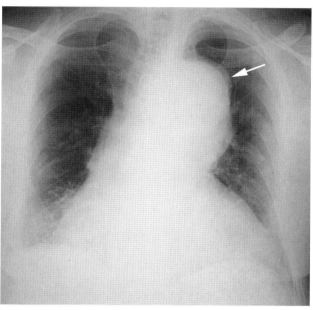

Fig 10-29. PA chest radiograph shows a markedly enlarged aorta with a dilated aortic arch (**arrow**).

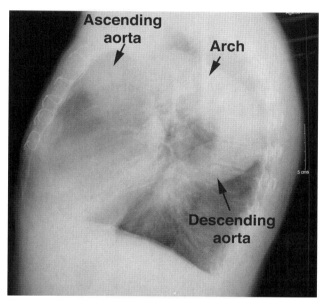

Fig 10-30. The lateral chest radiography demonstrates enlargement of the ascending aorta (retrosternal space is "filled") with a dilated and tortuous arch.

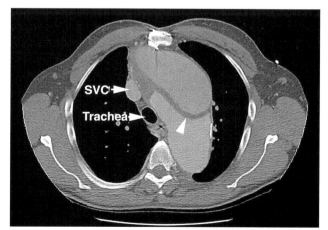

Fig 10-31. Chest CT without contrast shows the enlarged arch with displacement of the trachea to the right. There appears to be a less dense linear structure within the dilated arch (**arrowhead**), suggesting a dissection flap.

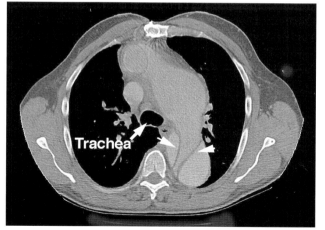

Fig 10-32. Another CT image of the aortic arch demonstrates a complex flap, resulting in marked narrowing of the true lumen (**arrows**) due to compression by the false lumen on both sides.

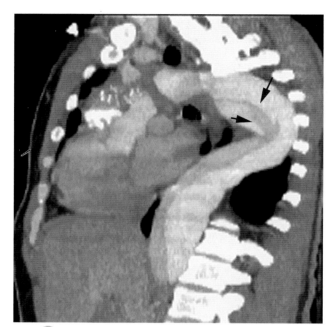

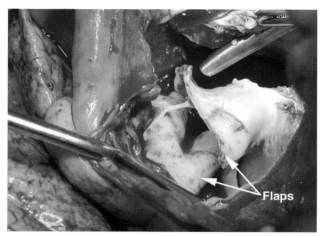

Fig 10-35. With the arch opened at surgery, the dissection flaps in the arch are seen.

DVD **Fig 10-33.** In this laterally reconstructed CT scan, the true lumen is again seen to be compressed by the complex dissection flap (**arrows**).

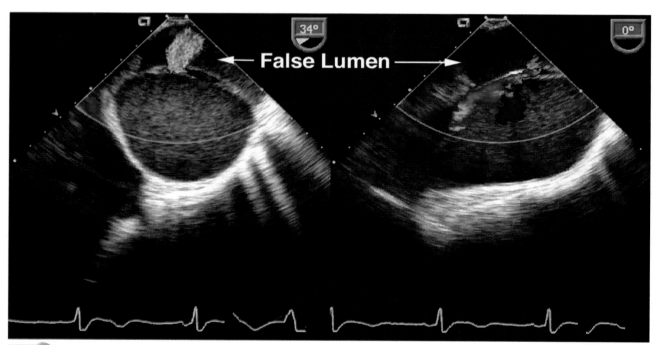

DVD **Fig 10-34.** Intraoperative TEE images of the aortic arch at 34 and 0 degrees rotation show the dissection flap with flow into the false lumen.

Comments

After surgical repair of an ascending aortic dissection, a persistent dissection flap persists in 81% of patients. In addition, more than mild aortic regurgitation is present in 25% of patients, and a persistent distal aneurysm >5 cm in diameter in 33%. However, these findings are usually present immediately after the surgical repair, requiring close clinical follow-up with periodic imaging studies.

The clinical presentation of a new dissection distal to the site of a previous repair suggests the possibility of an underlying connective tissue disorder, such as Marfan syndrome. In patients with Marfan syndrome, repair of the ascending aorta is lifesaving, but these patients are still at risk of dissection in other segments of the aorta and in more distal arteries. Thus, in patients with a previous dissection repair, any symptoms suggestive of progressive aortic disease require careful evaluation.

Suggested Reading

1. Dohmen G, Kuroczynski W, Dahm M et al. Value of echocardiography in patient follow-up after surgically corrected type A aortic dissection. Thorac Cardiovasc Surg 2001; 49:343–8.

2. Pyeritz RE. The Marfan syndrome. Annu Rev Med 2000; 51:481–510.

3. Alizad A, Seward JB. Echocardiographic features of genetic diseases: part 4. Connective tissue. J Am Soc Echocardiogr 2000; 13:325–30.

Case 10-5
Ascending Aortic Dissection

This 44-year-old woman, with a history of obesity, hypertension and diabetes, presented to the emergency department with chest pain.

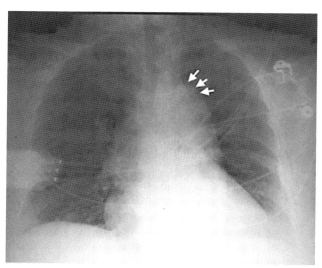

Fig 10-36. PA chest radiography shows a wide mediastinum with prominence of the aortic arch (**arrows**).

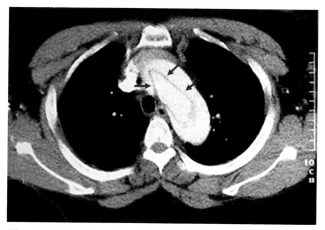

Fig 10-37. Chest CT with contrast demonstrates an enlarged aortic arch with a linear density within the lumen consistent with a dissection flap (**arrows**).

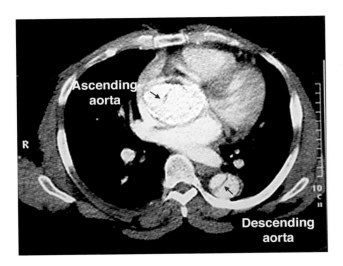

Fig 10-38. Chest CT at the level of the left atrium shows a dilated ascending aorta with a distorted contour and intraluminal density consistent with a dissection flap (**top arrow**). Although the descending thoracic aorta is normal in size, a linear dissection flap is present in the lumen (**bottom arrow**).

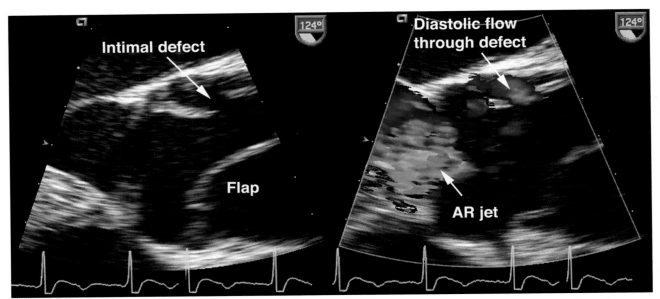

DVD ▶ **Fig 10-39.** Intraoperative TEE images in a magnified long-axis view of the ascending aorta show the dissection flap about 1 cm distal to the aortic valve leaflets. Along the posterior aspect of the aorta, an area of discontinuity in the flap is seen. Color flow imaging (*right*) shows flow into the false lumen via this defect and shows severe aortic regurgitation.

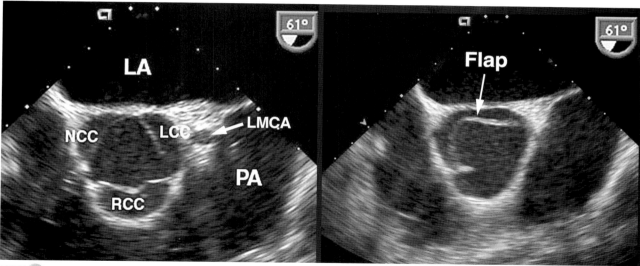

Fig 10-40. A short-axis TEE view of the aortic valve shows a normal trileaflet valve open in systole (*left*). The left main coronary artery (**LMCA**) is seen adjacent to the left coronary cusp (**LCC**). In diastole (*right*), the dissection flap prolapses proximally into the image plane. NCC = non-coronary cusp, RCC = right coronary cusp.

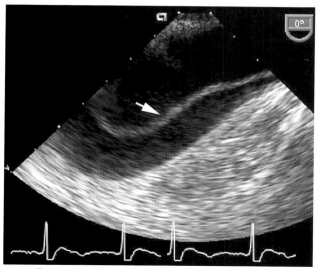

Fig 10-41. A high TEE view of the aortic arch shows the intraluminal flap (**arrow**). In real time, the motion of the intimal flap, independent from the motion of the aortic wall, can be appreciated.

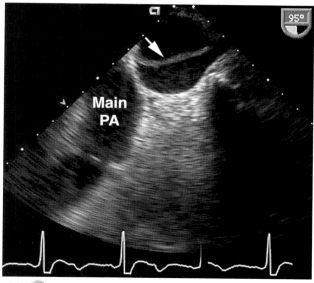

Fig 10-42. From the same transducer position as **Fig 10-41**, the image plane is rotated to 95 degrees to obtain this short-axis view of the aortic arch, with the intimal flap (**arrow**) seen.

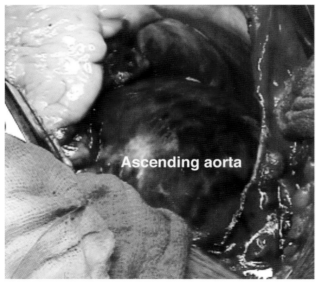

Fig 10-43. At surgery, the enlarged ascending aorta shows discoloration typical for a dissection.

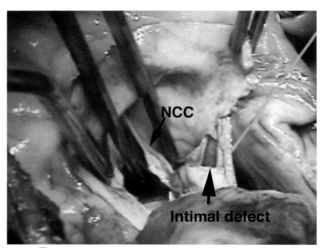

DVD **Fig 10-44.** After opening the aorta, the intimal defect (**arrow**) in close proximity to the aortic valve NCC is appreciated. The aortic valve was resuspended in a 28 mm Dacron tube graft replacement of the ascending aorta.

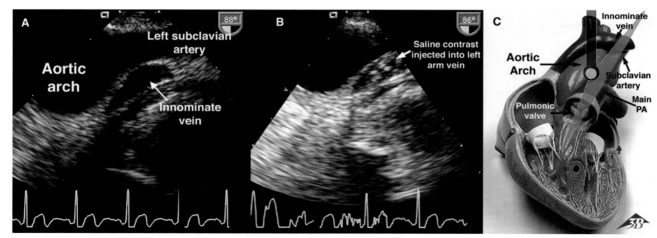

Fig 10-45. (*A*) A high esophageal view of the distal arch at 88 degrees, with the left subclavian artery clearly delineated. The innominate vein is anterior to the arch. The interface between the innominate vein and the arch may be mistaken for a dissection flap. (*B*) Agitated saline contrast injected through a left arm vein opacifies the innominate vein. (*C*) The anatomy is illustrated in a model. (Based on Economy Heart Model 3B Scientific.)

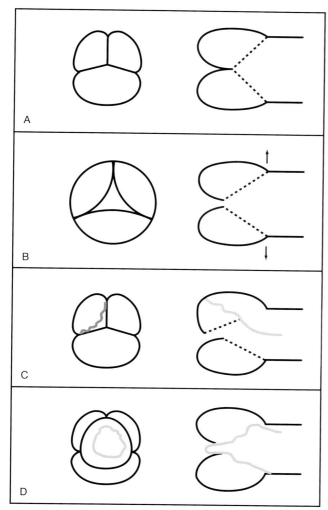

Fig 10-46. The different mechanisms of aortic regurgitation in type A aortic dissection. (Reproduced with permission from Movsowitz HD et al. Transesophageal echocardiographic description of the mechanisms of aortic regurgitation in acute type A aortic dissection: implications for aortic valve repair. J Am Coll Cardiol 2000; 36:884. ©Elsevier Inc.)

Comments

The echocardiographic diagnosis of aortic dissection is based on visualization of a linear mobile echogenic structure within the aortic lumen, e.g. the initial flap. It is particularly important to evaluate the ascending aorta because treatment of a dissection that involves the ascending aorta (type A) is surgery, whereas treatment of a dissection limited to the descending aorta (type B) is often medical.

On echocardiography, imaging artifacts may share some features of an aortic dissection; therefore, the echocardiographer should ensure that the mobile intraluminal echo is not due to reverberations. Dissection flaps may be missed if image quality is

poor or if there is limited visualization of any aortic segment. The interface between the innominate vein and the aortic arch may be mistaken for a dissection flap (see **Fig 10-45**). However, with a careful examination by an experienced echocardiographer, TEE has a sensitivity of about 98% and a specificity of 98% for diagnosis of aortic dissection. TEE has several advantages, including the ability to perform the examination at the bedside or in the operating room in unstable patients and the ability to assess valve regurgitation, ventricular function and the presence of a pericardial effusion at the time of the examination. Limitations of TEE are the limited definition of the distal extent of the dissection and the involvement of branch vessels.

Other imaging techniques for diagnosis of aortic dissection include chest CT and cardiac MRI. Both are equivalent to TEE in terms of sensitivity and specificity and both have the advantage of allowing evaluation of distal vessels and a wide field of view in the mediastinum. The choice of diagnostic modality in an individual patient often depends on the speed with which the study can be obtained and the expertise of each particular institution.

Figure 10-46 illustrates the different mechanisms of aortic regurgitation in type A aortic dissection. Compared to patients with normal aortic anatomy (a), aortic regurgitation may be due to (b) dilation of the sinuses of Valsalva with incomplete central coaptation of the leaflets, (c) extension of the dissection into the layers of the valve leaflet, resulting in a flail leaflet with severe regurgitation, or (d) distortion of the valve commissures by the dissection flap, leading to asymmetric leaflet closure and an eccentric regurgitant jet. Mechanisms b and d are usually managed with valve resuspension inside a prosthetic graft; mechanism c usually necessitates valve replacement, either in addition to a prosthetic graft, or as part of a valved aortic conduit.

Suggested Reading

1. Nienaber CA, Eagle KA. Aortic dissection: new frontiers in diagnosis and management: Part I: from etiology to diagnostic strategies. Circulation 2003; 108:628–35.

2. Moore AG, Eagle KA, Bruckman D et al. Choice of computed tomography, transesophageal echocardiography, magnetic resonance imaging, and aortography in acute aortic dissection: International Registry of Acute Aortic Dissection (IRAD). Am J Cardiol 2002; 89:1235–8.

3. Movsowitz HD, Levine RA, Hilgenberg AD, Isselbacher EM. Transesophageal echocardiographic description of the mechanisms of aortic regurgitation in acute type A aortic dissection: implications for aortic valve repair. J Am Coll Cardiol 2000; 36:884–90.

4. Nohara H, Shida T, Mukohara N et al.. Aortic regurgitation secondary to back-and-forth intimal flap movement of acute type A dissection. Ann Thorac Cardiovasc Surg 2004; 10(1):54–6.

Case 10-6
Chronic Descending Aortic Dissection

This 71-year-old man was found to have a thoraco-abdominal aneurysm during evaluation for prostate carcinoma. He denies all cardiac symptoms, although he does have a history of hypertension and hyperlipidemia.

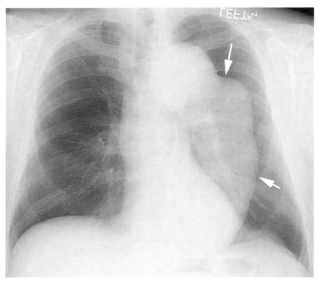

Fig 10-47. PA chest radiography demonstrates severe enlargement of the descending thoracic aorta (**arrows**).

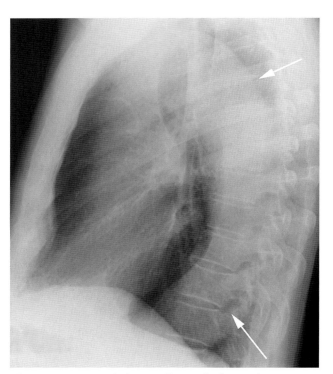

Fig 10-48. Lateral chest radiograph shows the extent of the descending thoracic aortic aneurysm from the left subclavian to the T10 level (**arrows**).

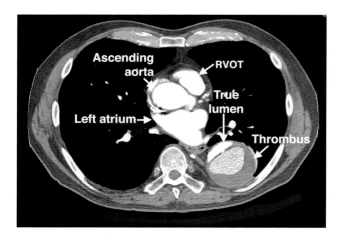

Fig 10-49. Chest CT with contrast shows the dissection flap and thrombus in the enlarged descending thoracic aorta; the smaller lumen with dense (white) contrast represents the true lumen, whereas the false lumen is larger but with less dense (gray) contrast and circumferential laminated thrombus. The ascending aorta is relatively normal in size.

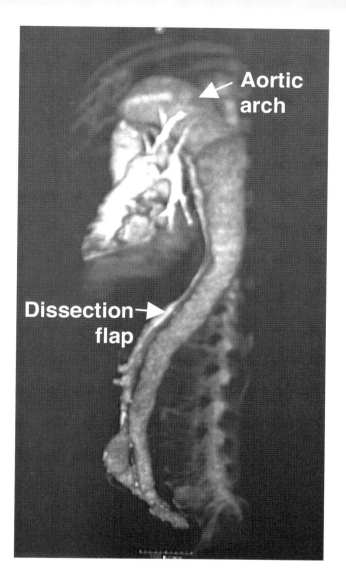

Fig 10-50. The 3D reconstruction of the CT images shows the extent of dilation and the dissection flap extending from the arch to the iliac bifurcation.

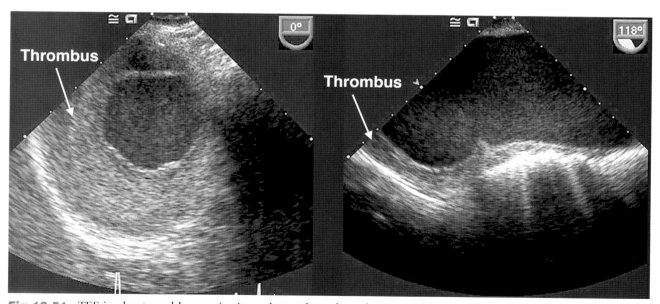

Fig 10-51. TEE in short- and long-axis views shows the enlarged aorta with extensively thrombosed false lumen.

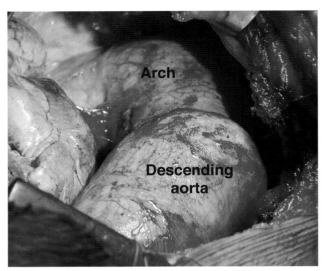

Fig 10-52. At surgery, this view taken from the foot of the patient, reveals the dilated descending aorta.

Comments

Aneurysms of the descending thoracic and abdominal aorta are typically diagnosed using CT imaging. TEE is of limited utility because it is not possible to evaluate the abdominal extent of the aneurysm. Risk factors for thoracic aneurysms are male gender (a 2–4 times increased risk), age and a history of hypertension. Most thoracic aortic aneurysms are associated with extensive atherosclerosis of the aorta. Many patients are asymptomatic at the time of diagnosis, as in this case. However, with large aneurysms there is a risk of rupture, compression of branch vessels and embolic events.

Suggested Reading

1. Kouchoukos NT, Dougenis D. Surgery of the thoracic aorta. N Engl J Med 1997; 336:1876–89.

Complications of Aortic Dissection

Case 10-7
Pericardial Effusion and Tamponade

This 60-year-old man presented with chest pain to an outside hospital 48 hours prior to transfer to our medical center. Coronary angiography was attempted, but the right coronary artery could not be identified and he became hypotensive. A chest CT showed an ascending aortic dissection and he was transferred for emergency surgery.

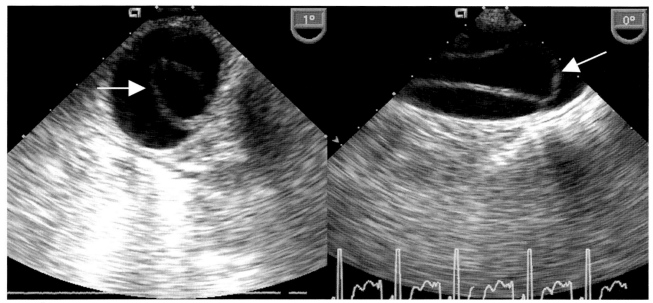

DVD **Fig 10-53.** TEE short- and long-axis views of the descending thoracic aorta show a prominent dissection flap (**arrows**).

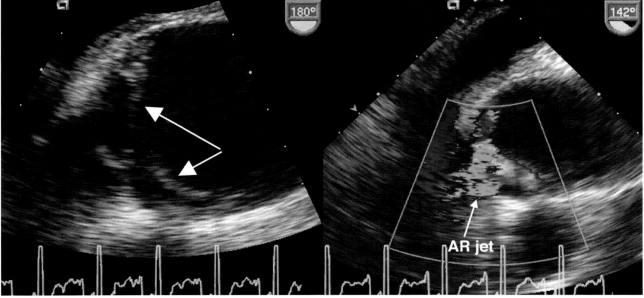

DVD **Fig 10-54.** Long-axis view at 180 degrees of the ascending aorta showing a complex dissection flap (**arrows**). Color Doppler (*right*) shows aortic regurgitation (**AR**).

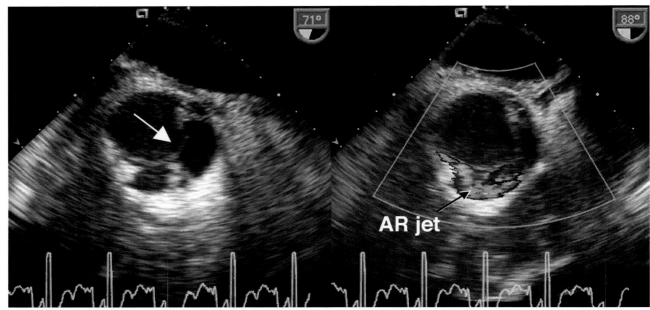

Fig 10-55. Rotation of the image plane to 71 degrees provides a short-axis view of the ascending aorta with a complex intimal flap (**arrow**) that on still-frame images might be mistaken for an aortic valve leaflet. Real-time images show the erratic motion characteristic of a dissection flap. Color flow (*right*) demonstrates AR.

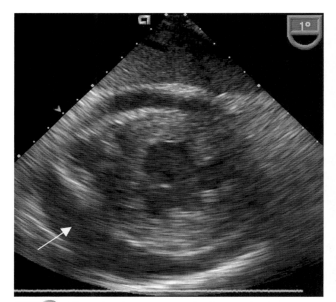

Fig 10-56. Transgastric short-axis view showing a circumferential pericardial effusion (**arrow**). In real time, there is right ventricular collapse.

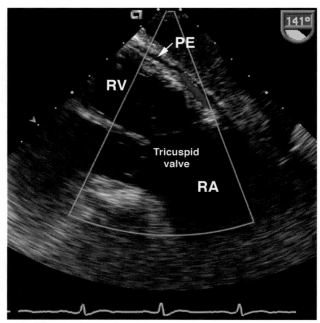

Fig 10-57. Transgastric long-axis imaging of the right-sided cardiac structures reveals color Doppler flow in the pericardial space. **PE** = pericardial effusion.

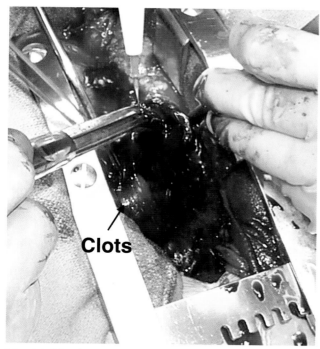

Fig 10-58. At surgery, the pericardium was tense and about 500–700 ml of old blood and clot were removed from the pericardial space.

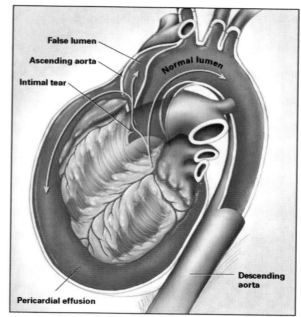

Fig 10-59. This drawing illustrates how blood entering the false lumen can enter the pericardial space via a defect in the aortic wall at its base. (Reproduced from Nallamothu B et al. Of nicks and time. N Engl J Med 2001; 345:359–63. ©Massachusetts Medical Society.)

Comments

An aortic dissection may cause a pericardial effusion by leakage from the aorta into the pericardium. The normal pericardium extends a small distance up the great vessels, with a potential pericardial space posterior to the aorta and pulmonary artery; this space is known as the transverse sinus of the pericardium. If the dissection extends into the base of the aorta, a small tear in the wall allows blood to enter the pericardial space via the transverse sinus (**Fig 10-59**). Thus, the finding of a pericardial effusion in a patient with suspected aortic dissection, especially in the presence of color Doppler flow in the pericardial space, is an ominous sign. If the leakage increases, pericardial tamponade may occur due to rapid accumulation of blood in the pericardial space.

Although women account for only about one-third of aortic dissections, they tend to be older, and most often have signs suggestive of rupture, including pericardial effusion, periaortic hematoma and pleural effusions. Women are more likely than men to be hypotensive and to have pericardial tamponade, and the surgical mortality in women is 32% compared with 22% in men.

Suggested Reading

1. Nienaber CA, Fattori R, Mehta RH et al; International Registry of Acute Aortic Dissection. Gender-related differences in acute aortic dissection. Circulation 2004; 109(24):3014–21.

Case 10-8
Right Coronary Artery Compromise

This 50-year-old man with a history of hypertension, presented with 4 days of intermittent chest pain. He was treated with a beta-blocker and heparin, and an ECG was obtained.

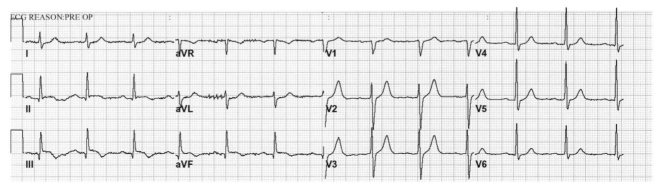

Fig 10-60. A 12-lead ECG with 1 mm ST elevation, T-wave inversion and small Q waves in leads II, III and aVF suggests inferior myocardial infarction. Because of these ECG changes, he was taken promptly to the catheterization laboratory.

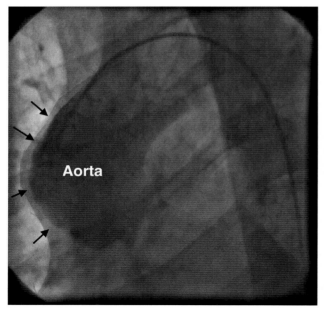

Fig 10-61. At catheterization, aortography shows an irregularity in the anterior contour of the ascending aorta (**arrows**) with contrast seen outside the aortic silhouette. Because of the concern for ascending aortic dissection, a chest CT study was performed.

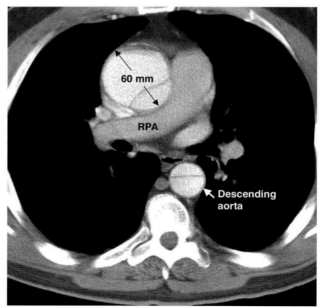

Fig 10-62. Chest CT with contrast at the level of the right pulmonary artery (**RPA**) shows a dilated ascending aorta (60 mm) with a prominent dissection flap. A flap is also seen in the descending aorta.

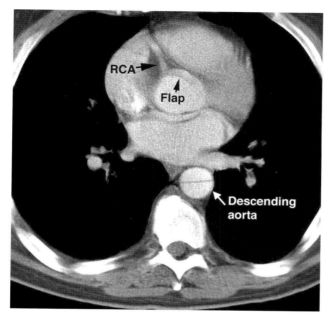

Fig 10-63. In this chest CT at the level of the right coronary artery (**RCA**), a dissection flap is seen in the descending thoracic aorta. The ascending aorta shows the dissection flap crossing the origin of the RCA, resulting in compromise of coronary blood flow.

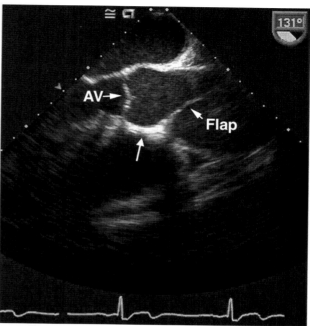

DVD **Fig 10-64.** Intraoperative long-axis TEE images of the ascending aorta demonstrate the enlarged aorta with an intimal flap that begins at the sinotubular junction, about 2 cm superior to the aortic valve (**AV**). Note the proximity of the flap to the site of origin of the right coronary artery (**arrow**).

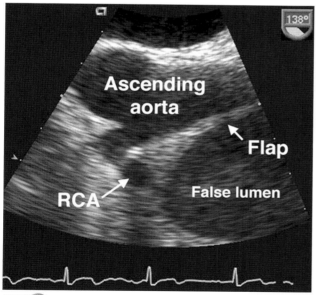

DVD **Fig 10-65.** Close-up of the long-axis TEE image better shows the relationship of the dissection flap and right coronary ostium.

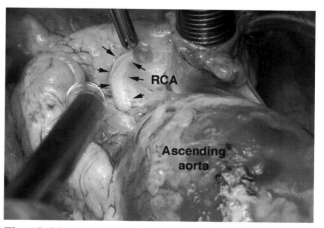

Fig 10-66. At surgery, the enlarged ascending aorta is at the bottom right side of the photograph. The right coronary artery (**RCA**) is of normal caliber.

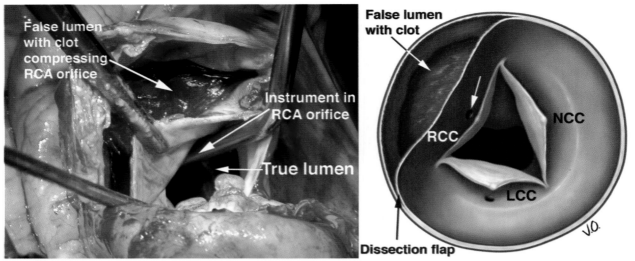

Fig 10-67. With the aorta opened, the false lumen with clot is seen compressing the aorta in the vicinity of the right coronary cusp (*left*). With slight retraction of the dissection flap, the distorted right coronary ostium is visualized (*right*) (**arrow**). The ascending aorta was replaced with a 28 mm Dacron graft, the aortic valve was resuspended and a saphenous vein graft was placed to the distal right coronary artery.

Comments

An aortic dissection may induce myocardial ischemia or infarction by compromising the blood flow in the coronary artery. The mechanism of impaired coronary blood flow may be extension of the dissection into the coronary artery itself or occlusion of the orifice by the dissection flap or a hematoma, as in this case. This case emphasizes the importance of considering aortic dissection in the differential diagnosis of chest pain, even when coronary ischemia is present.

Suggested Reading

1. Kawahito K, Adachi H, Murata S et al. Coronary malperfusion due to type A aortic dissection: mechanism and surgical management. Ann Thorac Surg 2003; 76(5):1471–6.

Case 10-9
Right Coronary and Aortic Valve Involvement

This 55-year-old man suddenly collapsed while at work. He was resuscitated by the emergency medical technicians but remained hypotensive and did not regain consciousness. Chest CT showed a type A aortic dissection and he was transferred to our medical center.

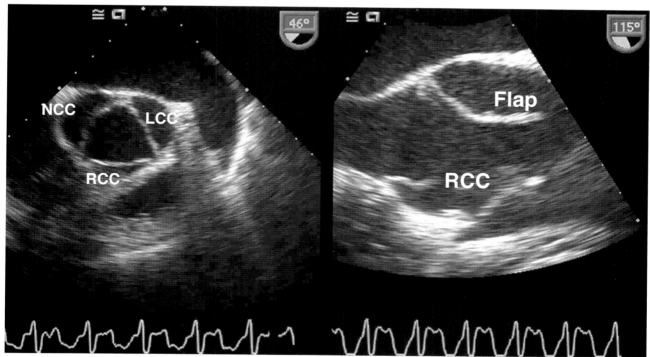

Fig 10-68. TEE images of the aortic valve show a trileaflet valve but, in real time, distortion of the shape of the non-coronary sinus of Valsalva is seen. In the long-axis view (*right*) the complex dissection flap is seen in close proximity to the valve leaflets.

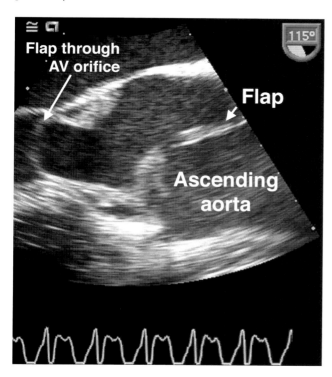

Fig 10-69. In a magnified long-axis view of the ascending aorta at 115 degrees, angulated medially, the dissection flap is seen to prolapse across the aortic valve in diastole.

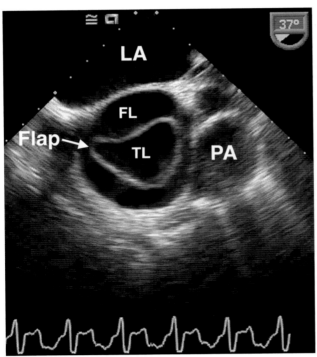

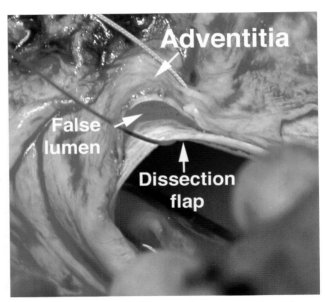

Fig 10-72. Close-up photograph of the aortic wall illustrating the dissection flap, the false lumen and the adventitia.

DVD ♪ **Fig 10-70.** A high TEE view of the ascending aorta shows a circumferential dissection flap. The true lumen (**TL**) is in the center. FL = false lumen.

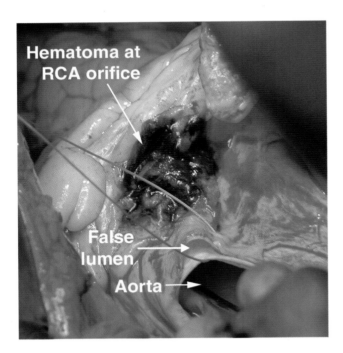

Fig 10-71. Surgical view of the opened aorta showing the extensive hematoma at the site of the right coronary orifice.

Comments

This patient had compromise of right coronary blood flow due to compression of the coronary artery by the aortic hematoma. Sudden collapse was due to ventricular fibrillation, most likely secondary to myocardial ischemia induced by the right coronary artery compression. The mild central aortic regurgitation was due to dilation of the sinuses of Valsalva, with relatively normal aortic leaflet motion despite the proximity of the dissection flap to the valve. Delineation of the origin and extent of the dissection flap may help the surgeon in planning the operative procedure, even with images obtained in the operating room by the anesthesiologist as the surgery is starting.

This case again demonstrates that the presence of a pericardial effusion in a patient with a suspected or known aortic dissection is an ominous sign, suggesting rupture into the pericardium and imminent tamponade physiology.

Aortic regurgitation is a second worrisome sign. The combination of a pericardial effusion and aortic regurgitation, even mild, signals the possibility of aortic dissection in a patient with chest pain. Aortic regurgitation in patients with an aortic dissection may be due to:

- dilation of the sinuses of Valsalva, with incomplete central coaptation of the leaflets
- distortion of the valve commissures by the dissection flap, leading to asymmetric leaflet closure and an eccentric regurgitant jet
- extension of the dissection into the layers of the valve leaflet, resulting in a flail leaflet with severe regurgitation.

Suggested Reading

1. Movsowitz HD, Levine RA, Hilgenberg AD, Isselbacher EM. Transesophageal echocardiographic description of the mechanisms of aortic regurgitation in acute type A aortic dissection: implications for aortic valve repair. J Am Coll Cardiol 2000; 36:884–90.

2. Nohara H, Shida T, Mukohara N et al. Aortic regurgitation secondary to back-and-forth intimal flap movement of acute type A dissection. Ann Thorac Cardiovasc Surg 2004; 10(1):54–6.

Other Aortic Pathology and Procedures

Case 10-10
Aortic Atheroma

This 78-year-old woman was referred for aortic valve replacement for severe aortic stenosis with congestive heart failure.

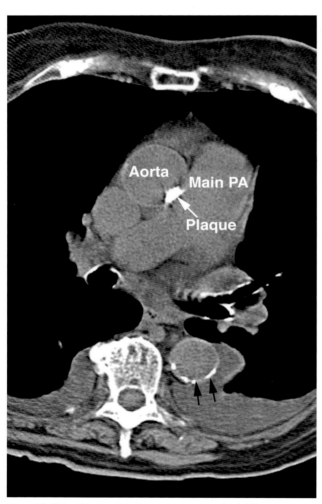

Fig 10-73. Chest CT shows an area of calcification, consistent with an atherosclerotic plaque along the posterior aspect of the descending aorta (**arrow**).

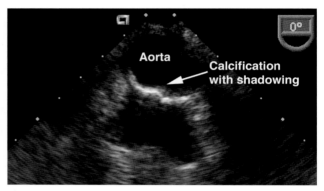

Fig 10-74. TEE imaging of the descending thoracic aorta shows prominent increased echogenicity with associated shadowing, typical for calcification.

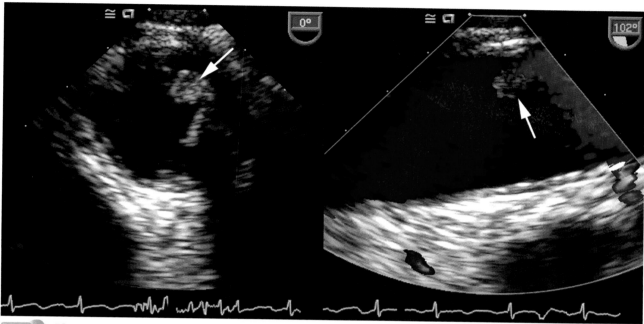

Fig 10-75. In a different segment of the descending thoracic aorta, a plaque that protrudes into the aortic lumen (**arrows**) is seen in short-axis (*left*) and long-axis (*right*) views.

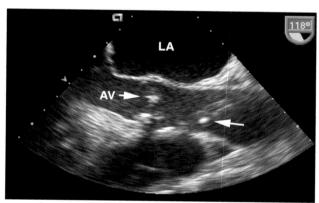

Fig 10-76. A long-axis view of the aortic valve and ascending aorta shows calcification of the aortic valve (**AV**) leaflets and an area of calcification in the ascending aorta (**arrow**).

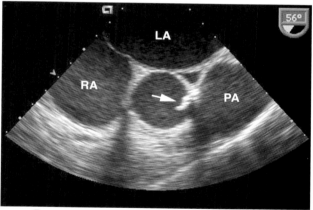

Fig 10-77. A short-axis view of the ascending aorta shows protruding atheroma (**arrow**).

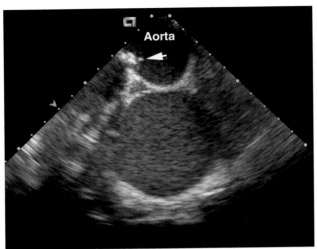

DVD **Fig 10-78.** The surgeon used sterile epiaortic scanning to carefully locate the area of atherosclerosis (**arrow**) in the ascending aorta. This allowed the surgeon to avoid this area during cannulation for cardiopulmonary bypass and to avoid placing a proximal vein graft anastomosis at this site.

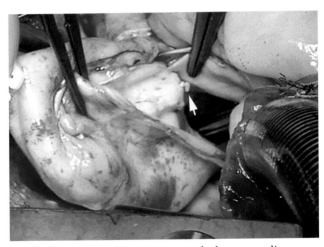

Fig 10-79. With the aorta opened, the protruding atheroma is visualized (**arrow**). The aortic valve was replaced with a biologic tissue prosthesis and the aortic atheroma was resected.

Comments

Aortic atheromas are identified on TEE imaging as irregular areas of variable echodensity that may follow the contour of the aortic wall or may protrude into the aortic lumen. Calcified areas in the plaques are identified by echodensity and shadowing. Atheromas that protrude into the lumen may rupture and be associated with localized thrombus formation.

The finding of aortic atheroma in the descending thoracic aorta is associated with the presence of coronary artery disease. In addition, plaque complexity predicts clinical outcome with a 15% annual risk of death or a cerebral embolic event in patients with a complex plaque (thickness ≥4 mm or any mobile components) compared with those with a non-complex plaque.

At the time of cardiac surgery, epiaortic scanning may be used, as in this case, to further delineate ascending aortic pathology, and thus avoid cross-clamping, cannulation or placement of bypass grafts in atherosclerotic regions of the vessel.

Suggested Reading

1. Bolotin G, Domany Y, de Perini L et al. Use of intraoperative epiaortic ultrasonography to delineate aortic atheroma. Chest 2005; 127(1):60–5.
2. Iglesias I, Bainbridge D, Murkin J. Intraoperative echocardiography: support for decision making in cardiac surgery. Semin Cardiothorac Vasc Anesth 2004; 8(1):25–35.

Case 10-11
Penetrating Ulcer with Pseudoaneurysm

This 75-year-old woman was sent from a skilled nursing facility for evaluation of a 2-week history of intermittent chest and back pain, and progressive lower extremity weakness limiting her ability to ambulate. Her cardiac and pulmonary physical examinations were normal. Her vascular examination was unremarkable with intact pulses. Laboratory data included a normal hematocrit.

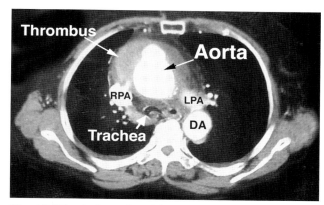

Fig 10-81. A chest CT with contrast shows the severely enlarged and distorted ascending aorta with a soft tissue density around the aorta consistent with thrombus. These findings are consistent with aortic rupture and pseudoaneurysm formation. Posteriorly, the trachea is compressed, but the descending thoracic aorta appears normal in caliber and shape. RPA = right pulmonary artery, LPA = left pulmonary artery, DA = descending aorta.

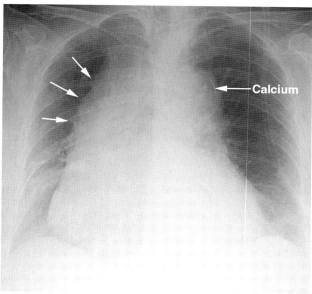

Fig 10-80. A chest radiograph shows a widened mediastinum, especially along the upper right mediastinal border (**arrows**), which is the region of the ascending aorta. The arch shows areas of calcification and the heart is enlarged. There is no pulmonary congestion.

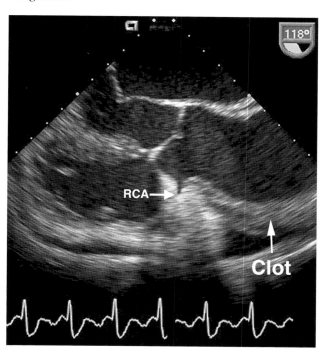

Fig 10-82. In a long-axis TEE view of the ascending aorta, the aortic valve, origin of the right coronary artery (**arrow**) and the sinuses of Valsalva appear normal. However, there is an echodensity anterior the ascending aorta suggestive of a clot (**arrow**).

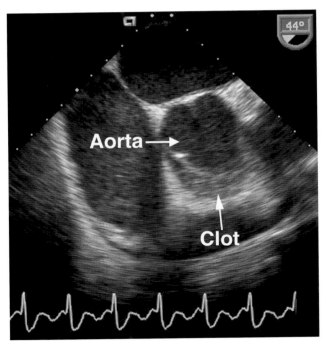

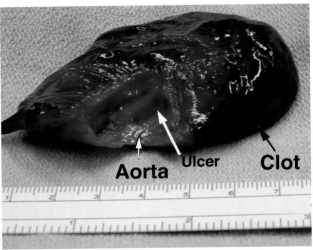

Fig 10-85. At surgery, the ascending aorta was resected from just distal the aortic valve to just proximal the right innominate artery, and replaced with a Dacron tube graft. Pathologic examination revealed cystic medial necrosis with chronic aneurysm formation and a penetrating ulcer with an attached large clot.

Fig 10-83. A TEE short-axis image just above the aortic valve shows the abnormal contour of the aorta with a crescent-shaped echodensity suggestive of a clot. Although a non-circular view of the aorta may be due to an oblique image plane, in this case careful rotation of the image plane showed that the aorta was not circular in cross section.

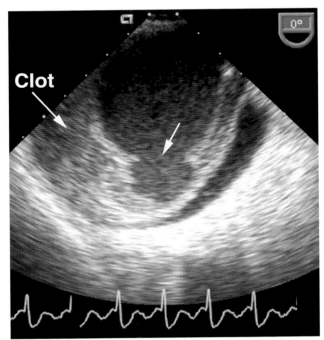

Fig 10-84. An oblique image of the ascending aorta at 0 degrees, corresponding to the image plane in the CT scan shown in **Fig 10-81**, shows the distorted shape of the lumen (**arrow**), with thrombus surrounding the aortic arch.

Comments

Instead of the classic presentation of an aortic dissection, a limited tear in the aortic wall may allow hematoma formation in the wall of the aorta, termed an aortic intramural hemorrhage. On echocardiography, an aortic intramural hemorrhage appears as a crescent-shaped area of increased echodensity around the aorta. The prognosis and treatment of aortic intramural hematoma is similar to aortic dissection.

Another clinical variant is weakening of the aortic wall at the site of an atherosclerotic plaque with a contained rupture of the aorta into the surrounding tissue, termed a penetrating aortic "ulcer." The contained rupture, or pseudoaneurysm, is identified as an irregular blood-filled space adjacent to the aorta, with or without a demonstrable connection between the aorta and the pseudoaneurysm. Treatment is surgical to replace the ruptured segment of the aorta.

Suggested Reading

1. Mohr-Kahaly S, Erbel R, Kearney P et al. Aortic intramural hemorrhage visualized by transesophageal echocardiography: findings and prognostic implications. J Am Coll Cardiol 1994; 23:658–64.

2. Vilacosta I, San Roman JA, Ferreiros J et al. Natural history and serial morphology of aortic intramural hematoma:

a novel variant of aortic dissection. Am Heart J 1997; 134:495–507.

3. Pepi M, Campodonico J, Galli C et al. Rapid diagnosis and management of thoracic aortic dissection and intramural haematoma: a prospective study of advantages of multiplane vs. biplane transoesophageal echocardiography. Eur J Echocardiogr 2000; 1:72–9.

4. Ganaha F, Miller DC, Sugimoto K et al. Prognosis of aortic intramural hematoma with and without penetrating

atherosclerotic ulcer: a clinical and radiological analysis. Circulation 2002; 106:342–8.

5. Moizumi Y, Komatsu T, Motoyoshi N, Tabayashi K. Clinical features and long-term outcome of type A and type B intramural hematoma of the aorta. J Thorac Cardiovasc Surg 2004; 127:421–9.

Case 10-12
Traumatic Aortic Rupture

The patient, a 35-year-old female, was the driver involved in a head-on collision. On examination, there was obvious chest trauma, with bruising from the shoulder strap of her seatbelt.

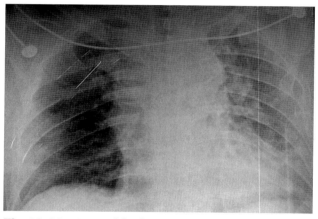

Fig 10-86. A portable chest radiograph shows a wide mediastinum.

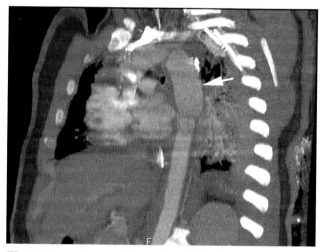

Fig 10-87. A coronal CT view of the thoracic aorta shows localized dilation of the aorta (**arrow**) just beyond the left subclavian artery.

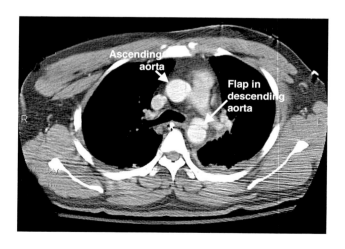

Fig 10-88. A cross-sectional CT image with contrast shows a dissection flap in the descending thoracic aorta. The ascending aorta is normal in caliber.

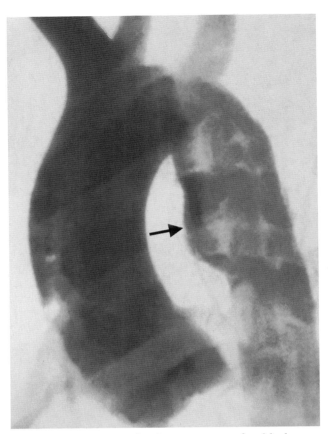

Fig 10-89. Aortography demonstrates a focal bulge (**arrow**) in the aortic contour beyond the left subclavian artery.

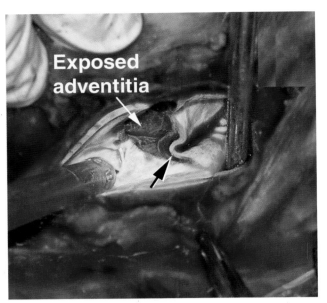

Fig 10-91. The patient was taken to surgery. A left thoracotomy was performed and the descending thoracic aorta exposed. With aortic clamps applied, the descending thoracic aorta was opened and the intraluminal flap (**arrow**) exposed. (Courtesy of Robert Maggisano, MD).

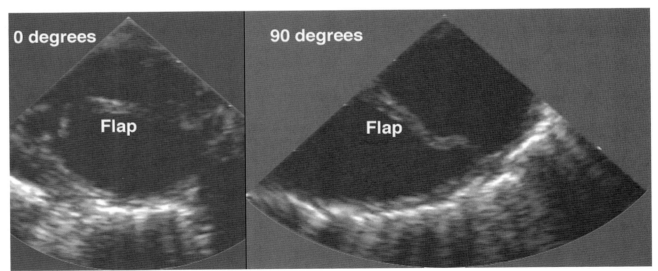

DVD   **Fig 10-90.** TEE imaging of the descending thoracic aorta shows a thick intraluminal flap in views at 0 degrees (*left*) and at 90 degrees (*right*).

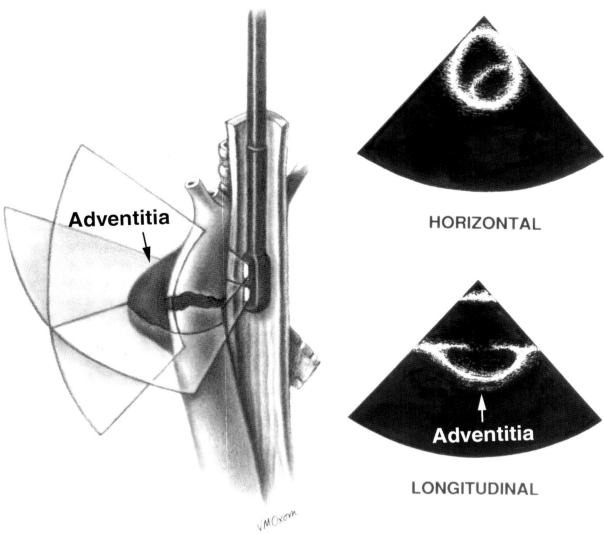

HORIZONTAL

LONGITUDINAL

Fig 10-92. This illustration shows biplane interrogation of the descending thoracic aorta demonstrating aortic disruption, with adventitial containment. (Reproduced with permission from Oxorn D, Edelist G, Smith MS. An introduction to transoesophageal echocardiogaphy: II. Clinical applications. Can J Anaesth 1996; 43:278–94.)

Comments

The most common cardiac injury with blunt chest trauma or deceleration injury (e.g. motor vehicle accidents) is disruption of the thoracic aorta just beyond the left subclavian. This patient had a subadventitial aortic disruption based on the echocardiographic appearance of a thick flap, the presence of aortic isthmus deformity and the pathologic diagnosis. Other manifestations that may be seen are traumatic aortic intimal tears, which, because of their small and superficial nature, are not associated with isthmus deformity, and are clinically less worrisome, and localized intramural hematomas. Diagnosis can be made with TEE imaging but chest CT is more commonly used in the acute setting as it allows concurrent evaluation of other thoracic trauma.

With chest wall trauma, other cardiac injuries include myocardial contusion, rupture of the aortic or tricuspid valve with acute severe regurgitation and pericardial effusion.

Suggested Reading

1. Pretre R, Chilcott M. Blunt trauma to the heart and great vessels. N Engl J Med 1997; 336:626–32.

2. Smith MD, Cassidy JM, Souther S et al. Transesophageal echocardiography in the diagnosis of traumatic rupture of the aorta. N Engl J Med 1995; 332:356–62.

3. Vignon P, Guéret, P, Vedrinne JM. Role of transesophageal echocardiography in the diagnosis and management of traumatic aortic disruption. Circulation 1995; 92:2959–68.

Case 10-13
Aortic Valve Resuspension

This 40-year-old man with a diagnosis of probable Marfan syndrome was followed with annual echocardiography for 5 years with a stable maximum aortic dimension of 4.8 cm, at the level of the sinuses of Valsalva. However, his most recent echocardiogram showed a maximum aortic dimension of 5.3 cm, with a CT scan confirming a dimension of 5.4 cm. He was referred for replacement of the ascending aorta because of progression aortic dilation in the setting of probable Marfan syndrome.

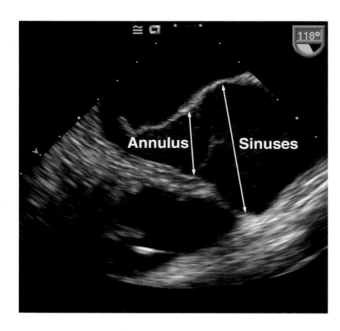

Fig 10-93. A TEE long-axis view of the ascending aorta shows the marked dilation of the sinuses of Valsalva with a maximum dimension of 5.1 cm. However, the dimension of the annulus is relatively normal at 3.0 cm.

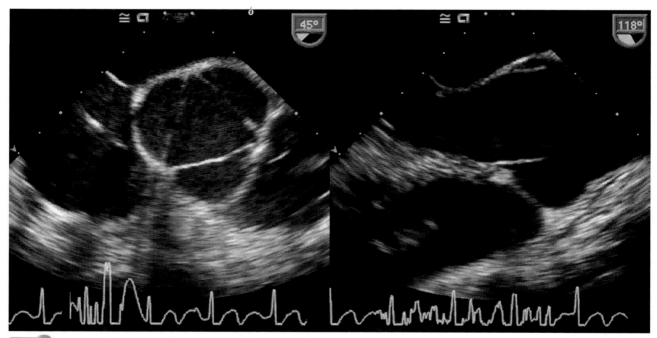

DVD **Fig 10-94.** Magnified short- (*left*) and long-axis (*right*) views of the aortic valve in systole show a normal trileaflet valve with thin, mobile (but stretched) leaflets.

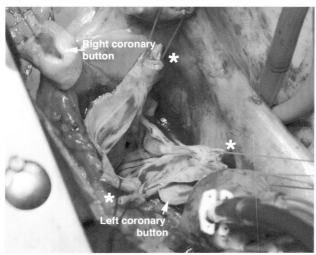

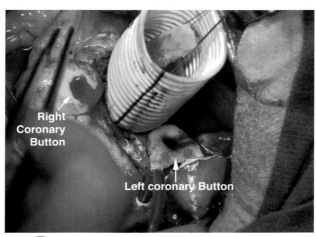

DVD **Fig 10-95.** At surgery, the ascending aorta was resected, with preservation of the aortic valve, including small "posts" of the ascending aorta (**asterisks**) corresponding to the three commissures of the aortic valve. The right and left coronary ostia were isolated with a small circle of aortic tissue, called "buttons."

DVD **Fig 10-96.** A Dacron tube graft replacement for the ascending aorta has been positioned around the valve. The aortic annulus end of the graft is scalloped to provide "neo-sinuses."

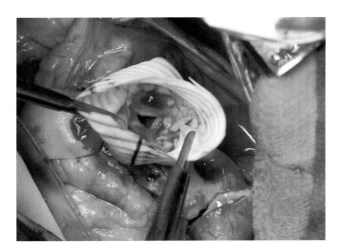

DVD **Fig 10-97.** A view of the valve inside the graft with the commissural posts positioned for resuspension of the valve. After the valve procedure is complete, the coronary buttons are then reimplanted onto the graft.

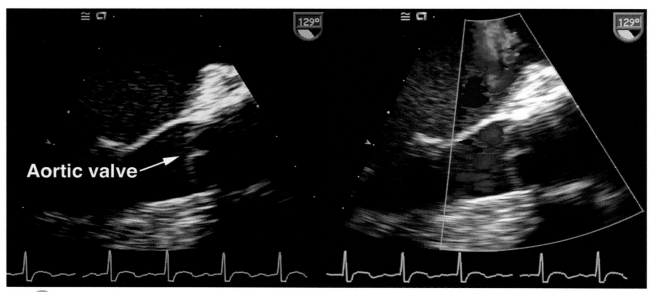

DVD   **Fig 10-98.** Post-bypass TEE long-axis images of the aortic valve show normal closure in diastole (*left*) with no aortic regurgitation on color Doppler imaging (*right*). Note the diameter of the sinuses has been markedly reduced compared with the baseline image in **Fig 10-93**.

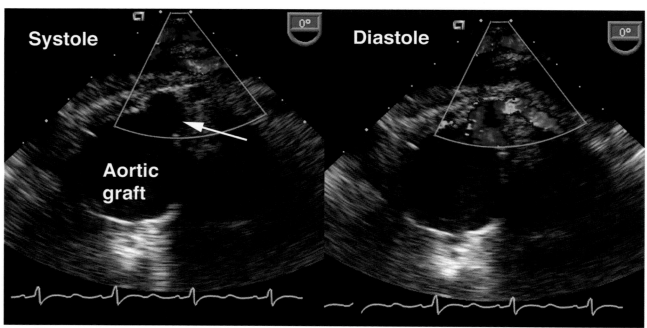

DVD   **Fig 10-99.** A short-axis view of the aortic graft at the level of the left coronary reimplantation shows the "button" (*left*, **arrow**), with color flow showing normal diastolic coronary blood flow (*right*).

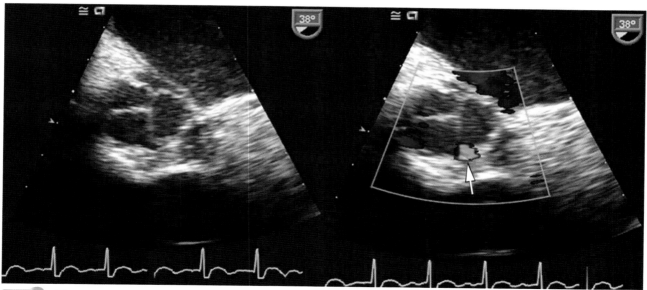

Fig 10-100. A short-axis view of the aortic valve at 38 degrees shows the trileaflet native valve (*left*) in diastole with only a small amount of aortic regurgitation at the commissure between the left and right coronary cusps (*right*, **arrow**).

Comments

The pattern of aortic dilation in patients with Marfan syndrome is characterized by loss of the normal contour of the sinotubular junction, with dilation extending from the aortic annulus without interruption into the ascending aorta. Because the genetic defect affects the entire aorta, the surgical procedure includes resection and replacement of the sinuses of Valsalva all the way down to the annulus level. This necessitates reimplantation of the coronary arteries.

When the aortic valve leaflets are abnormal, a valved conduit is used. However, if the aortic valve appears anatomically normal, many surgeons prefer to retain the native aortic valve. The normal relationships of the commissures and leaflets are restored by resuspension of the valve within the aortic conduit. The combination of a smaller diameter at the level of the commissures, along with stabilization of the aortic annulus, results in a competent valve, and the leaflets are no longer stretched across an enlarged annulus. Because of the redundancy of leaflet tissue, the resuspended valve often does not look classically trileaflet.

Suggested Reading

1. Lai DT, Miller DC, Mitchell RS et al. Acute type A aortic dissection complicated by aortic regurgitation: composite valve graft versus separate valve graft versus conservative valve repair. J Thorac Cardiovasc Surg 2003; 126(6):1978–86.

2. Aybek T, Sotiriou M, Wohleke T et al. Valve opening and closing dynamics after different aortic valve-sparing operations. J Heart Valve Dis 2005; 14(1):114–20.

Pulmonary Artery Pathology

Case 10-14
Pulmonary Thromboendarterectomy

This 51-year-old man had a 7-year history of dyspnea and was found to have recurrent pulmonary emboli. He had progressive symptoms and a decline in func-tional status, despite appropriate anticoagulation and placement of an inferior vena cava filter. He was now referred for pulmonary thromboembolectomy surgery.

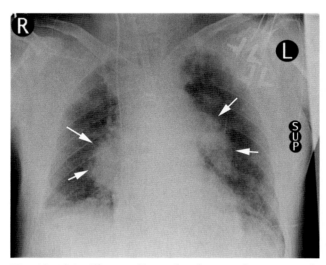

Fig 10-101. Chest radiography shows enlargement of the right and left pulmonary arteries consistent with chronic pulmonary hypertension (**arrows**).

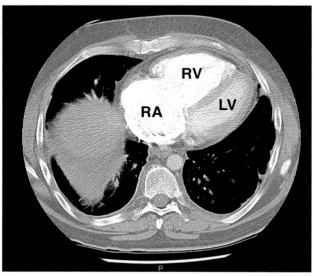

Fig 10-102. A chest CT with contrast at the level of the ventricles shows severe right ventricular and right atrial enlargement.

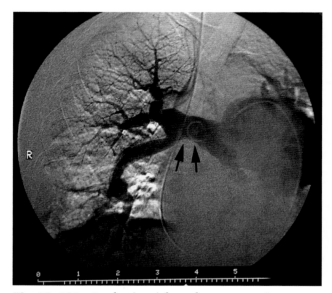

Fig 10-103. A selective right pulmonary angiogram shows an irregular contour along the inferior aspects of the dilated artery (**arrows**) consistent with intraluminal thrombus. Other areas of irregularity and stenosis are seen distally in the pulmonary vascular bed.

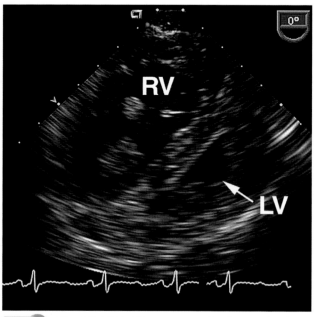

DVD **Fig 10-104.** The transgastric short-axis view shows the severely enlarged and hypokinetic right ventricle with septal flattening consistent with right ventricular pressure and volume overload.

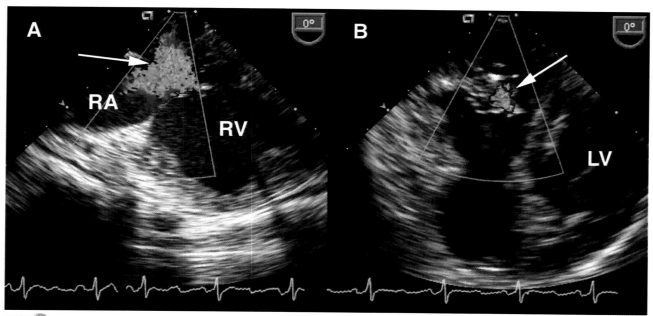

Fig 10-105. A view of the right ventricle (**RV**) and right atrium (**RA**) at 0 degrees (*A*) shows moderate tricuspid regurgitation (**arrow**), in addition to severe right ventricular dilation. The right ventricular free wall is thickened, consistent with long-standing pulmonary hypertension. Transgastric imaging of the tricuspid valve in short axis shows the tricuspid regurgitation jet to be central (*B*).

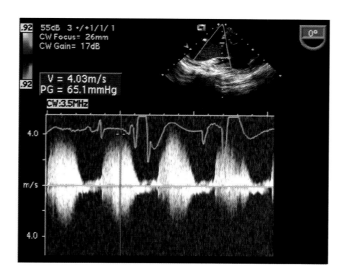

Fig 10-106. Continuous wave Doppler interrogation of the tricuspid regurgitation jet shows a velocity of 4 m/s. Although this may be an underestimate due to a non-parallel intercept angle, this velocity indicates a right ventricular to right atrial pressure difference of 64 mmHg in systole. If right atrial pressure is 10 mmHg, estimated pulmonary artery systolic pressure is 74 mmHg.

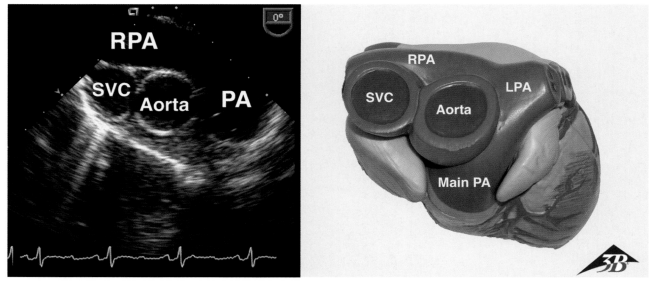

Fig 10-107. A high TEE view at 0 degrees in a normal subject shows the pulmonary artery (**PA**), right pulmonary artery (**RPA**), superior vena cava (**SVC**) and aorta (*left*). A model shows the relevant areas in more detail (*right*). (Based on Economy Heart Model 3B Scientific.)

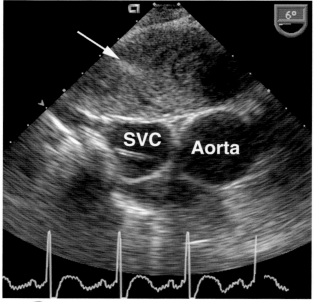

DVD ▶ **Fig 10-108.** In this patient, the same TEE view shows a severely dilated right pulmonary artery with spontaneous contrast (**arrow**) consistent with stasis of blood flow. A catheter is present in the superior vena cava (**SVC**).

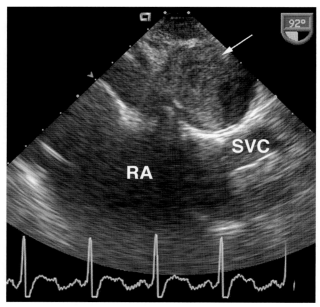

Fig 10-109. Rotating the image plan to 92 degrees, a large thrombus is seen in the enlarged right pulmonary artery (**arrow**).

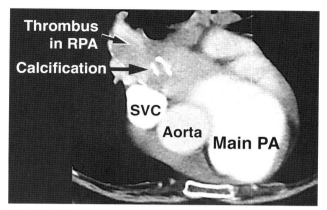

Fig 10-110. A CT scan with contrast, with the image oriented to correspond to the TEE view in **Fig 10-109**, shows the severe dilated pulmonary artery with chronic thrombus (and calcification) in the RPA.

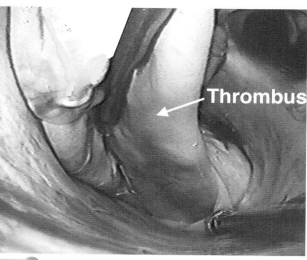

DVD **Fig 10-112.** With the pulmonary artery opened, a chronic thrombus was identified and an endarterectomy of the right pulmonary vascular bed was performed. The left pulmonary artery was also opened and an endarterectomy performed.

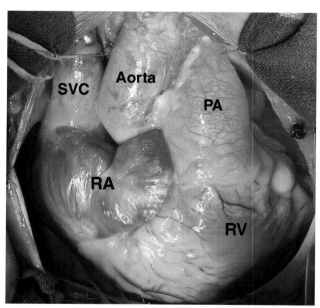

Fig 10-111. This intraoperative view of the heart shows the relationships between the great vessels. All of the right-sided structures are dilated.

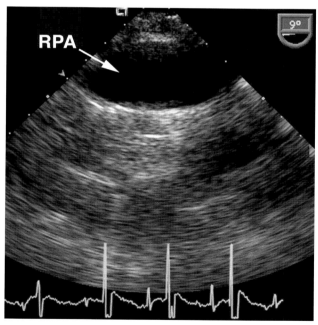

Fig 10-113. The TEE view of the right pulmonary artery (**RPA**) after completion of the procedure. Note the absence of thrombus.

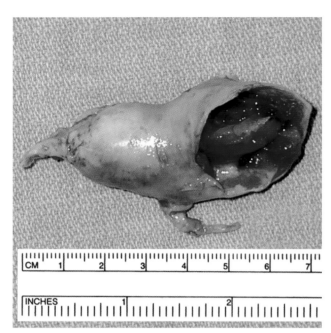

Fig 10-114. The resected thrombus corresponding to the area seen on TEE imaging. Histologic examination revealed laminated thrombotic material with focal areas of atherosclerosis.

Comments

TEE is not used as a primary diagnostic approach to evaluation of pulmonary embolism. It is unusual to directly visualize thrombi in the pulmonary arteries, even with TEE imaging, although these findings have a high specificity when present, as in this case.

However, echocardiography provides indirect evidence of pulmonary vascular disease and is often the first test to suggest that pulmonary emboli be considered in the differential diagnosis. In patients with pulmonary hypertension, typical findings include right ventricular dilation, hypertrophy and systolic dysfunction with a characteristic pattern of septal motion towards the right ventricle (instead of towards the center of the left ventricle) in systole. With right-sided pressure overload, the reversed contour of the ventricular septum persists in both systole and diastole. In contrast, with right-sided volume overload, the reverse curvature of the septum is most prominent in diastole.

Echocardiography provides reliable estimates of pulmonary systolic pressure based on the velocity in the tricuspid regurgitation jet (right ventricular to right atrial systolic pressure difference equals four times the tricuspid regurgitant velocity squared) plus the estimated right atrial pressure (based on the size and respiratory variation of the inferior vena cava).

In patients undergoing pulmonary thrombo-endarterectomy, TEE is useful for detection of extra-pulmonary thrombi; for example, in the SVC or IVC, the right atrium or right ventricle. Detection of extra-pulmonary thrombi altered surgical management in 10% of cases in a surgical series of 50 patients.

Suggested Reading

1. Rosenberger P, Shernan SK, Mihaljevic T, Eltzschig HK. Transesophageal echocardiography for detecting extrapulmonary thrombi during pulmonary embolectomy. Ann Thorac Surg 2004; 78(3):862–6.

2. Rosenberger P, Shernan SK, Body SC, Eltzschig HK. Utility of intraoperative transesophageal echocardiography for diagnosis of pulmonary embolism. Anesth Analg 2004; 99(1):12–16.

3. Jamieson SW, Kapelanski DP, Sakakibara N et al. Pulmonary endarterectomy: experience and lessons learned in 1,500 cases. Ann Thorac Surg 2003; 76:1457–62.

Case 10-15
Pulmonary Artery Obstruction after Heart Transplantation

This 51-year-old women with class III/IV heart failure due to restrictive cardiomyopathy underwent heart transplantation. However, while attempting to wean from cardiopulmonary bypass, she was noted to have a right ventricular pressure of 70/40 mmHg and the right heart catheter could not be advanced into the pulmonary artery.

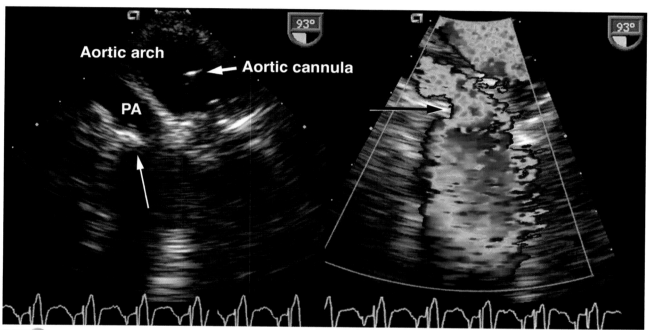

Fig 10-115. In this view, a posterior ridge at the pulmonary artery (**PA**) anastomosis is seen (*left*, **arrow**) causing narrowing of the main pulmonary artery. Color Doppler shows an increase in velocity at the ridge level (*right*, **arrow**).

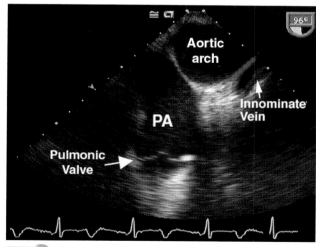

Fig 10-116. In this upper esophageal aortic arch short-axis view from a normal patient, the pulmonary artery (**PA**), pulmonic valve, aortic arch, and innominate vein can be seen. For a description of how this view was obtained, see Case 6-1, **Fig 6-8** and DVD.

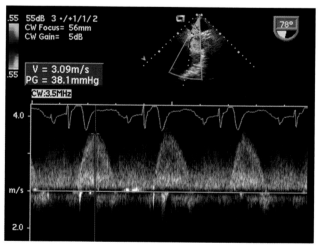

Fig 10-117. Continuous wave Doppler shows a velocity of 3.1 m/s across the pulmonic annulus, consistent with a maximum systolic gradient of 38 mmHg.

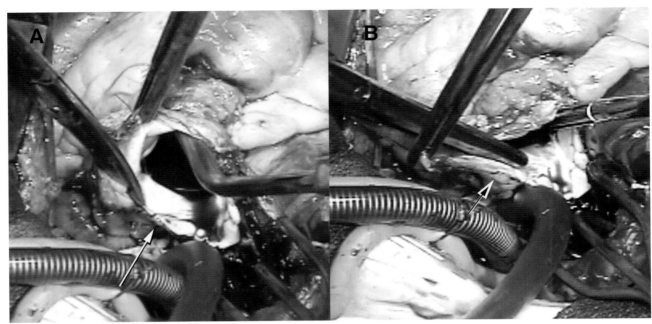

DVD ▶ **Fig 10-118.** At surgery, after reopening the PA anastomosis the pulmonic valve was normal but a posterior shelf of tissue was distorting the shape of the pulmonary artery (**arrow**, *A*). After this tissue was removed (**arrow**, *B*), right ventricular pressures were normal as cardiopulmonary bypass was weaned.

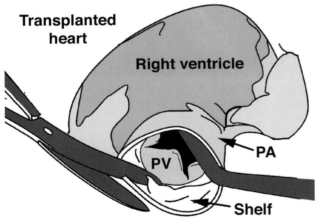

DVD ▶ **Fig 10-119.** This illustration demonstrates resection of the shelf. PV = pulmonic valve, PA = pulmonary artery.

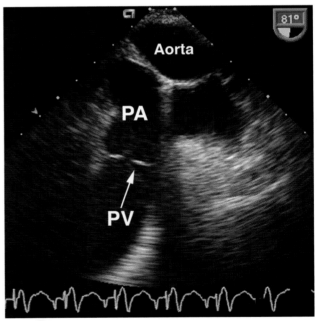

DVD ▶ **Fig 10-120.** After the surgical repair, the same view as **Fig 10-116** shows a normal diameter of the pulmonary artery.

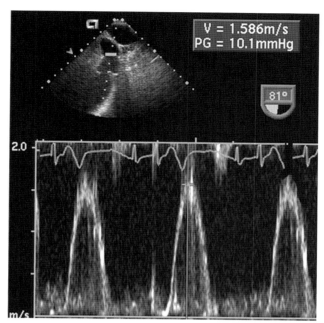

Fig 10-121. Pulsed Doppler interrogation of pulmonary artery flow shows a laminar flow signal with a maximum velocity of only 1.6 m/s.

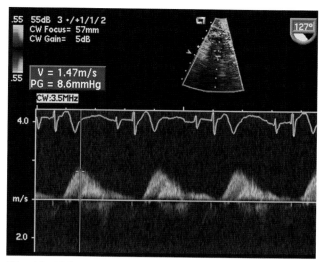

Fig 10-122. Continuous wave Doppler recordings confirm a velocity of 1.5 m/s.

Comments

In this patient the pliable pulmonary artery had normal flow after the transplant procedure. However, when the chest wall was closed, the pulmonary artery was pushed posteriorly against a ridge of tissue, result-ing in apparent pulmonary artery obstruction. The possibility of extrinsic compression causing pseudo-stenosis should be considered when there is an acute change in hemodynamics, particularly in the immediate perioperative period.

11
Masses

Normal variants

Thrombi and vegetations

Primary cardiac tumors

Secondary tumors

Normal Variants

Case 11-1
Left Atrial Appendage

Normal view of the left atrial appendage in a patient undergoing coronary artery bypass grafting surgery.

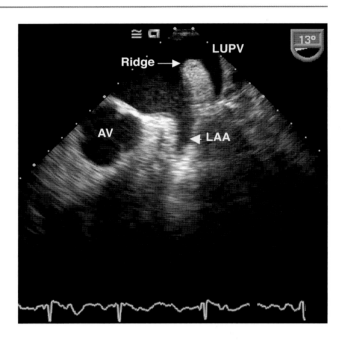

DVD **Fig 11-1.** In this high TEE view, the aortic valve (**AV**) is seen in short axis, adjacent to the left atrial appendage (**LAA**). Note the normal curved triangular shape of the atrial appendage and the prominent ridge of tissue between the appendage and left upper pulmonary vein (**LUPV**). It is important to recognize the normal variation in the size and appearance of this normal ridge so that it is not mistaken for an atrial mass.

Case 11-2
Eustachian Valve

In a patient undergoing cardiopulmonary bypass, baseline echocardiographic images were obtained before cannulation of the inferior vena cava via the right atrium.

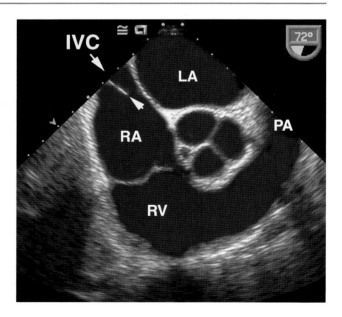

Fig 11-2. In a short-axis image plane at 72 degrees rotation, a linear structure (**arrow**) is seen at the junction of the inferior vena cava (**IVC**) and right atrium (**RA**).

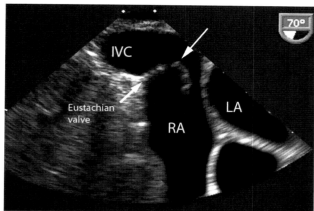

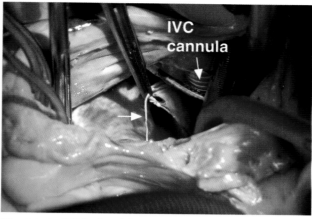

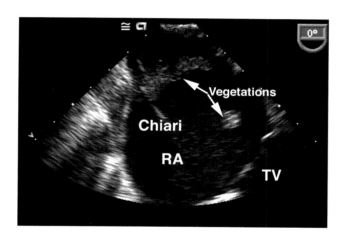

DVD **Fig 11-3.** By advancing the probe in the esophagus, in the same image plane, a view of the IVC is obtained with better visualization of the Eustachian valve originating at the IVC–RA junction and extending into the right atrium. The linear strand (**arrow**) extending from the valve is part of a Chiari network, which sometimes has several strands of tissue extending from the IVC to SVC junction with chaotic motion on echocardiography that mimics the appearance of echo-contrast microbubbles.

Fig 11-4. With the right atrium opened for placement of the IVC cannula, the forceps are grasping the edge of the Eustachian valve. A portion of the Chiari network (**arrow**) is also seen.

DVD **Fig 11-5.** In this short-axis image, the Chiari network has become a nidus for infective endocarditis.

Case 11-3
Lipomatous Hypertrophy of the Interatrial Septum

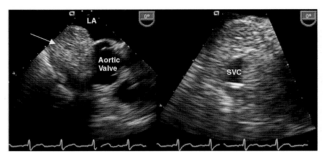

Fig 11-6. In this mid-esophageal view, marked thickening of the interatrial septum is seen in an anteriorly angulated four-chamber view, with the aortic valve in an oblique tomographic view (*left*). A view of the superior vena cava (**SVC**) shows a mass encircling the vein (*right*).

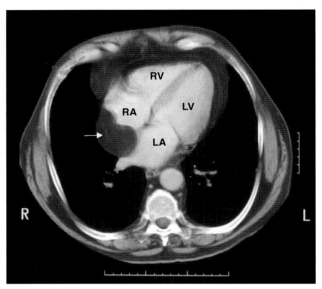

Fig 11-8. A CT scan with contrast shows a hypodense mass (**arrow**) adjacent to the right atrium, extending into the superior part of the atrial septum. This tissue density is consistent with adipose tissue, with additional hypodense tissue seen within the pericardial space (epicardial adipose tissue).

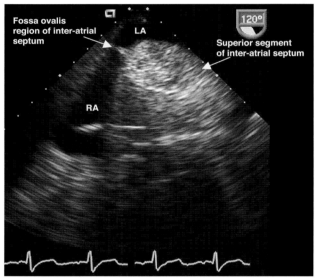

DVD **Fig 11-7.** Rotation of the image plane to the bicaval view of the right atrium shows that the fossa ovalis region of the interatrial septum is normal despite severe thickening of the superior segment of the atrial septum.

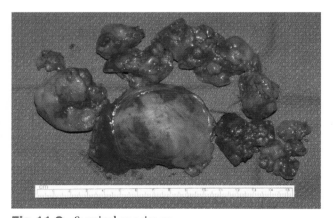

Fig 11-9. Surgical specimen.

Comments (for Cases 11.1, 11.2 and 11.3)

The differential diagnosis of a cardiac mass on echo-cardiography is:

- normal structure
- thrombus
- vegetation
- tumor.

Because echocardiography is poor at defining tissue structure, these conditions are differentiated largely by the location of the mass, associated structural heart disease and the clinical presentation. Thus, a detailed understanding of normal cardiac anatomy and variants of normal structures is needed for correct echo-cardiographic interpretation.

There are many variations of normal cardiac anatomy that may appear as a mass, as shown by these three examples. Normal variants that are commonly mistaken for an abnormal intracardiac mass include the crista terminalis in the right atrium, the ridge between the left superior pulmonary vein and left atrial appendage in the left atrium, and a Eustachian valve in the right atrium, aberrant trabeculations in the left ventricle and Lambl's excrescences on the aortic valve.

In this case a large amount of adipose tissue in the interatrial septum is seen. Lipomatous hypertrophy of the interatrial septum (LHIAS) is a benign condition that typically spares the fossa ovalis region of the septum. In a series of almost 1300 patients undergoing multislice chest computed tomography, LHIAS was present in 2%, with a mean age of 72 years in affected patients. There are usually no adverse clinical consequences of this condition, although an increased incidence of atrial arrhythmias has been suggested and extreme hypertrophy rarely causes hemodynamic obstruction.

Suggested Reading

1. Heyer CM, Kagel T, Lemburg SP et al. Lipomatous hypertrophy of the interatrial septum: a prospective study of incidence, imaging findings, and clinical symptoms. Chest 2003; 124:2068–73.

2. Kindman LA, Wright A, Tye T et al. Lipomatous hypertrophy of the interatrial septum: characterization by transesophaegeal and transthoracic echocardiography, magnetic resonance imaging, and computed tomography. J Am Soc Echocardiogr 1988; 1:450–4.

3. Oxorn DC, Edelist G, Goldman BS, Joyner CD. Echocardiography and excision of lipomatous hypertrophy of the interatrial septum. Ann Thorac Surg 1999; 67(3):852–54.

Case 11-4
Inverted Left Atrial Appendage

About 2 weeks after aortic valve and root replacement for acute aortic dissection, this 44-year-old woman presented with a transient neurologic event. A transthoracic echocardiogram showed a left atrial mass and she was referred for cardiac surgery.

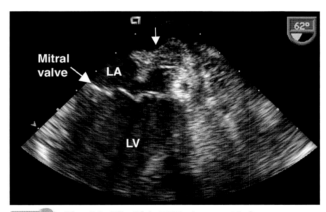

Fig 11-10. This TEE view at 62 degrees shows an irregular loculated mass protruding into the left atrial chamber (arrow). On **DVD**, the motion of this mass is seen. Despite careful angulation, the left atrial appendage could not be visualized. The report from the previous operation did not indicate that the atrial appendage was resected.

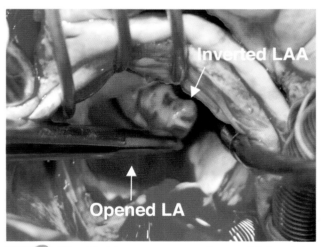

Fig 11-11. At surgery, an inverted left atrial appendage was found. Because the atrial appendage could not be returned to its normal configuration, it was resected due to concern for thrombus formation.

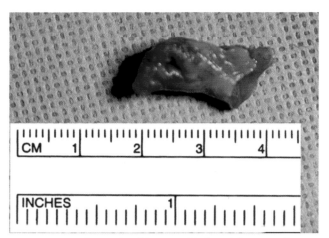

Fig 11-12. The excised inverted left atrial appendage with normal trabeculation.

Comments

During cardiac surgery, some surgeons invert the left atrial appendage to avoid retention of air in the appendage during the procedure. When weaning the patient off cardiopulmonary bypass, the appendage usually spontaneously returns to its normal con- figuration. In this patient, the atrial appendage remained inverted and was initially misinterpreted as a mass. The clues to the diagnosis were the finding of a left atrial mass after recent cardiac surgery that was not present before the procedure, the inability to visualize the atrial appendage and the apparent origin of the mass in the region of the normal left atrial appendage. Although uncommon, this finding will be seen occasionally at most cardiac surgery centers. It is unclear whether the woman's neurologic symptoms were related to the inverted atrial appendage but excision was appropriate as it could serve as a nidus for thrombus formation in the long term.

Suggested Reading

1. Toma DM, Stewart RB, Miyake-Hull CY, Otto CM. Inverted left atrial appendage mimicking a left atrial mass during mitral valve repair. J Am Soc Echocardiogr 1995; 8:557–9.

2. Aronson S, Ruo W, Sand M. Inverted left atrial appendage appearing as a left atrial mass with transesophageal echocardiography during cardiac surgery. Anesthesiology 1992; 76:1054–5.

3. Cohen AJ, Tamir A, Yanai O et al. Inverted left atrial appendage presenting as a left atrial mass after cardiac surgery. Ann Thorac Surg 1999; 67:1489–91.

Case 11-5
Spinal Cord

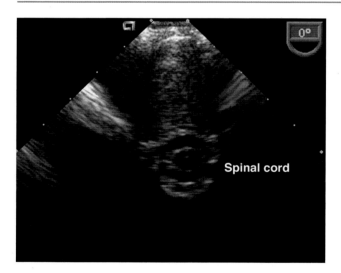

Spinal cord

DVD ▶ Fig 11-13. With the TEE probe rotated posteriorly to image the descending thoracic aorta, the spinal cord may be seen and should not be mistaken for an abnormal finding.

Case 11-6
Lambl's Excrescence

This 71-year-old woman presented for aortic valve replacement because of severe aortic insufficiency.

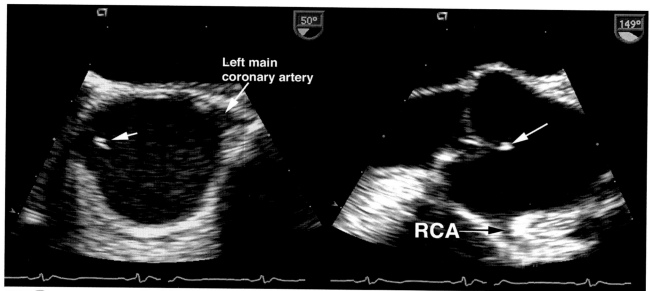

Fig 11-14. Preoperative TEE in long- and short-axis views revealed a small mobile density (**arrows**) approximately 3 mm in diameter, which appeared to be attached to the edge of one of the valve leaflets.

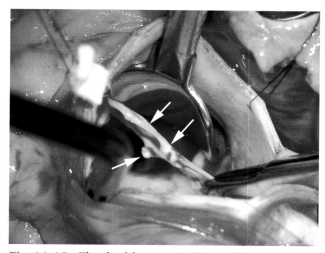

Fig 11-15. The double arrow indicates the non-coronary cusp of the aortic valve. The single arrow indicates the mass seen on TEE.

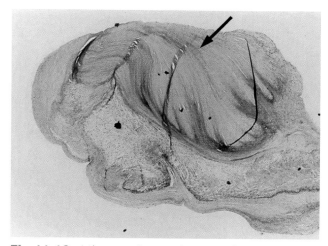

Fig 11-16. Microscopic examination of one of the aortic leaflets shows fibroelastic thickening of the free edge, with sheets of fibroelastic tissue (**arrow**), consistent with long-standing aortic regurgitation.

Comments

Small valve strands that microscopically are fibro-elastic tissue are normal components of the aortic and mitral valve that increase in frequency with age. These small strands, often called Lambl's excrescence, appear as small, linear mobile echoes that are most often attached to the upstream side of the valve (ventricular side of the aortic and atrial side of the mitral valve). However, they are also seen attached to the nodules of Arantius at the tip of the valve cusps, on the aortic side of the valve, as in this case. The clinical importance of valve strands is unclear, with some studies suggesting an association with stroke but other data suggesting that these are an incidental finding associated with age but without clinical consequences.

Suggested Reading

1. Menzel T, Mohr-Kahaly S, Arnold KJ et al. Detection of strands in native aortic valves by transesophageal echocardiography. Am J Cardiol 1997; 79(11):1549–52.

2. Homma S, Di Tullio MR, Sciacca RR et al; PICSS Investigators. Effect of aspirin and warfarin therapy in stroke patients with valvular strands. Stroke 2004; 35(6):1436–42.

Thrombi and Vegetations

Case 11-7
Left Atrial Appendage Thrombus

This 52-year-old man was diagnosed with severe three-vessel coronary artery disease, a left ventricular ejection fraction of 10% and chronic atrial fibrillation. He was referred for coronary bypass grafting surgery with a concurrent Maze procedure to treat atrial fibrillation.

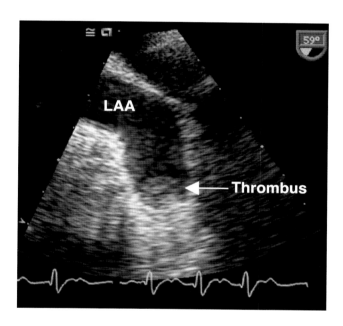

Fig 11-17. Intraoperative echocardiography from a high esophageal position at about 60 degrees rotation, with careful angulation and rotation to optimize the image of the left atrium, shows an echodensity consistent with a thrombus. Spontaneous contrast is also present in the appendage. The sensitivity of TEE for detection of left atrial thrombus is highest when a high-frequency transducer (typically 7 MHz) and the instrument's magnification (or resolution) mode is utilized.

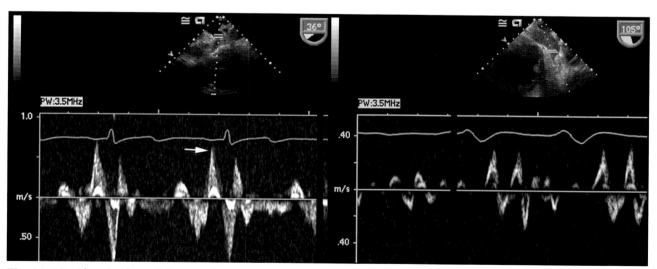

Fig 11-18. Flow in the atrial appendage is examined by placing a pulsed Doppler sample volume about 1 cm from the mouth of the appendage. In normal sinus rhythm (*left*), a flow velocity following atrial contraction of at least 0.4 cm/s towards the transducer is normal (**arrow**). In atrial fibrillation, as in this case, lower-velocity, more-frequent flow signals are seen (*right*).

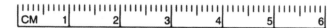

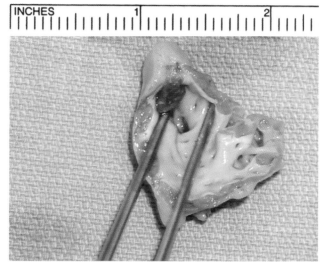

Fig 11-19. Because of the presence of an atrial appendage thrombus in a patient undergoing the Maze procedure, the left atrial appendage was resected. The surgical specimen shows the red thrombus and the paler normal trabeculation of the atrial appendage, which must be distinguished from thrombus on TEE imaging.

Comments

Patients with atrial fibrillation are at risk of systemic embolic events due to thrombus formation in the fibrillating left atrium. Most left atrial thrombi occur in the atrial appendage, which is not well visualized on transthoracic imaging. The sensitivity of transthoracic echocardiography for detection of left atrial thrombus is only about 50%. TEE provides high-resolution images of the left atrium and, with an experienced operator, has a sensitivity and specificity of nearly 100% for detection of atrial thrombi.

Imaging of the left atrial appendage should be performed in at least two orthogonal views, typically at 0 and 90 degrees of rotation of the image plane, using a high-frequency transducer and the resolution imaging mode. Careful angulation and rotation from this image plane is needed to distinguish normal appendage trabeculations, which move with and connect with the atrial wall, from thrombi, which often protrude and have independent motion. Less often, thrombi occur in the body of the atrium, so that careful examination in multiple image planes of the entire atrium, including the atrial septal region, is needed.

Suggested Reading

1. Tolat AV, Manning WJ. The role of echocardiography in atrial fibrillation and flutter. In: Otto CM, ed. The Practice of Clinical Echocardiography, 2nd edn. Philadelphia: WB Saunders, 2002: 829–44.

2. Zabalgiotia M, Halperin JL, Pearce LA et al. Transesophageal echocardiographic correlates of clinical risk of thromboembolism in nonvalvular atrial fibrillation. J Am Coll Cardiol 1998; 31:1622–66.

Case 11-8
Embolization of Valve Vegetation

This 35-year-old woman, with a remote history of Hodgkin's disease treated with radiation, presented with abdominal pain due to ischemic bowel. Echocardiography showed a large mitral valve vegetation and severe mitral regurgitation. Multiple blood cultures grew *Enterococcus faecalis*. Due to recurrent systemic emboli, she was referred for mitral valve surgery 6 days after hospital admission.

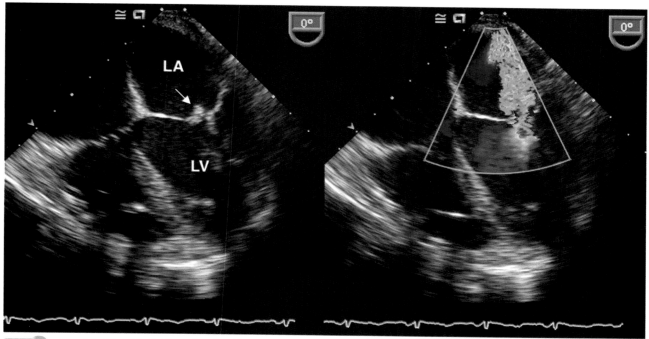

Fig 11-20. 2D (*left*) and color flow (*right*) images at 0 degrees from a high esophageal position show a mass on the left atrial side of the anterior mitral leaflet (**arrow**) and mitral regurgitation with a posteriorly directed jet. These findings are consistent with endocarditis, with a valvular vegetation and leaflet destruction.

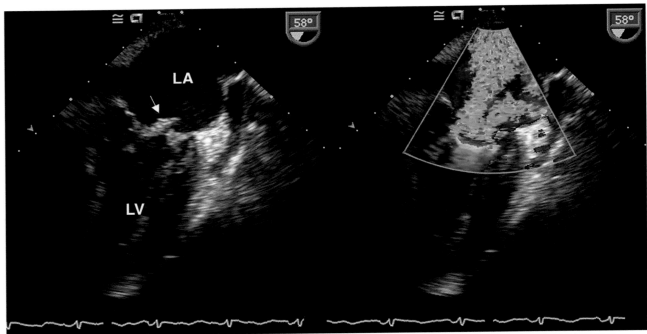

DVD **Fig 11-21.** Rotation of the image plane to 58 degrees, a two-chamber view, adds information on the extent of leaflet involvement (**arrow**) and the size of the color regurgitant jet. At surgery, mitral valve endocarditis was seen with inflammation of the anterior leaflet and perforation of the posterior leaflet. Due to the extensive valve destruction, the mitral valve was replaced with a mechanical prosthesis, with preservation of the posterior chordal apparatus. She was weaned from cardiopulmonary bypass without difficulty.

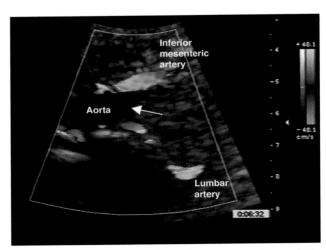

Fig 11-22. However, in the early postoperative period, an absence of peripheral pulses in both legs was noted. From a transcutaneous approach, color Doppler flow and 2D imaging of the abdominal aorta demonstrate an occluded abdominal aorta (black lumen, arrow) with flow preservation in the inferior mesenteric and lumbar arteries.

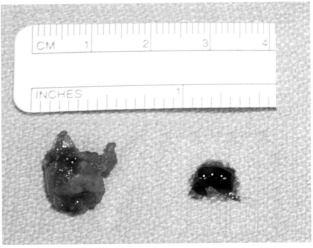

DVD **Fig 11-23.** The surgically removed material from the aorta included several pieces of tissue, with the largest measuring 1 cm in diameter, as shown on the left. The smaller red mass on the right is consistent with fresh thrombus. Pathologic examination confirmed poorly organized thrombus with bacteria present, consistent with an embolized vegetation. It is important to alert the pathologist to the underlying diagnosis, as the microscopic appearance of thrombi and vegetations is similar. The presence of bacteria in the thrombus and the valve involvement support the diagnosis of vegetation. In this case, bacteria were seen on the embolized mass but not the valve tissue.

Comments

Valvular vegetations are identified on echocardiography as mobile masses attached to the upstream side of a valve with independent motion. The risk of embolization is highest with large (>1 cm), mobile vegetations in the mitral positions, and embolization is more likely with some organisms (such as fungi). The risk of embolization decreases with the duration of antibiotic therapy. However, as this case illustrates, embolization can occur at any time, even in the operating room. Comparing the baseline intraoperative TEE with the surgical observations, this vegetation probably embolized early in the surgical procedure.

Suggested Reading

1. Villacosta I, Graupner C, San Roman JA et al. Risk of embolization after institution of antibiotic therapy for infective endocarditis. J Am Coll Cardiol. 2002; 39:1489–95.

Case 11-9
Pericardial Thrombus with Compression of Right Atrium

This 71-year-old woman was transferred from another hospital for rapid atrial fibrillation and hypotension 5 days after coronary bypass grafting and aortic valve replacement. Transthoracic echocardiography showed a large mass with obstruction to the right atrial flow stream. It was not clear if the mass was intracavity or external to the right atrium.

Surgical exploration revealed a large extra-atrial clot adjacent to the right atrium. This thrombus was removed, with a prompt improvement in hemodynamics.

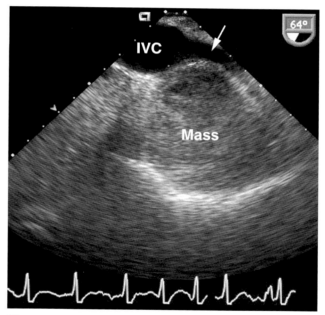

Fig 11-24. From a transgastric view, a mass is seen compressing the inferior vena cava (**IVC**) at its junction with the right atrium (**arrow**).

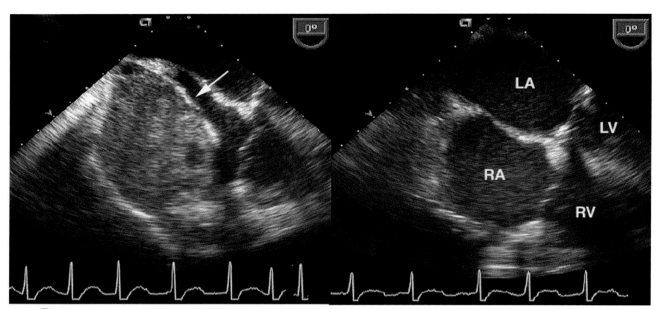

DVD **Fig 11-25.** In a TEE four-chamber view, a large mass is seen that appears to be in the right atrium. However, closer examination shows the increased echogenicity and slight irregularity of the contour along the inner edge of the mass (**arrow**); this is the inverted right atrial wall. Thus, this mass is most likely a pericardial hematoma that is localized to the region of the right atrium with compression of the right atrial chamber. The postoperative image on the right shows the normal appearance of the right atrium after removal of the hematoma. Note the slight normal irregularity in the "roof" of the right atrium, which corresponds to the uninverted free wall.

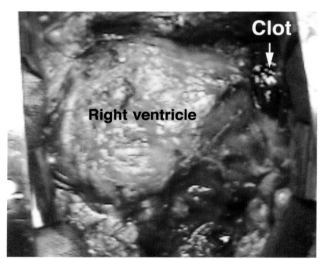

DVD **Fig 11-26.** Clot. This video clip shows the opened chest with the beating heart exposed. The base of the heart is to the lower right of the image with the apex towards the upper left. The anterior surface of the heart is the right ventricle, with the right atrium towards the right of the screen. The surgeon reaches around the right atrium, in the pericardial space, and removes the large hematoma as a single mass.

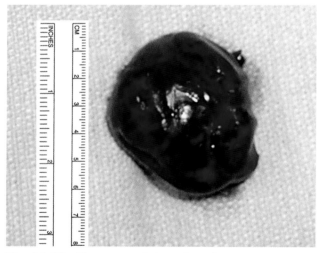

Fig 11-27. The removed thrombus demonstrates a slightly heterogeneous surface, consistent with a subacute process.

Comments

Pericardial effusion or hematoma is a well-recognized complication of cardiac surgery and most patients have a small amount of pericardial fluid or thrombus seen on an early postoperative echocardiogram. Persistent bleeding can lead to a large circumferential pericardial effusion, with development of tamponade physiology (see Chapter 9).

However, localized thrombus formation can also be seen and may cause compression of a cardiac chamber, with hemodynamic compromise, as illustrated by this case. With a localized thrombus, there is little or no free pericardial fluid, and echocardiographic signs of tamponade are not always present. In patients with hypotension in the early postoperative period, the possibility of localized hematoma should be considered, with a diligent search on transthoracic or transesophageal imaging for abnormal extracardiac masses.

Suggested Reading

1. Russo AM, O'Connor WH, Waxman HL. Atypical presentations and echocardiographic findings in patients with cardiac tamponade occurring early and late after cardiac surgery. Chest 1993 ; 104:71–8.

2. Schoebrechts B, Herregods MC, Van de Werf F, De Geest H. Usefulness of transesophageal echocardiography in patients with hemodynamic deterioration late after cardiac surgery. Chest 1993 ; 104:1631–2.

Primary Cardiac Tumors

Case 11-10
Atrial Myxoma

This 52-year-old woman with endometrial stromal sarcoma, who had been treated with radiation therapy, underwent a chest CT scan and MRI as part of the evaluation before surgical resection of the endometrial tumor. A 4 cm left atrial mass was noted and confirmed on TEE. She had no other evidence of metastatic disease and was referred for cardiac surgery.

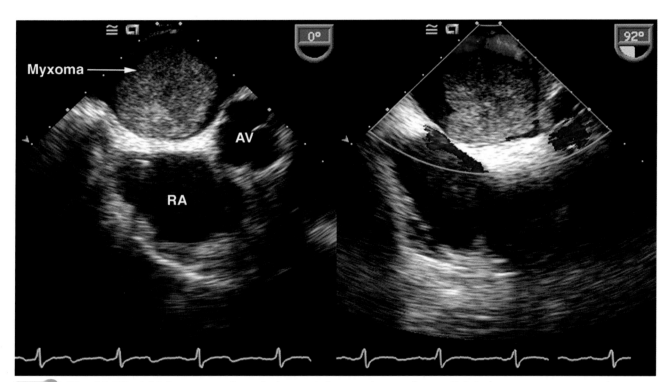

DVD **Fig 11-28.** A high transesophageal view at 0 degrees shows a large, slightly heterogeneous mass that appears to arise from the fossa ovalis region of the atrial septum (*left*). Color Doppler shows flow around the mass but without significant obstruction to blood flow (*right*).

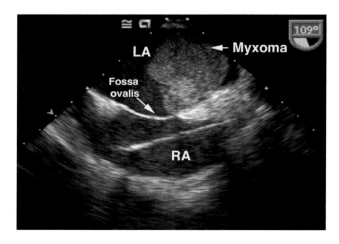

DVD **Fig 11-29.** Rotation of the image plane to 109 degrees provides better visualization of the attachment of the mass, via a narrow base, to the superior aspect of the fossa ovalis.

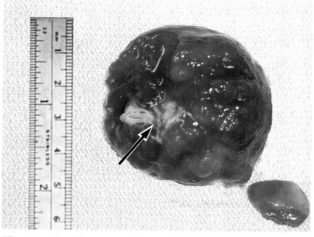

Fig 11-30. The MRI scan shows the mass in the left atrium. **LPVs** = left pulmonary veins.

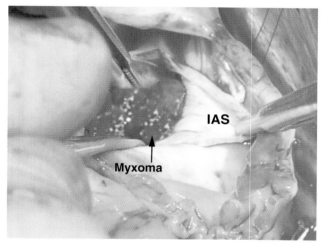

Fig 11-31. The surgical approach was via the right atrium, with an incision from the right atrium through the fossa ovalis after careful palpation to identify the base of the tumor. The entire base in the atrial septum was excised, along with the mass, and the atrial septum was repaired. The postoperative TEE showed no residual tumor or atrial septal defect. IAS = interatrial septum.

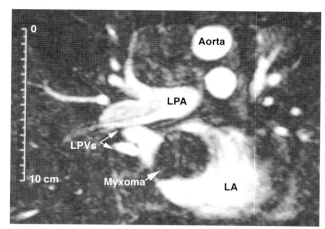

Fig 11-32. The excised mass is typical for an atrial myxoma, which has a relatively smooth surface with a gelatinous appearance. The arrow indicates the attachment site of the tumor to the fossa ovalis.

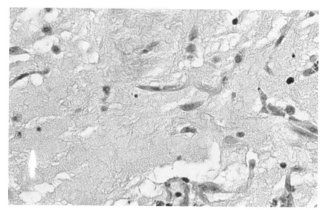

Fig 11-33. Microscopic examination with a hematoxylin and eosin (**H&E**) stain is typical for a myxoma, which has scattered cells with abundant intercellular material.

Comments

Most primary cardiac tumors are benign, with myxomas accounting for 27% of them. Cardiac myxomas originate in the left atrium in 75% of cases, with less common sites including the right atrium (18%), left ventricle (4%) and right ventricle (4%). Atrial myxomas are usually attached to the fossa ovalis region of the interatrial septum. An atrial myxoma may present with systemic symptoms such as fever, malaise and embolic events. However, even a pathologically benign tumor may be hemodynamically malignant if there is obstruction to intracardiac blood flow. Large left atrial tumors may obstruct left ventricular filling, with a clinical presentation that mimics mitral stenosis. With the increasing use of non-invasive imaging techniques, cardiac tumors are more often diagnosed earlier in the disease course, on studies ordered for other indications, as in this case.

Suggested Reading

1. Salcedo EE, Cohen GI, White RD, Davison MB. Cardiac tumors: diagnosis and management. Curr Probl Cardiol 1992; 17:75–137.

2. Grebenc ML, Rosado de Christenson ML, Green CE et al. Cardiac myxoma: imaging features in 83 patients. Radiographics 2002; 22:673–89.

Case 11-11
Obstruction of LV Filling by Myxoma

Example of a left atrial myxoma resulting in obstruction of left ventricular inflow.

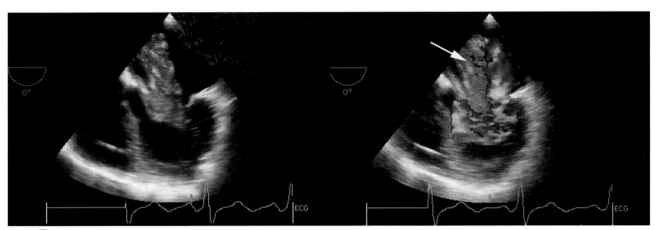

DVD **Fig 11-34.** 2D (*left*) and color Doppler (*right*) imaging in a four-chamber view shows a large mobile left atrial mass (**arrow**) that prolapses into the mitral orifice in diastole with reduction in the flow stream from the left atrium to ventricle.

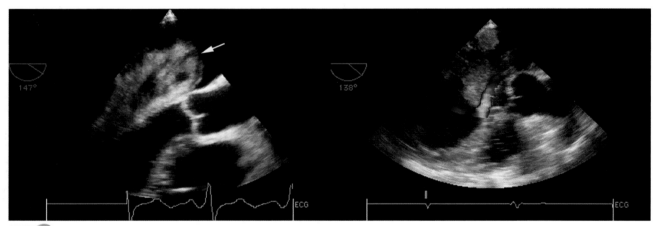

DVD **Fig 11-35.** A long-axis view further demonstrates the obstruction to left ventricular filling due to the left atrial mass (**arrow**) partially occluding the mitral valve orifice.

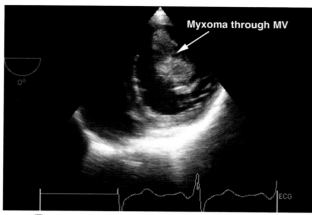

DVD **Fig 11-36.** A transgastric short-axis view at the level of the mitral leaflets shows the mass prolapsing into the valve orifice in diastole.

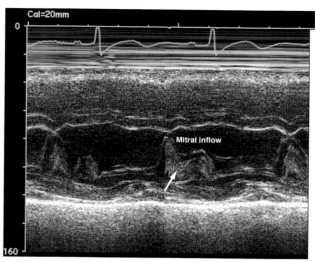

Fig 11-37. An M-mode tracing at the level shown in **Fig 11-36** illustrates the typical appearance of a myxoma (**arrow**) on M-mode.

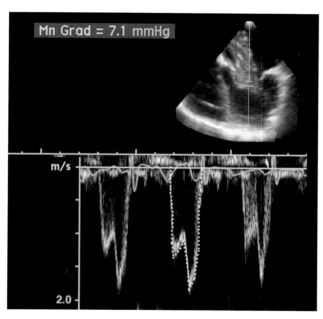

Fig 11-38. Pulsed Doppler recording of transmitral flow from a four-chamber view shows a mild increase in flow velocity with a mean diastolic gradient of 7 mmHg, consistent with mild mitral stenosis.

Comments

Even though this tumor is a pathologically benign atrial myxoma, from a physiologic point of view the mass is malignant because it obstructs left ventricular inflow. Any further increase in size of the tumor will result in hemodynamics similar to mitral valve stenosis with an elevated left atrial pressure and pulmonary pressures resulting in symptoms of shortness of breath, decreased exercise tolerance and pulmonary edema. Thus, it is important for the echocardiographer to evaluate the physiologic consequences of an intracardiac mass, in addition to defining the anatomy.

Tumors can cause cardiovascular compromise by several mechanisms:

- obstruction to flow (as in this case)
- compression of cardiac chambers
- production of pericardial fluid with tamponade physiology
- invasion of myocardium
- tumor embolization.

Case 11-12
Left Ventricular Myxoma

This 78-year-old woman presented to her primary care physician with symptoms consistent with a transient ischemic attack. As part of her work-up, she was referred for echocardiography. A mass was noted in the LV cavity, and she was referred for a surgical opinion.

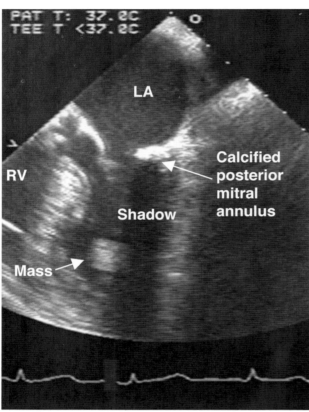

DVD **Fig 11-39.** In this four-chamber view, there is extensive calcification of the posterior mitral leaflet, with shadowing in the LV cavity. There is an apical mass seen, which in real time moves in a random fashion.

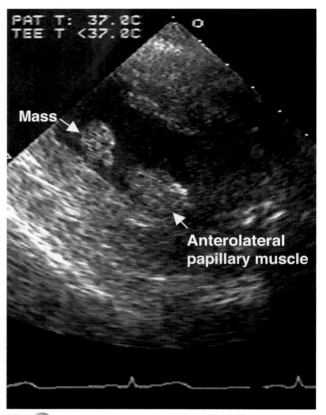

DVD **Fig 11-40.** In this transgastric long-axis view of the LV, the mass is seen more apically than the anterolateral papillary muscle. In real time its random movement is in contrast to the stable position of the papillary muscle.

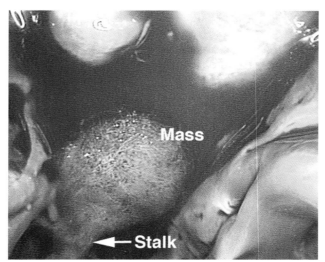

DVD **Fig 11-41.** With the introduction of a fiberoptic scope through the aortic valve, the mass and its stalk are seen in the apex of the LV cavity.

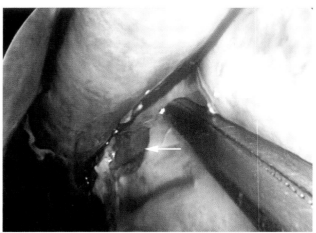

DVD **Fig 11-42.** The mass was resected with instruments introduced through the aortic valve. Afterwards, an area of denuded LV endothelium is seen where the tumor was attached (**arrow**). Pathology was consistent with a myxoma.

Comments

Although most myxomas are single and located in the left atrium, some arise from other locations, including the left ventricle, as in this case. Echocardiography demonstrated that this left ventricular mass was separate from the papillary muscle (i.e. it was not a normal structure). These findings might be consistent with thrombus, but thrombus typically occurs when there is regional or global systolic dysfunction leading to blood stasis. The appearance did not help distinguish between a benign and malignant tumor. Because the woman had a neurologic event and a cardiac mass, resection was indicated, regardless of the histology of the mass. There is a low risk of recurrence (about 5%), so her prognosis is good after removal of a myxoma.

Suggested Reading

1. Selkane C, Amahzoune B, Chavanis N et al. Changing management of cardiac myxoma based on a series of 40 cases with long-term follow-up. Ann Thorac Surg 2003; 76(6):1935–8.

2. Pinede L, Duhaut P, Loire R. Clinical presentation of left atrial cardiac myxoma. A series of 112 consecutive cases. Medicine (Baltimore) 2001; 80(3):159–72.

Case 11-13
Interatrial Septal Hemangioma

This 48-year-old woman presented with palpitations. Physical examination was normal but an echocardiogram showed a thickened interatrial septum. Magnetic resonance scanning indicated that the atrial thickening was not fat density, so she was referred for surgical excision.

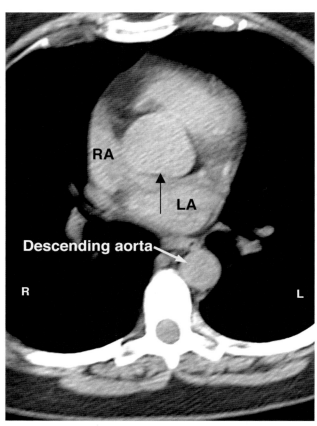

Fig 11-43. CT scan at the level of the atrial septum showing a large, tissue density, globular mass (**arrow**).

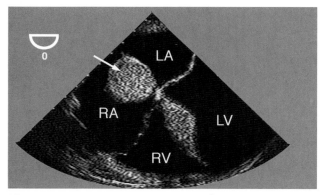

Fig 11-44. Intraoperative TEE in a four-chamber view shows a large mass in the interatrial septum (**arrow**).

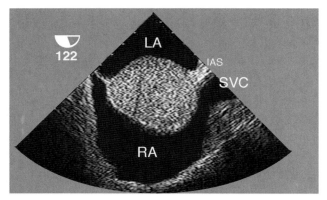

Fig 11-45. Rotation to the bicaval long-axis view at 122 degrees demonstrates the symmetric shape of the mass, filling the fossa ovalis region of the interatrial septum (**IAS**).

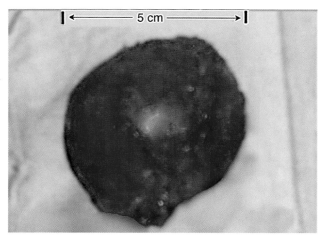

Fig 11-46. At surgery, a large encapsulated tumor in the atrial septum was excised in its entirety.

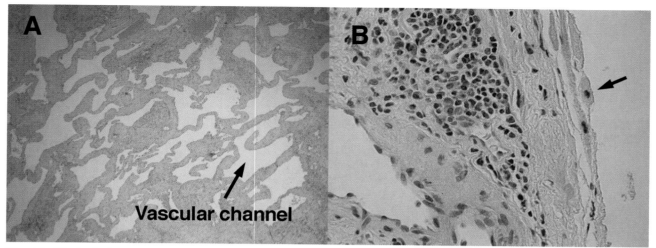

Fig 11-47. Pathologic examination. (*A*) A low-power hematoxylin and eosin (**H&E**) section with multiple vascular channels consistent with a hemangioma. (*B*) A higher resolution showing occasional muscle cells (**arrow**).

Comments

The TEE images show a symmetric mass in the fossa ovalis region of the interatrial septum that is unusual for lipomatous hypertrophy, which typically spares the fossa ovalis. However, the appearance of lipomatous hypertrophy can vary, so that evaluation by CT is helpful to determine whether the mass is adipose tissue. The appearance is also atypical for a myxoma, which usually has a narrow base or stalk. Surgical exploration is indicated unless the mass is clearly adipose tissue. In this case, the benign tumor was completely excised so that recurrence is unlikely. Cardiac hemangiomas are rare (1–3% of all benign primary cardiac tumors). Typically, these tumors are asymptomatic, but cases of pericardial tamponade and symptoms of dyspnea and palpitations have been reported.

Suggested Reading

1. Verunelli F, Amerini A, D'Alfonso A et al. Left atrial cardiac hemangioma: a report of two cases. Ital Heart J 2004; 5:299–301.

2. Sata N, Moriyama Y, Hamada N et al. Recurrent pericardial tamponade from atrial hemangioma. Ann Thorac Surg 2004; 78:1472–5.

3. Kamiya H, Yasuda T, Nagamine H et al. Surgical treatment of primary cardiac tumors: 28 years' experience in Kanazawa University Hospital. Jpn Circ J 2001; 65:315–19.

Case 11-14
Aortic Valve Fibroelastoma

This 60-year-old woman was referred for placement of a mitral annuloplasty ring for treatment of severe mitral regurgitation due to a dilated cardiomyopathy with congestive heart failure symptoms.

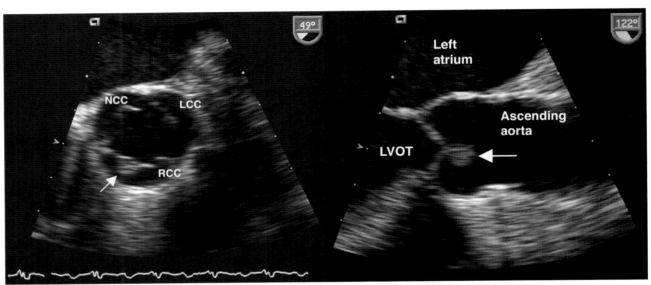

Fig 11-48. An incidental finding on intraoperative TEE, shown in short-axis (*left*) and long-axis (*right*) views of the aortic valve, was a small, globular mass on the tip of the right coronary cusp (**arrows**).

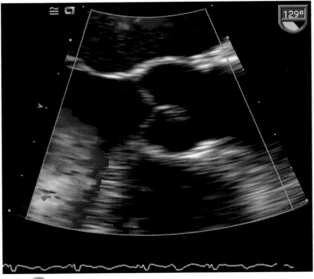

Fig 11-49. Color flow imaging in a long-axis view shows no aortic regurgitation.

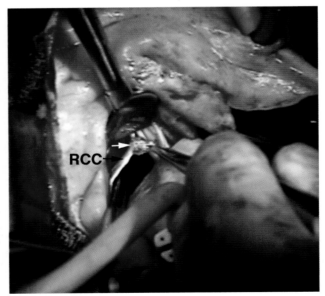

Fig 11-50. At surgery, a small verrucous mass (**arrow**) was excised from the right coronary cusp of the aortic valve. There was no injury to the valve leaflets and no aortic regurgitation on post-pump TEE. The pathology was consistent with a papillary fibroelastoma.

Comments

A papillary fibroelastoma is a benign cardiac tumor that typically occurs on the aortic or mitral valve. Unlike valvular vegetations, these tumors tend to be located on the downstream (instead of upstream) side of the valve and are not associated with destruction of the underlying valve disease. The macroscopic appearance of these tumors is a frond-like mass, sometimes with superimposed thrombus (see **Fig 6-53**). Microscopically, there is abundant elastic and fibrous tissue—similar to the normal component of the valve leaflet. The prevalence of papillary fibroelastomas increases with age, although the gender distribution is about equal. The most common valve sites (in order of prevalence) are aortic (44%), mitral (35%), tricuspid (13%) and pulmonic (8%) valves, with size at the time of detection ranging from 2 to 70 mm.

The optimal management of these tumors is controversial; many are found incidentally on echocardiography requested for other reasons, as in this case. In others, the tumor appears to be related to cerebrovascular events, myocardial infarction, sudden death or peripheral embolic events. Clearly, in patients with embolic events or other symptoms, excision is appropriate. With smaller asymptomatic masses, there is disagreement about optimal management, although risk factors for events include size and mobility of the mass. As echocardiographic image quality improves, it is likely that more, smaller fibroelastomas will be detected as incidental findings.

Suggested Reading

1. Klarich KW, Enriquez-Sarano M, Gura GM et al. Papillary fibroelastoma: echocardiographic characteristics for diagnosis and pathologic correlation. J Am Coll Cardiol 1997; 30:784–90.

2. Vander Salm TJ. Unusual primary tumors of the heart. Semin Thorac Cardiovasc Surg 2000; 12:89–100.

3. Gowda RM, Khan IA, Nair CK et al. Cardiac papillary fibroelastoma: a comprehensive analysis of 725 cases. Am Heart J 2003; 146:404–10.

Case 11-15
Atypical Papillary Fibroelastoma

This 33-year-old woman with a history of mediastinal radiation therapy for Hodgkin's disease presented during pregnancy with congestive heart failure. Evaluation showed severe aortic stenosis and severe mitral stenosis and regurgitation and she was managed medically. She is now 1 month postpartum and is referred for valve surgery. A preoperative TEE showed a left atrial mass. She has not been documented to have atrial fibrillation.

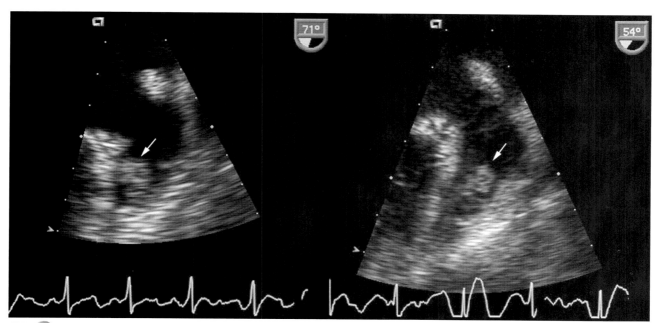

Fig 11-51. Images of the left atrial appendage at 71 and 54 degrees show a mobile mass (**arrows**) in the left atrial appendage that is consistent with thrombus. It is clearly separate from the trabeculations of the appendage wall and moves independently.

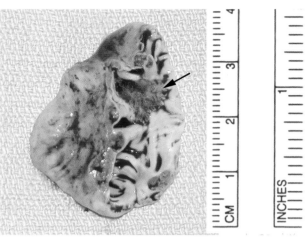

Fig 11-52. The left atrial appendage was removed at surgery. The excised specimen shows the normal trabeculated appearance with a verrucous mass (**arrow**) that on microscopic examination was a papillary fibroelastoma.

Comments

Although typically attached to a valve, fibroelastomas may be seen in atypical locations in 13% of all papillary fibroelastoma cases. Non-valvular sites include the left ventricle, left atrium, and the left atrial appendage, as in this case. Papillary fibroelastomas have also been reported attached to the right atrial wall, right atrial appendage, Eustachian valve and right ventricle. A complete examination is essential, as multiple tumors are found in 6% of cases.

Case 11-16
Angiosarcoma

This 33-year-old man presented with hemoptysis and dyspnea and was found to have a pericardial effusion and diffuse pulmonary nodules on chest CT imaging. Echocardiography shows a right atrial mass with apparent involvement of the right atrial free wall. He was referred for surgical intervention for a tissue diagnosis and resection of the mass.

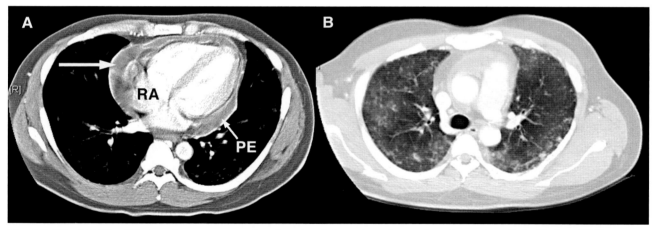

Fig 11-53. (*A*) The CT scan shows a mass abutting the right atrium (**arrow**) and a pericardial effusion (**PE**). (*B*) The lungs show diffuse, widespread pulmonary ground-glass opacities in a miliary nodular pattern, most consistent with hematogenous spread of metastases.

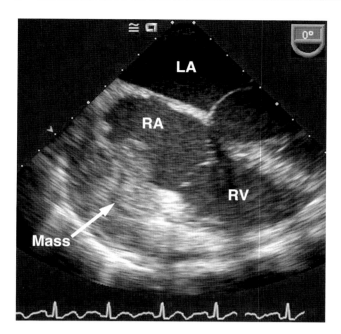

Fig 11-54. Mid-esophageal four-chamber TEE shows a mass infiltrating the right atrial wall, with intracavitary extension. The tricuspid valve appears uninvolved.

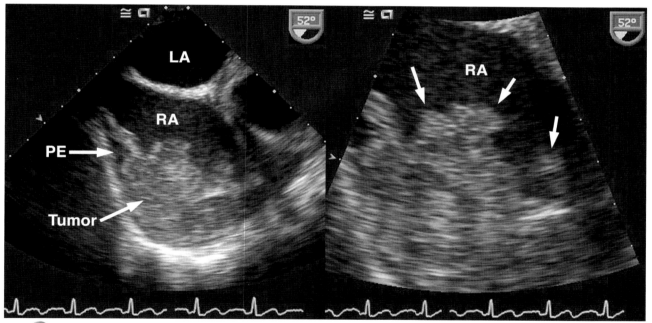

Fig 11-55. Rotating the probe to 52 degrees shows the mass again. In real time, the intracavitary components are quite mobile (**arrows**). The mass is densely adherent to the right atrial wall, and is surrounded by a pericardial effusion.

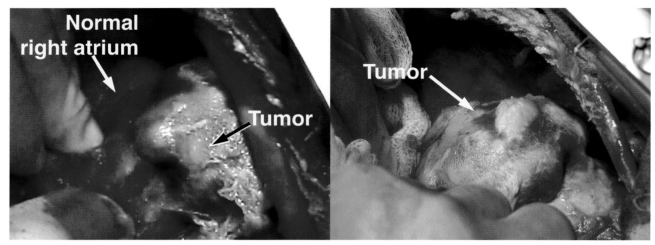

Fig 11-56. After sternotomy, medial retraction of the heart reveals a densely adherent tumor. Further retraction of the heart reveals the full extent of the tumor.

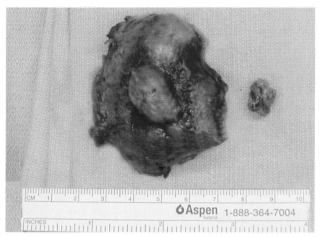

Fig 11-57. Two components of the tumor are shown—the tumor itself on the left, and a smaller mass on the right, which was one of the mobile components within the RA on TEE.

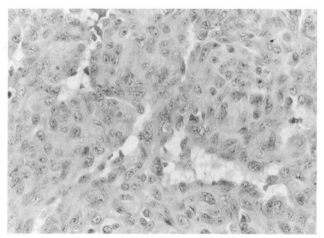

Fig 11-58. Microscopic examination of the tumor using hematoxylin and eosin (**H&E**) shows spindled to epithelioid cells with oval to elongated, enlarged, hyperchromatic nuclei with prominent nucleoli. The cells are arranged in sheets that form anastomosing, slit-like vascular spaces.

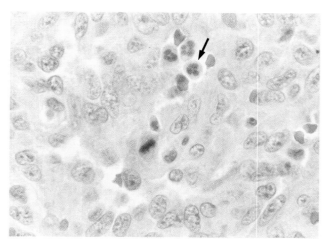

Fig 11-59. A high-power view of the histology shows a mitotic figure (**arrow**). There were up to 41 mitotic figures per 10 high-power fields. Approximately 50% of the neoplasm was necrotic.

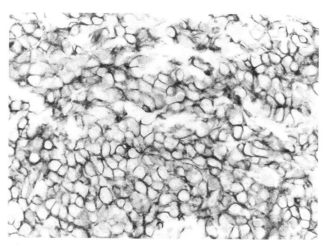

Fig 11-60. Using a specific immunohistochemical stain marker for vascular endothelial cells (**CD31**) shows prominent vascular tissue consistent with an angiosarcoma.

Comments

The differential diagnosis of a right atrial mass includes thrombus, either of local origin or in transit from a peripheral vein, an atypical infected vegetation or a tumor. Tumors may represent direct extension from a non-cardiac primary tumor (most often lung, breast or lymphoma) or may be cardiac in origin. Most primary cardiac tumors are benign, with 18% of cardiac myxomas presenting in the right atrium. Malignant cardiac tumors account for only about one-quarter of all primary cardiac tumors, with the percent of all cardiac tumors about 9% for angiosarcomas, 5% for rhabdosarcomas, 4% for mesotheliomas, and 3% for fibrosarcomas.

In patients with a cardiac tumor, the echo-cardiographic examination focuses on the location and extent of the tumor, the physiologic consequences (e.g. valve obstruction or regurgitation), and any associated findings, such as pericardial effusion. The appearance of this mass was suggestive of a primary malignant cardiac tumor. The mass appeared to invade the right atrial free wall, had an irregular appearance within the right atrium and was associated with a pericardial effusion. However, this tumor did not result in hemodynamic compromise; instead, clinical manifestations were related to pulmonary embolic events.

Suggested Reading

1. Piazza N, Chughtai T, Toledano K et al. Primary cardiac tumours: eighteen years of surgical experience on 21 patients. Can J Cardiol. 2004; 20(14):1443–8.

2. Meng Q, Lai H, Lima J et al. Echocardiographic and pathologic characteristics of primary cardiac tumors: a study of 149 cases. Int J Cardiol 2002; 84(1):69–75.

Secondary Tumors

Case 11-17
Renal Cell Carcinoma with Extension to Right Atrium

This 55-year-old male with renal cell carcinoma extending into the right atrium underwent surgery for en bloc removal of the right kidney and mass with cooperation of urologic, liver and cardiac surgeons.

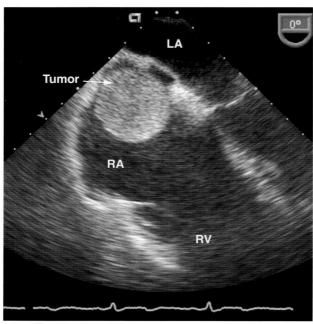

Fig 11-61. TEE images in a four-chamber view show a large spherical mass in the right atrium that appears adjacent, but not attached, to the atrial septum.

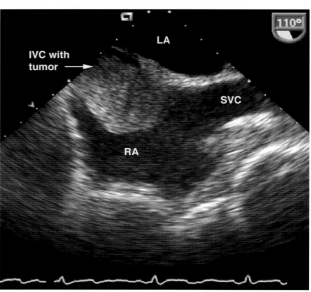

Fig 11-62. As the image plane is rotated to a long-axis view of the right atrium (**RA**) and superior vena cava (**SVC**), the mass is seen extending from the inferior vena cava (**IVC**) into the RA.

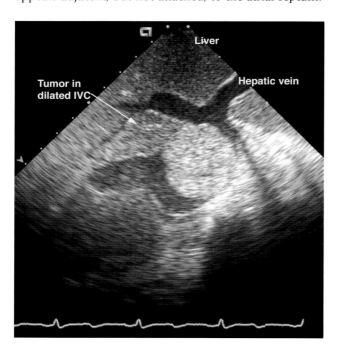

Fig 11-63. Placing a sterile sheathed surfaced probe directly on the liver provides an image of the tumor mass filling the inferior vena cava. The hepatic veins are also dilated.

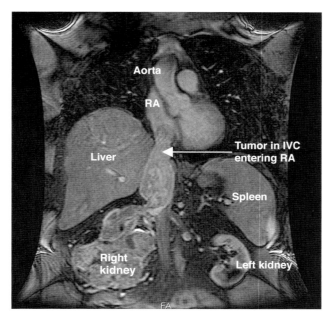

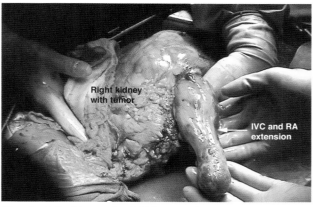

Fig 11-65. The excised kidney with tumor extension into the IVC and RA was removed en bloc.

Fig 11-64. A sagittal plane MR image demonstrated the extent of the tumor from the right kidney into the inferior vena cava and right atrium.

Case 11-18
Renal Cell Carcinoma with Tumor Embolization to Pulmonary Artery

This 54-year-old man with a right renal tumor with extensive vena caval thrombosis presented with pulmonary embolism. At baseline in the operating room for en bloc resection of renal tumor, a mobile tumor was seen in the right atrium extending from the inferior vena cava into the right atrium, with diastolic prolapse into the right ventricle. During the procedure, the extension of tumor into the heart disappeared.

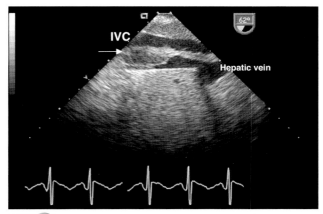

Fig 11-66. Transgastric images of the inferior vena cava (**IVC**) show a mass (**arrow**) extending along the length of the vessel.

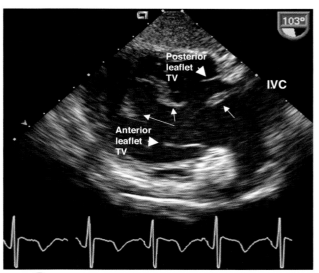

Fig 11-67. A transgastric right ventricular inflow view shows that the mass (**arrows**) extends from the inferior vena cava (**IVC**), across the right atrium, and crosses the tricuspid valve (**TV**) into the right ventricle.

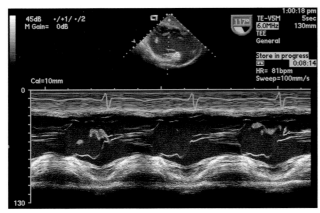

Fig 11-68. M-mode from this position confirms that the mass moves independently (i.e. with a different pattern of motion) from the tricuspid valve, with motion that varies from beat to beat.

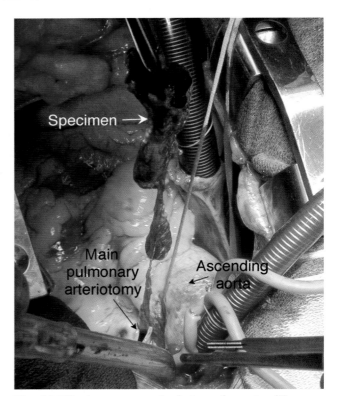

Fig 11-70. At surgery, a single irregular string-like mass was removed en bloc: it extended from the inferior vena cava, through the right heart, and into the pulmonary artery.

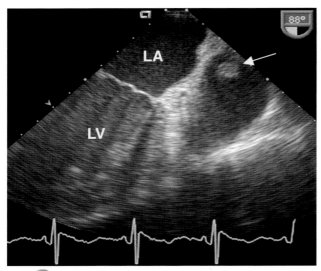

DVD **Fig 11-69.** A TEE two-chamber view shows that a mass (**arrow**) is also present in the pulmonary artery.

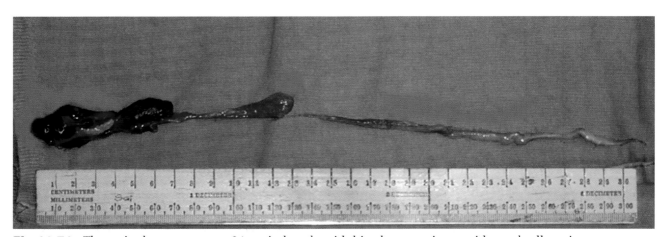

Fig 11-71. The excised mass was over 24 cm in length, with histology consistent with renal cell carcinoma.

Comments (for cases 11-17 and 11-18)

Renal cell carcinoma may spread by direct extension up the inferior vena cava into the right atrium. Tumor extension into the right atrium demonstrates a typical appearance, as illustrated by these two cases. TEE allows precise delineation of the size and location of tumor extension into the right atrium and allows confirmation that the tumor does not attach to the atrial wall or involve the tricuspid valve. With a complete anatomic definition of the tumor, the surgical resection is often performed "en bloc", with collaboration between the renal and cardiac surgeons. Intraoperative TEE is essential for guiding the surgical approach and documenting the absence of tumor and normal right heart function after resection.

Suggested Reading

1. Allen G, Klingman R, Ferraris VA et al. Transesophageal echocardiography in the surgical management of renal cell carcinoma with intracardiac extension. J Cardiovasc Surg (Torino) 1991; 32:833–6.

2. Chatterjee T, Muller MF, Carrel T et al. Images in cardiovascular medicine. Renal cell carcinoma with tumor thrombus extending through the inferior vena cava into the right cardiac cavities. Circulation 1997; 96:2729–30.

3. Chiappini B, Savini C, Marinelli G et al. Cavoatrial tumor thrombus: single-stage surgical approach with profound hypothermia and circulatory arrest, including a review of the literature. J Thorac Cardiovasc Surg 2002; 124:684–8.

Case 11-19
Chondrosarcoma Embolism to Pulmonary Artery

While undergoing hemipelvectomy for high-grade chondrosarcoma of the right pelvis, this 32-year-old woman became hypotensive and unresponsive to volume infusion.

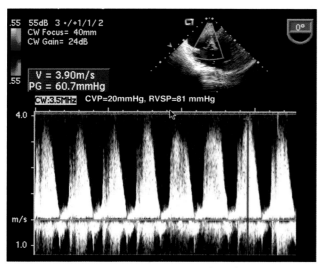

Fig 11-72. Continuous wave Doppler of the tricuspid regurgitant jet shows a maximum velocity of 3.9 m/s, which corresponds to a right ventricular to right atrial pressure difference of 61 mmHg. Central venous pressure (**CVP**) was 20 mmHg, so that estimated pulmonary systolic pressure is 81 mmHg.

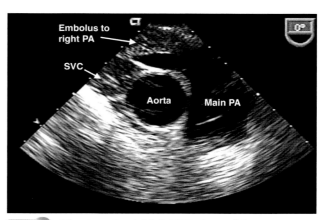

Fig 11-73. A high TEE view of the pulmonary artery shows a mass obstructing the right pulmonary artery (**arrow**).

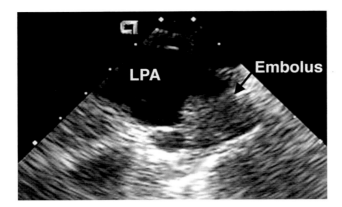

Fig 11-74. Rotation of the image plane towards the patient's left side shows the left pulmonary artery (**LPA**) completely occluded by a mass.

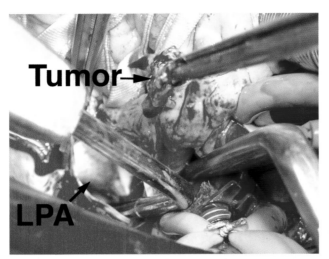

Fig 11-75. The patient underwent pulmonary tumor embolectomy. A mass is shown after removal from the LPA.

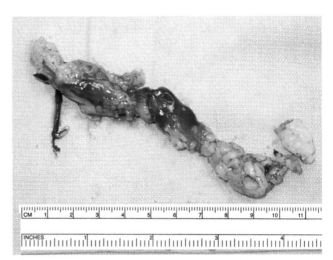

Fig 11-76. The mass excised from the right pulmonary artery. Pathology was consistent with metastatic high-grade osteosarcoma, chondroblastic subtype.

Comments

In a patient with a right-sided cardiac mass, acute hypotension during the surgical procedure should prompt evaluation for embolization of the mass. First, the tomographic planes where the mass was visible can be checked to ascertain if the mass is still visualized. Then, the pulmonary artery bifurcation can be imaged from a high TEE view to evaluate for obstruction. A sudden rise in pulmonary pressures is also an indicator of possible embolization. The absence of diagnostic images does not exclude the possibility of pulmonary embolism, so that other imaging procedures should be considered, as appropriate.

Suggested Reading

1. Chen H, Ng V, Kane CJ, Russell IA. The role of transesophageal echocardiography in rapid diagnosis and treatment of migratory tumor embolus. Anesth Analg 2004; 99:357–9.
2. Newkirk L, Vater Y, Oxorn D et al. Intraoperative TEE for the management of pulmonary tumour embolism during chondroblastic osteosarcoma resection. Can J Anaesth 2003; 50:886–90.

Case 11-20
Lung Cancer Invading Superior Vena Cava

This 37-year-old woman presented with superior vena caval syndrome due to a large primary mediastinal carcinoma. She was initially treated with chemotherapy and radiation therapy due to the large size and location of the tumor, which precluded resection.

Subsequent evaluation with CT imaging showed resolution of disease progression, except for a localized area in the region of the superior vena cava (SVC). She was referred for resection and reconstruction of the SVC.

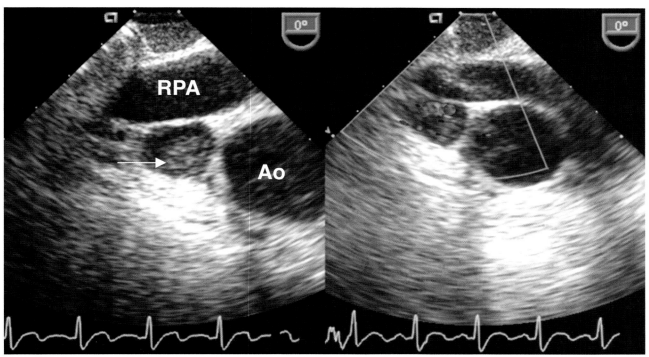

Fig 11-77. Echocardiographic images from a high TEE position show a poorly defined opacity in the superior vena cava (**arrow**) adjacent to the right pulmonary artery (**RPA**) and aorta (**Ao**). Doppler color flow (*right*) shows the obstruction to flow due to this mass.

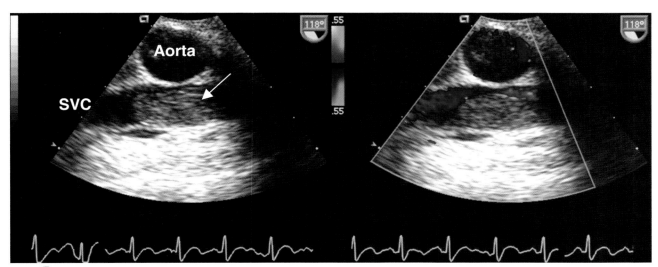

Fig 11-78. Longitudinal views of the superior vena cava (**SVC**) and mass were obtained by rotating the image plane to 118 degrees. In real time, the tumor appears adherent to the anterior wall of the SVC.

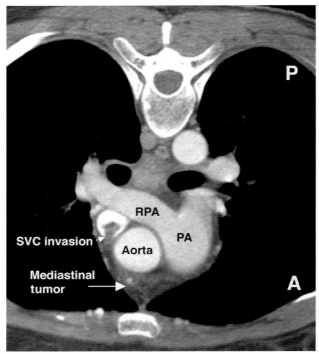

Fig 11-79. A CT scan at the level of the pulmonary artery has been oriented to match the orientation of the echocardiographic images in **Fig 11-77**. The mediastinal tumor and invasion of the SVC are seen.

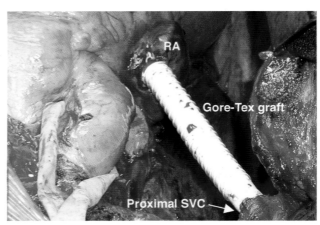

Fig 11-81. Reconstruction was performed using an end-to-end anastomosis of azygos into SVC and a 10 mm Gore-Tex graft from the right innominate vein to the right atrial appendage.

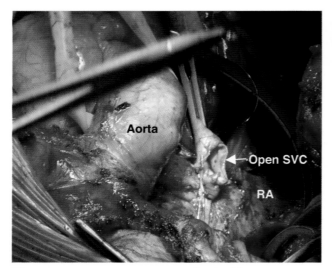

Fig 11-80. At surgery, an area of palpable tumor was found in the mid-SVC, but with a normal caval margin of 2–3 cm between this region and the junction with the right atrium. The tumor and section of SVC were resected.

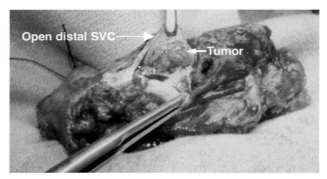

Fig 11-82. The pathology of the resected tumor was consistent with metastatic adenocarcinoma.

Comments

Direct extension or metastasis of a non-cardiac tumor to the heart is 20 times more common than a primary cardiac tumor. The most common tumors metastatic to the heart, in order of frequency, are lung, lymphoma, breast, leukemia, stomach, melanoma, liver and colon cancer. Although melanoma has the highest rate of metastasis to the heart, this tumor is much less common than other tumors so does not account for a very large percentage of cardiac metastases overall. In autopsy studies of patients with malignant disease, about 11% have cardiac involvement. Metastatic disease typically involves the epicardium and often leads to a pericardial effusion. Myocardial involvement is less common and extension into the cardiac chambers is rare.

Suggested Reading

1. Abraham KP, Reddy V, Gattuso P. Neoplasms metastatic to the heart: review of 3314 consecutive autopsies. Am J Cardiovasc Pathol 1990; 3:195–8.

2. Klatt EC, Heitz DR. Cardiac metastases. Cancer 1990; 65:1456–9.

3. Odim J, Reehal V, Laks H et al. Surgical pathology of cardiac tumors. Two decades at an urban institution. Cardiovasc Pathol 2003; 12:267–70.

Case 11-21
Pericardial Mass

This 71-year-old man, with an ice pick cardiac perforation 13 years previously, presented with congestive heart failure and left extremity edema, with worsening symptoms over the last year.

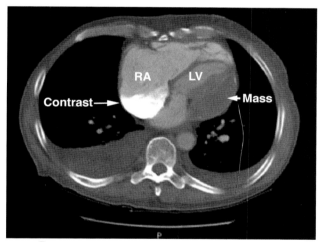

DVD **Fig 11-83.** Chest CT shows a large mass (3 × 5 × 7 cm) lateral to the left ventricle (**LV**), with a small LV chamber and a large right atrium (**RA**). Bilateral pleural effusions are also present. Residual contrast is seen in the RA.

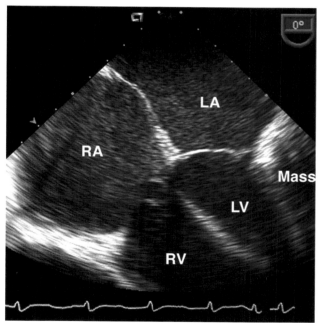

DVD **Fig 11-84.** In a TEE four-chamber view, there is an ill-defined echodensity lateral to the left ventricle (**LV**) with compression of the LV chamber. The right and left atrium are markedly enlarged, with evidence of spontaneous echo contrast seen in both atria in real time.

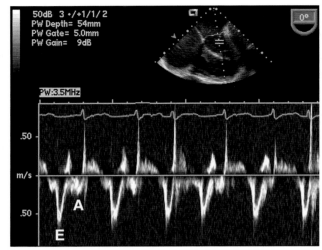

Fig 11-85. The Doppler LV inflow velocity curve shows a prominent early diastolic velocity (**E**) with a small atrial contribution (**A**) to ventricular filling. This pattern of diastolic filling is consistent with decreased diastolic compliance or constrictive pericarditis.

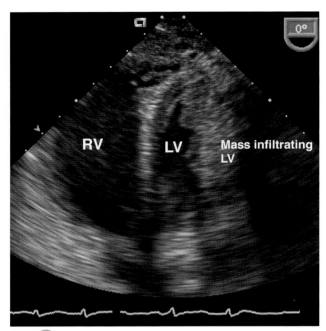

DVD **Fig 11-86.** The transgastric apical view shows better definition of an echodense mass adjacent to the lateral wall of the LV with a small LV chamber.

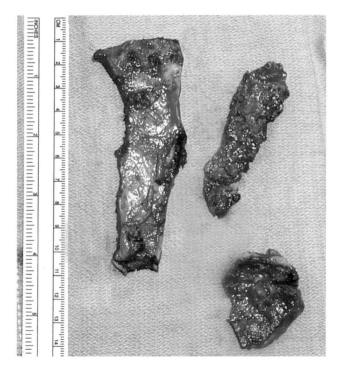

DVD **Fig 11-87.** Surgical findings were a large firm mass on lateral aspect of LV. The pericardium was incised and an old hematoma expressed and irrigated. The roof of this cavity was dissected free, with the pathology showing fibroadipose tissue consistent with an old hematoma and an inflamed fibrous wall.

Comments

A chronic pericardial hematoma is a rare, but reported, complication after cardiac trauma or cardiac surgery. The diagnosis can be challenging, as a chronic hematoma presents as a mass. If cardiac compression is present, differentiation of an extracardiac from intracardiac mass can be difficult. Acute pericardial hematoma can have an atypical clinical presentation and the hematoma may be localized to one region of the pericardium, rather than symmetrically filling the pericardial space. TEE allows recognition of the mass and evaluation of the effects of compression on cardiac hemodynamics. In some cases, wide-angle tomographic imaging approaches, such as chest CT or cardiac MR, may be needed for complete evaluation of the mass.

Suggested Reading

1. Hirai S, Hamanaka Y, Mitsui N et al. Chronic expanding hematoma in the pericardial cavity after cardiac surgery. Ann Thorac Surg 2003; 75:1629–31.

2. Gologorsky E, Gologorsky A, Galbut DL, Wolfenson A. Left atrial compression by a pericardial hematoma presenting as an obstructing intracavitary mass: a difficult differential diagnosis. Anesth Analg 2002; 95:567–9.

3. Fukui T, Suehiro S, Shibata T et al. Retropericardial hematoma complicating off-pump coronary artery bypass surgery. Ann Thorac Surg 2002; 73(5):1629–31.

12

Catheters and Devices

Catheters

Devices

Catheters

Case 12-1
Venous Cannula

In preparation for cardiopulmonary bypass, cannulas are placed to direct the systemic venous return into the bypass pump and then return the oxygenated blood into the ascending aorta. One approach is to place separate cannulas in the superior vena cava (SVC) and inferior vena cava (IVC). Alternatively, one cannula can be placed in the right atrium via the atrial appendage. The choice of cannulation is dependent on the specific surgical procedure.

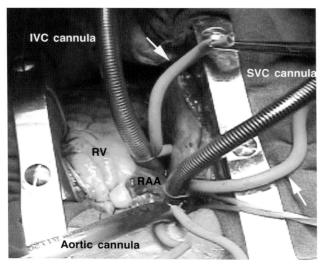

Fig 12-1. This view of the opened chest at the start of cardiopulmonary bypass shows separate cannulation of the superior vena cava (**SVC**) and inferior vena cava (**IVC**) for collection of systemic venous return, which drains by gravity into the bypass pump and oxygenator. The pump output is directed into the aortic cannula. The red flexible tubes (**arrows**) secure the purse-string sutures around the insertion of each cannula into the cardiac chamber or vessel.

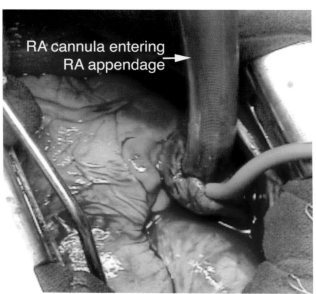

Fig 12-2. In this patient, a single straight right atrial cannula, inserted via the right atrial appendage, is used for the inflow into the cardiopulmonary bypass pump.

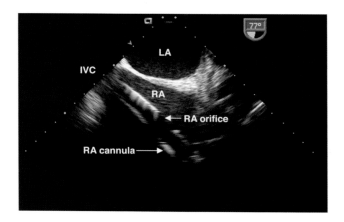

Fig 12-3. On bicaval TEE imaging of the cannulation in **Fig 12-2**, the distal end of the cannula is seen in the **IVC**, which it drains. The side-hole **RA orifice** drains blood entering the **RA** from the SVC and coronary sinus.

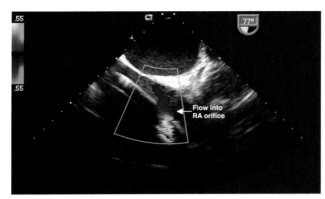

Fig 12-4. Color Doppler demonstrates continuous flow into the cannula during cardiopulmonary bypass.

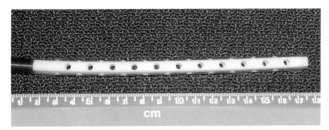

Fig 12-5. When access to the cardiac structure is difficult or stabilization of the patient prior to sternotomy is needed, venous return can also be directed to the bypass pump via the femoral vein. This multiple side-hole catheter is inserted via the femoral vein with the tip advanced to the level of the right atrium.

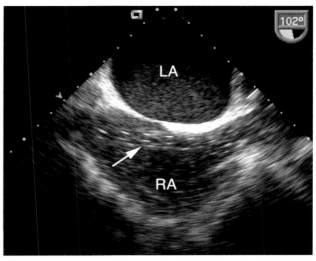

Fig 12-6. On the TEE bicaval view, the femoral venous catheter is seen correctly positioned in the right atrium (**arrow**).

Comments

Venous cannula flow may be decreased if the entry sites are too close to the vessel or chamber walls, if the cannula is kinked or if air from a loose connection blocks blood flow. Usually these problems are recognized and corrected visually, but the TEE images are helpful in ensuring optimal positioning of the venous cannula at the start of the procedure.

Case 12-2
Coronary Sinus Catheter

A catheter is placed in the coronary sinus when retrograde cardioplegia is used. TEE may be helpful in ensuring correct placement of this catheter.

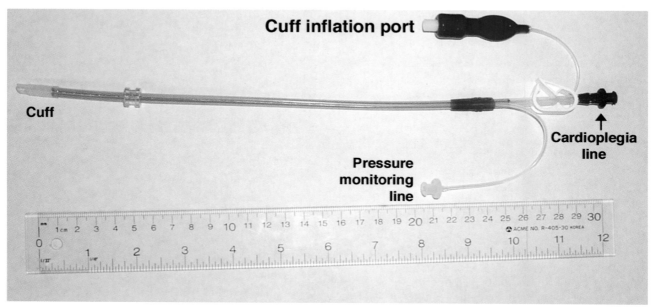

Fig 12-7. Photograph of a typical coronary sinus catheter. The cuff, just proximal to the catheter tip, is inflated after positioning to improve retrograde delivery of cardioplegia solution to the myocardium. The pressure monitoring line allows the perfusionist to keep the cardioplegia infusion pressure low enough to avoid coronary sinus injury.

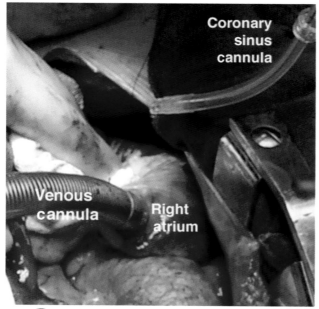

DVD ▶ **Fig 12-8.** The surgeon's finger indicates the point where the right atrium will be punctured, and the catheter passed through the right atrium and into the coronary sinus orifice.

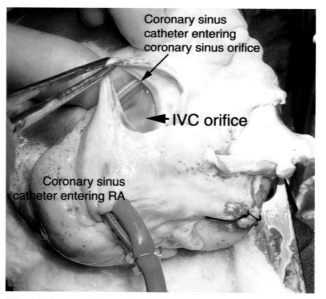

Fig 12-9. In a donor heart being prepared for implantation at the time of transplantation, the coronary sinus catheter is seen entering the right atrium. The path of the catheter as it crosses the atrium towards the coronary sinus orifice is seen through the orifice of the inferior vena cava (**IVC**).

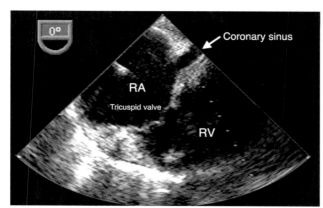

Fig 12-10. A standard view for TEE imaging of the coronary sinus is to start from the high TEE four-chamber view, turn the image plane towards the right heart and then advance the probe until the coronary sinus is seen entering the right atrium adjacent to the tricuspid annulus.

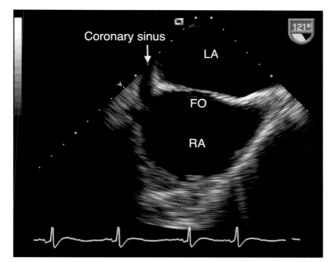

Fig 12-11. Rotation to an angle of about 120 degrees provides a second view of the coronary sinus entry into the right atrium. The fossa ovalis (FO) of the interatrial septum is seen.

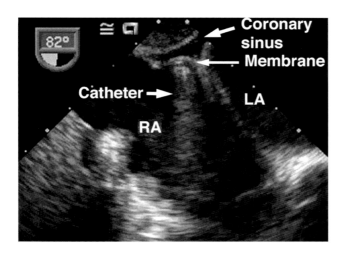

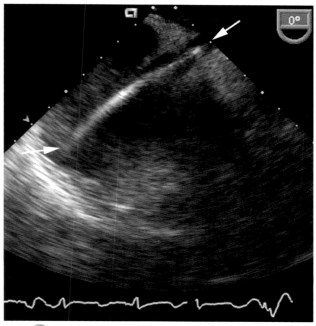

DVD 🔊 Fig 12-12. In a patient with a coronary sinus catheter, the position of the catheter (arrow) is seen in the 0 degrees view.

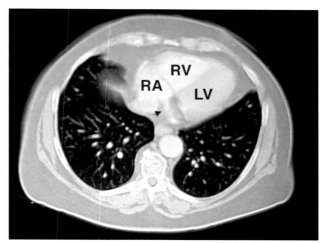

Fig 12-13. A chest CT scan demonstrates the position of the coronary sinus relative to the right atrium (RA) and the right (RV) and left ventricles (LV).

DVD 🔊 Fig 12-14. This example is taken from a case where the surgeon was unable to pass the catheter into the coronary sinus orifice. TEE revealed a membrane (also known as the Thebesian valve) covering the orifice and blocking catheter entry (arrows).

Case 12-3
Pulmonary Vein Cannula for Partial Bypass

Cannulas may be placed via a left pulmonary vein into the left atrium for partial heart bypass, with a portion of the pulmonary venous return directed through the bypass pump and returned to the aorta, usually via the femoral artery. With partial bypass, the right heart continues to pump blood normally through the lungs.

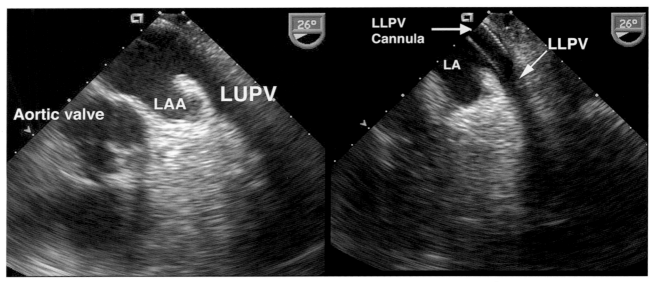

Fig 12-15. The left upper pulmonary vein (**LUPV**) is easily visualized adjacent to the left atrial appendage (**LAA**) from a high TEE view at 0–30 degrees of rotation (*above*). As the probe is advanced, the left lower pulmonary vein (**LLPV**) with the cannula in position comes into view (*below*).

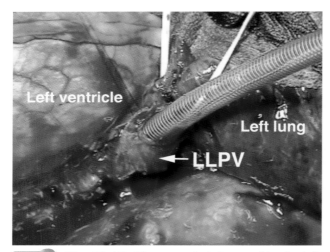

DVD **Fig 12-16.** The cannula is inserted in the left lower pulmonary vein (**LLPV**).

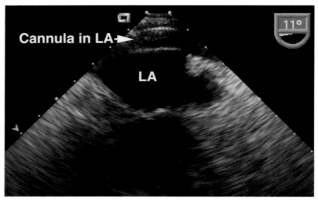

Fig 12-17. View of the cannula in the left atrium (**LA**). It is important to ensure that the inflow segment of the cannula is correctly positioned in the center of the LA (and is not advanced into another pulmonary vein).

Case 12-4
Left Ventricular Vent

In situations where there is persistent blood flow into the left ventricle during cardiopulmonary bypass, a vent may be placed to return this blood to the bypass pump and thereby avoid left ventricular distention. This is most commonly done in patients with a significant degree of aortic regurgitation. The vent may be placed via the left ventricular apex, or now, more commonly, via a pulmonary vein and then across the mitral valve.

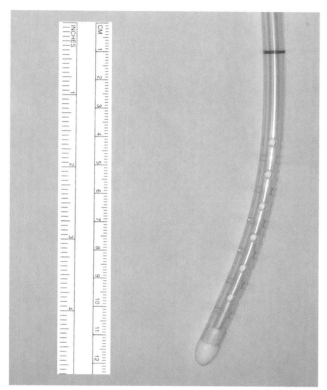

Fig 12-18. Photograph of a typical LV vent catheter with a soft tip and multiple side holes.

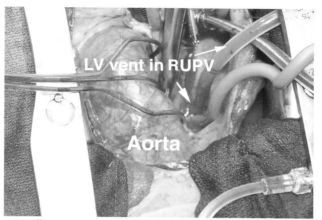

Fig 12-19. Intraoperative photograph of the left ventricular (**LV**) vent positioned via the right upper pulmonary vein (**RUPV**).

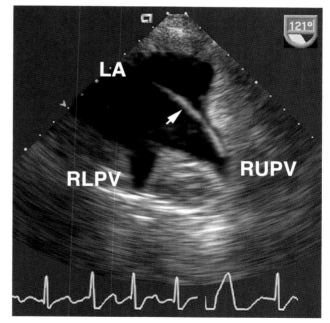

Fig 12-20. TEE imaging of the right pulmonary veins shows the vent passing into the left atrium via the right upper pulmonary vein (**arrow**).

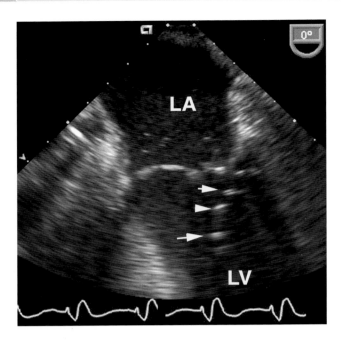

DVD **Fig 12-21.** The TEE four-chamber view shows the catheter positioned across the mitral valve with the side holes (**arrows**) in the left ventricle. The right heart is not well seen, as it is both relatively empty and obscured by shadowing by the right heart cannula during cardiopulmonary bypass.

Case 12-5
Aortic Cannula

The aortic cannula is placed in the ascending aorta to allow oxygenated blood to be pumped to the patient from the bypass machine and supply arterial blood to the tissues.

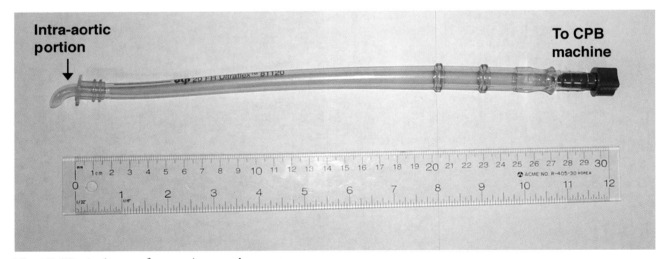

Fig 12-22. A picture of an aortic cannula.

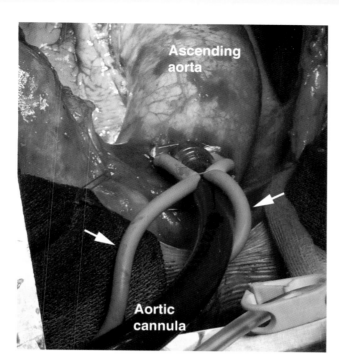

Ascending
aorta

Aortic
cannula

DVD **Fig 12-23.** The aortic cannula is seen placed in the ascending aorta. The red flexible tubes (**arrows**) secure the purse-string sutures that help to prevent the cannula from dislodging.

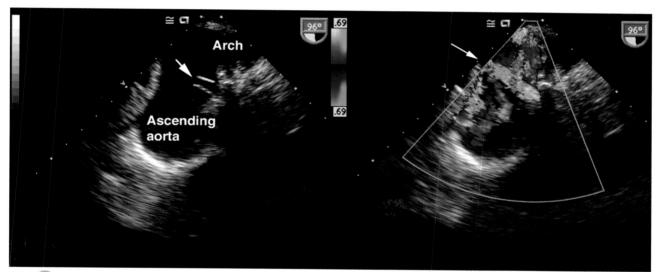

DVD **Fig 12-24.** On the left, the cannula (**arrow**) is seen entering the ascending aorta. On the right, an intense stream of continuous color flows from the cannula and strikes the opposite wall of the aorta (**arrow**).

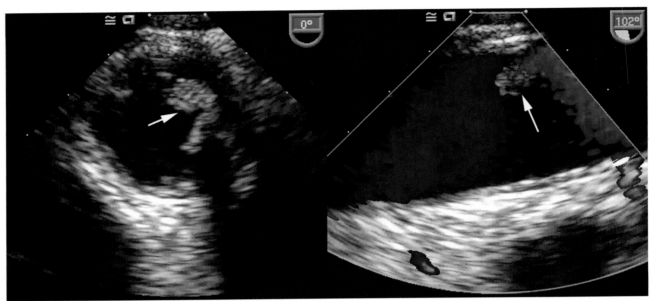

DVD **Fig 12-25.** In this patient, TEE examination of the descending aorta revealed mobile atheroma (**arrows**) in the 0-degree (*left*) and 102-degree (*right*) planes. Color is seen to go around the lesion.

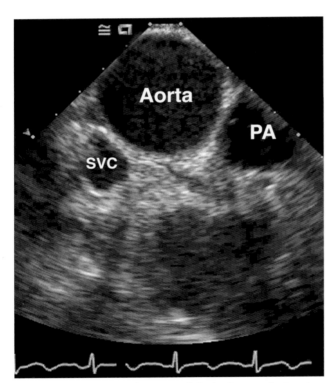

Fig 12-26. Because the area of desired cannulation is often not well visualized by TEE, an epiaortic scan was performed, which helped to identify an area of the ascending aorta suitable for cannulation.

Comments

Complications of cannulation of the aorta include bleeding, embolization of atherosclerotic plaque and aortic dissection. With cannulation of the ascending aorta for cardiopulmonary bypass, an aortic atheroma can be dislodged at the cannulation site. Some cardiac surgeons use an epicardial ultrasound probe to evaluate for aortic atheroma before cannulation. Evidence of atherosclerosis on TEE imaging of the ascending aorta on the baseline images should be promptly reported to the surgeon. Dissection is rare, but is most likely with femoral artery cannulation, either for bypass or for placement of an intra-aortic balloon pump. The aorta can easily be evaluated for the possibility of dissection by TEE when femoral cannulation has been performed.

Suggested Reading

1. Wareing TH, Davila-Roman VG, Barzilai B et al. Management of the severely atherosclerotic ascending aorta during cardiac operations. A strategy for detection and treatment. J Thorac Cardiovasc Surg 1992; 103:453–62.

Devices

Case 12-6
Intra-aortic Balloon Pump

An intra-aortic balloon pump (IABP) may be positioned before surgery in patients with hemodynamic compromise or with critical coronary artery disease or may be placed at the end of the procedure to facilitate weaning from cardiopulmonary bypass in patients with severely impaired left ventricular systolic function. The catheter is inserted via a femoral artery, and positioned in the descending thoracic aorta, with the catheter tip just distal to the left subclavian artery. The balloon inflates during diastole and deflates during systole, with timing based on an arterial pressure waveform and/or the electrocardiogram. Balloon inflation in diastole improves coronary artery blood flow, which occurs mainly in diastole, by increasing the coronary perfusion pressure. Balloon deflation in systole effectively decreases left ventricular afterload.

An IABP is contraindicated in patients with significant aortic regurgitation, as diastolic balloon inflation increases the volume of backflow across the aortic valve.

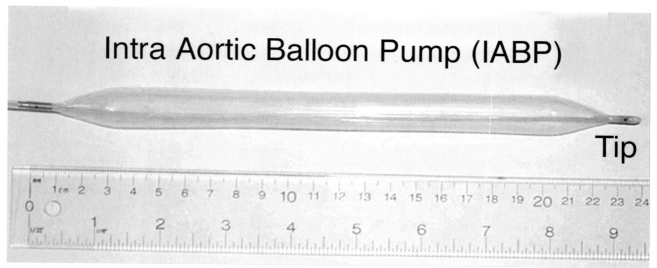

Fig 12-27. A photograph of an intra-aortic balloon pump (**IABP**), demonstrating the tip and the length of the balloon that is placed in the descending aorta and the tip. The IABP tip has a radiopaque marker to aid in positioning. The proximal end of the catheter is off the image to the left.

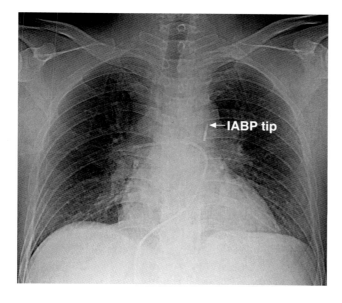

Fig 12-28. Chest radiograph demonstrating the tip of the IABP just distal to the aortic arch. A right heart catheter is also present.

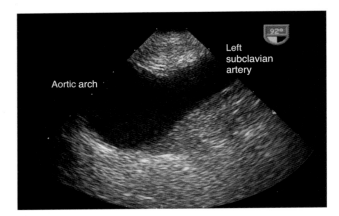

Fig 12-29. This view of the aortic arch and left subclavian artery is obtained from a very high TEE position, with the probe turned to the patient's left side and the image plane rotated to about 90 degrees. This view is helpful for confirming correct positioning of the IABP, which will be seen if the tip is advanced too far into the aorta.

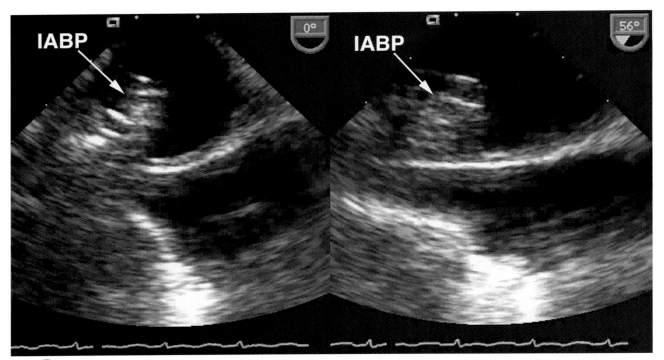

Fig 12-30. This view of the descending thoracic aorta reveals the typical appearance in short-axis view (*left*) and long-axis view (*right*) of the intra-aortic balloon pump. In real time, the device is seen to pulsate in synchrony with the heart beat.

Case 12-7
Biventricular Assist Device

A ventricular assist device bypasses the right heart with systemic venous return from the right atrium directed through the assist device and back into the pulmonary artery. The left heart assist device intake is from the left ventricular apex, with blood returned to the ascending aorta. DVD

It is important to rule out significant AR or PR as this will lead to ventricular distention when the device is active. It is also important to exclude the presence of a PFO with a left ventricular assist device, as the negative pressure created in the left side of the heart may suck desaturated blood from the RA to the LA.

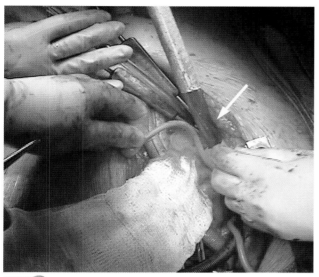

DVD **Fig 12-31.** Photograph of the right atrial cannula being positioned.

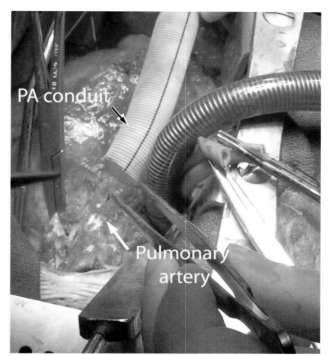

DVD **Fig 12-33.** Photograph of the pulmonary artery cannula anastomosis with the main pulmonary artery.

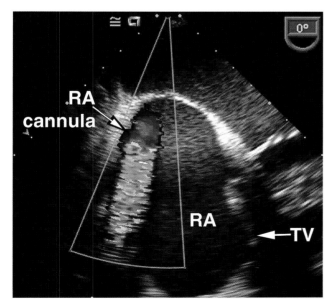

Fig 12-32. TEE view in a four-chamber orientation showing color Doppler interrogation of the right atrial cannula.

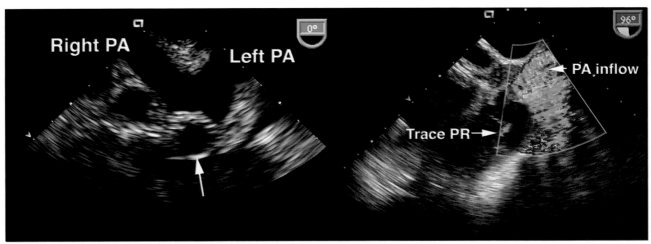

Fig 12-34. TEE view of the pulmonary artery bifurcation at 0 degrees showing the site of the PA cannula (**arrow**) (*left*). At 96 degrees (*right*), color flow into the PA produces only trace pulmonic regurgitation (**PR**). This is important, as severe degrees of PR will lead to right ventricular distention.

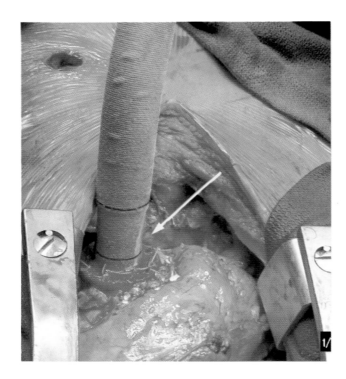

Fig 12-35. Photograph of the apical position of the left ventricular cannula (**arrow**).

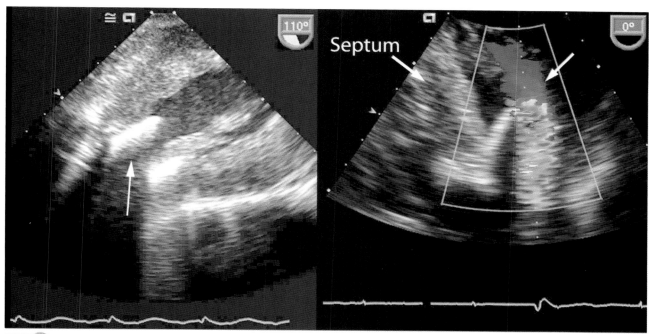

Fig 12-36. TEE transgastric long-axis view of the left ventricle with the apical cannula (**arrow**) (*left*). At 0 degrees, color Doppler indicates flow from the left ventricle into the cannula (**arrow**) (*right*).

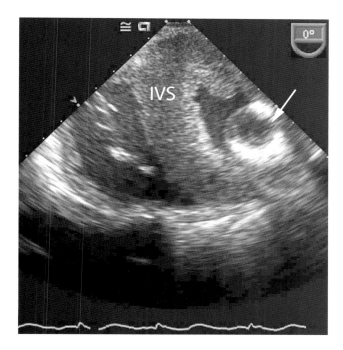

Fig 12-37. TEE transgastric short-axis view of the left and right ventricles with the apical cannula (**arrow**). It is important to determine that the left ventricular cannula does not abut on the interventricular septum (**IVS**), as this would interfere with drainage.

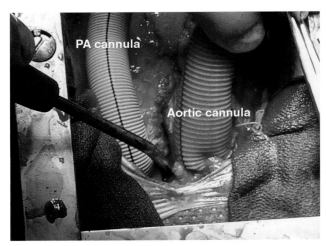

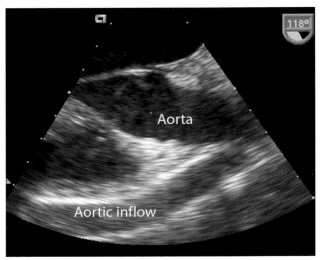

Fig 12-38. Photograph of the placement of the aortic cannula, adjacent to the pulmonary artery cannula.

DVD **Fig 12-39.** TEE long-axis view of the ascending aorta showing the aortic cannula. In real time, aortic inflow produces no aortic regurgitation (**AR**). This is important, as severe degrees of AR will lead to left ventricular distention. Note the aortic valve does not open though the mitral valve does.

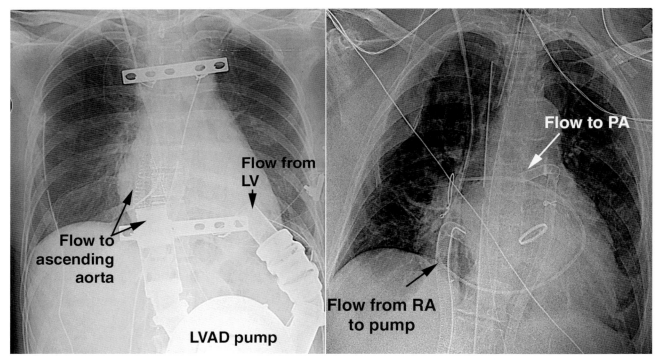

Fig 12-40. In another patient with only a left-sided assist device, a chest X-ray (*left*) reveals the pump implanted in the abdominal wall, the left ventricular cannula in the apex of the left ventricle and a cannula leaving the pump destined for the ascending aorta. In another patient with only a right-sided assist device, a chest X-ray (*right*) reveals the right atrial cannula and the pulmonary artery cannula.

Case 12-8
Inferior Vena Cava Filter Migration

This 49-year-old man had a Greenfield inferior vena cava filter (Boston Scientific, Natick, MA) placed at the IVC–RA junction after pulmonary tumor endarterectomy for renal cell carcinoma embolization bilaterally to his pulmonary arteries. Two weeks later, during surgery for radical nephrectomy and resection of his vena caval tumor, the IVC filter embolized to the right atrium as the abdominal mass was mobilized.

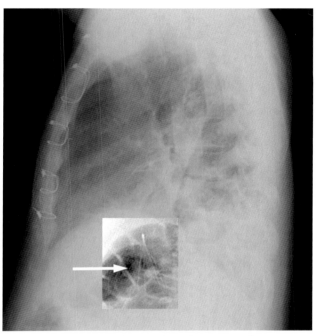

Fig 12-41. Chest radiograph with image enhancement and magnification to show the vena caval filter.

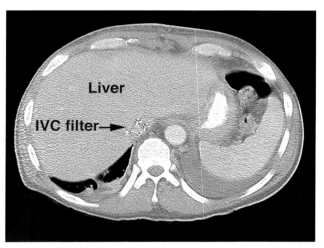

Fig 12-42. Abdominal CT scan showing the inferior vena caval (**IVC**) filter in position before the procedure.

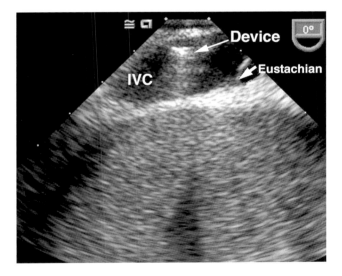

Fig 12-43. TEE view at 0 degrees with the probe at the gastroesophageal junction and turned toward the IVC. The filter is seen in position, with a Eustachian valve at the junction with the right atrium.

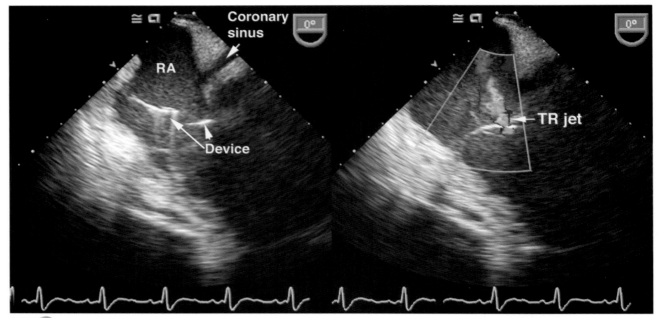

Fig 12-44. During the procedure, the IVC filter disappeared from view. Repositioning the TEE probe to a four-chamber view, angulated posteriorly to include the coronary sinus, demonstrates embolization of the filter into the right atrium. There is only mild tricuspid regurgitation.

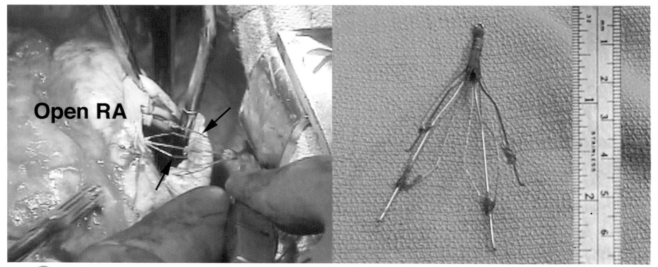

Fig 12-45. The patient was placed on cardiopulmonary bypass. The filter was trapped in the tricuspid valve but was gently explanted via a right atrial incision without damage to the valve leaflets.

Case 12-9
Atrial Septal Defect Closure Device

This 42-year-old woman was referred for mitral valve repair for severe mitral regurgitation due to mitral valve prolapse. She had undergone a percutaneous closure of a PFO about 1 year earlier using a CardioSEAL device (NMT Medical, Boston, MA).

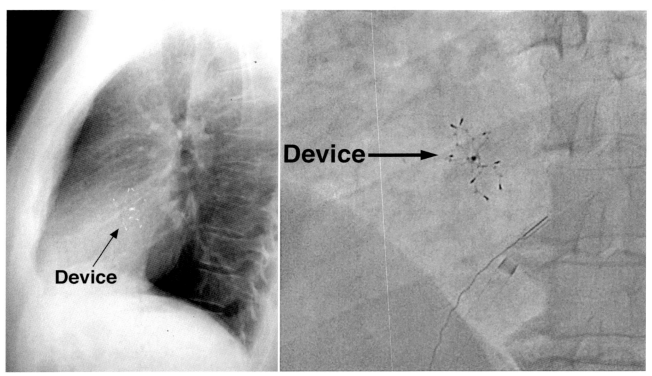

Fig 12-46. Preoperative chest radiography shows multiple echodensities in the region of the atrial septum (**arrow**). An enlarged view (*right*) is seen in this still from cardiac catheterization (**arrow**).

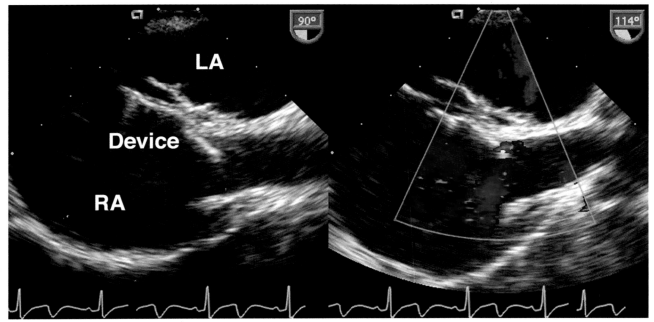

DVD   **Fig 12-47.** The baseline TEE image in the bicaval view at 90 degrees demonstrates the two "wings" of the device on both sides of the atrial septum. Color Doppler (*right*) shows no evidence for flow across the atrial septum.

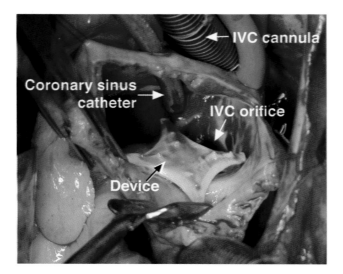

Fig 12-48. At surgery, the device was removed as part of the approach to the mitral valve repair. This view shows the opened right atrium with the inferior vena cava (**IVC**) orifice and cannula, the coronary sinus catheter and the device.

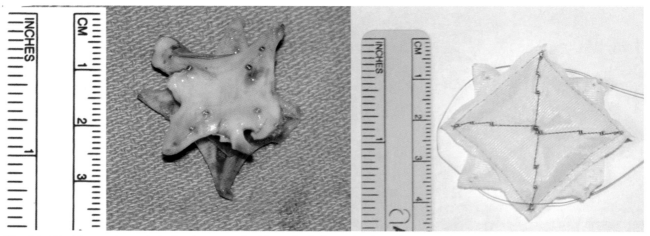

Fig 12-49. The explanted device is covered with endothelium (*left*) with a new device in the same orientation shown for reference (*right*).

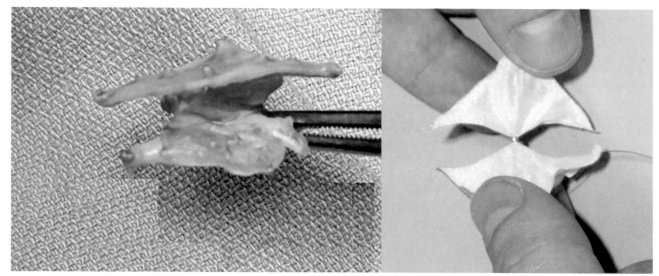

Fig 12-50. A side view of the explanted device shows how it straddles the atrial septum via the patent foramen ovale (*left*), with the opening of the "wings" that allow the device to fit inside a catheter, shown on the right.

Case 12-10
Prolapsing Atrial Septal Defect Closure Device

The patient is a 59-year-old man with two previous neurologic events. The first was 5 years prior to admission and was described as 1 minute of aphasia. This was treated with aspirin. Then 3 months prior to admission he had left leg weakness that lasted approximately 3 minutes.

Upon eventual work-up of this, he was found to have a PFO with an enlarged right atrium and ventricle, and mildly decreased right ventricular function, with mildly elevated pulmonary pressures of 30 mmHg.

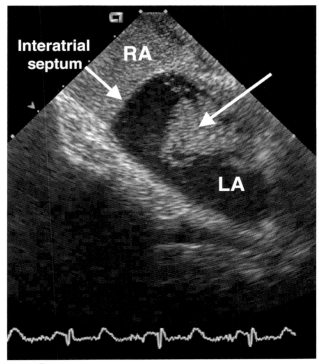

Fig 12-51. Intracardiac echocardiography reveals saline contrast appearing in the left atrium (**LA**) (**arrow**). In real time, an interatrial septal aneurysm is appreciated.

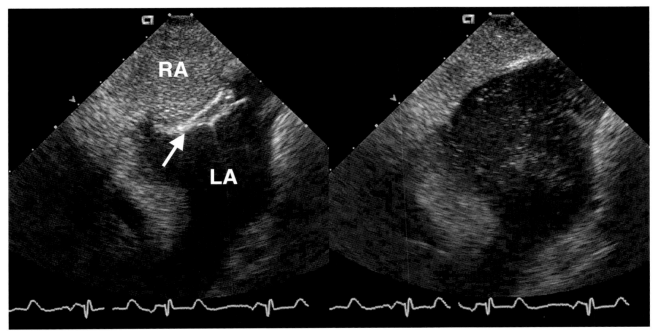

Fig 12-52. Following deployment of the device (CardioSEAL), the amount of saline contrast was significantly decreased. However, upon Valsalva, the superior limb of the occluder device prolapsed into the PFO (**arrow**). There was some passage of echo-contrast from right to left atrium noted in association with the device prolapse.

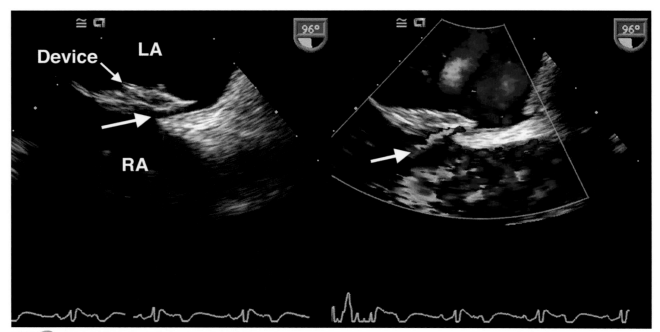

DVD ▶ **Fig 12-53.** The patient was taken to the operating room for surgical removal of the device and complete closure of the ASD and septal aneurysm. Intraoperative TEE revealed the device in the interatrial septum, with a rim of PFO that appeared open and was confirmed by color flow Doppler (**arrow**).

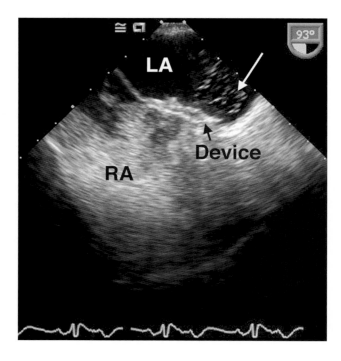

DVD ▶ **Fig 12-54.** Injected saline contrast appeared in the left atrium (**arrow**).

Case 12-11
Right Atrial Pacing Lead

Right atrial pacing leads are generally positioned in the right atrial appendage.

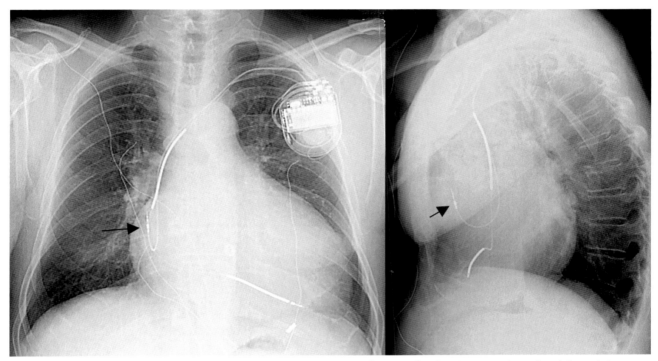

Fig 12-55. These PA and lateral chest X-rays show the right atrial pacing lead as it curves into the right atrial appendage (**arrows**).

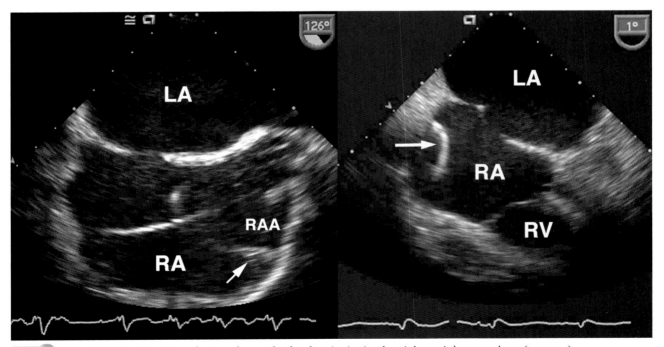

Fig 12-56. This bicaval view shows the lead as it sits in the right atrial appendage (**arrows**).

Index